W9-AKC-525

Cardiovascular Disorders
SOURCEBOOK

SEVENTH EDITION

Health Reference Series

Cardiovascular Disorders
SOURCEBOOK

SEVENTH EDITION

Basic Consumer Health Information about Heart and Blood Vessel Disorders, Such as Cardiomyopathy, Heart Attack, Heart Failure, Heart Rhythm Disorders, Heart Valve Disease, Aneurysms, Atherosclerosis, Stroke, Peripheral Arterial Disease, Varicose Veins, and Deep Vein Thrombosis, with Details about Risk Factors, Prevention, Diagnosis, and Treatment

Along with Information about Cardiovascular Concerns of Special Significance to Children, Women, Men, and Minority Populations, a Glossary of Related Medical Terms, and a Directory of Resources for Further Help and Information

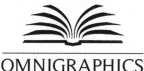

OMNIGRAPHICS

615 Griswold, Ste. 520, Detroit, MI 48226

Library of Congress Cataloging-in-Publication Data

Names: Omnigraphics, Inc., issuing body.

Title: Cardiovascular disorders sourcebook: basic consumer health information about
heart and blood vessel disorders, such as cardiomyopathy, heart attack, heart failure,
heart rhythm disorders, heart valve disease, aneurysms, atherosclerosis, stroke,
peripheral arterial disease, varicose veins, and deep vein thrombosis, with details
about risk factors, prevention, diagnosis, and treatment; along with information
about cardiovascular concerns of special significance to children, men, women, and
minority populations, a glossary of related medical terms, and a directory of resources
for further help and information.

Description: Seventh edition. | Detroit, MI: Omnigraphics, Inc., [2019] | Series:
Health reference series | Includes bibliographical references and index.

Identifiers: LCCN 2019013868 (print) | LCCN 2019014308 (ebook) | ISBN
9780780817081 (ebook) | ISBN 9780780817074 (hard cover: alk. paper)

Subjects: LCSH: Cardiovascular system--Diseases--Popular works.

Classification: LCC RC672 (ebook) | LCC RC672.C35 2019 (print) | DDC 616.1--dc23

LC record available at https://lccn.loc.gov/2019013868

Table of Contents

Part IV: Cardiovascular Disorders in Specific Populations

Part V: Diagnosing Cardiovascular Disorders

Part VI: Treating Cardiovascular Disorders

Part VII: Preventing Cardiovascular Disorders

Part VIII: Additional Help and Information

Preface

About This Book

Cardiovascular disease is the leading cause of death in the United States. According to the Centers for Disease Control and Prevention (CDC), 735,000 Americans suffer a heart attack and 610,000 people die of heart disease in the United States every year. Additionally, coronary heart disease (CHD) is the most common type of heart disease, killing over 370,000 people annually. Yet, cardiovascular disease is often preventable. With careful attention to diet; an active lifestyle; and control of contributing factors, such as diabetes, cholesterol levels, blood pressure, tobacco use, and weight, Americans can reduce their chances of facing heart disease, stroke, or other blood vessel disorders. Furthermore, advances in our understanding of how to treat cardiovascular conditions make it possible to reduce the disabling health consequences frequently associated with these disorders.

Cardiovascular Disorders Sourcebook, Seventh Edition provides information about the symptoms, diagnosis, and treatment of disorders of the heart and blood vessels, including cardiomyopathy, heart attack, heart rhythm disorders, heart valve disease, atherosclerosis, stroke, peripheral arterial disease, and deep vein thrombosis. It offers details about the conditions associated with increased risks, explains the methods used to diagnose and treat them, and offers suggestions for steps men and women can take to decrease their likelihood of developing these disorders. The book also includes a discussion of cardiovascular concerns specific to men, women, children, and minority populations, and it concludes with a glossary and a directory of resources for further help and information.

How to Use This Book

This book is divided into parts and chapters. Parts focus on broad areas of interest. Chapters are devoted to single topics within a part.

Part I: Understanding Cardiovascular Risks and Emergencies describes how the heart works, explains the known risk factors for cardiovascular disease, and offers details about the conditions that make it more likely that a person will develop a cardiovascular disorder. It describes recent research regarding the genetic links and risk factors for cardiovascular disease, and it explains how to recognize a cardiac emergency and what to do when one occurs.

Part II: Heart Disorders provides basic information about the types of disorders that affect the heart. These include problems with the heart's blood supply, problems with the heart's rhythm, heart valve disease, and certain infectious diseases, as well as heart attack, sudden cardiac arrest, cardiomyopathy, and heart failure. Individual chapters include information about the development, symptoms, diagnosis, and treatment of each disorder.

Part III: Blood Vessel Disorders discusses the types of disorders that affect the arteries and veins, including atherosclerosis, carotid artery disease, stroke, disorders of the peripheral arteries and veins, and aortic disorders. It explains how these disorders arise, what their symptoms are, how they are diagnosed, and how they are treated.

Part IV: Cardiovascular Disorders in Specific Populations describes the unique ways that cardiovascular disease affects men, women, and children. It also offers some statistics on the occurrence of cardiovascular disorders in each of these populations, and it concludes with a discussion of cardiovascular disease among minority populations in the United States.

Part V: Diagnosing Cardiovascular Disorders explains the methods used to diagnose disorders of the heart and blood vessels. It describes diagnostic tests, including blood tests, electrocardiography and echocardiography, angiography, stress testing, and Holter and event monitors, and it explains how to prepare, what to expect, and which risks are associated with each test.

Part VI: Treating Cardiovascular Disorders discusses medications and procedures used to treat these disorders, including antiarrhythmic and anticoagulant medications, catheterization, coronary artery bypass grafting, stenting, and pacemakers. It also includes a discussion of aneurysm and heart defect repair, heart transplant, and the use of the total artificial heart. The section concludes with a discussion of cardiac and stroke rehabilitation techniques.

Part VII: Preventing Cardiovascular Disorders describes the things that can be done to help prevent heart and blood vessel disease. It explains how to control risk factors, such as high blood pressure, high cholesterol, diabetes, and stress, and it offers suggestions for increasing healthy behaviors, such as maintaining a heart-healthy diet, managing weight, incorporating physical activity into a daily routine, and quitting smoking.

Part VIII: Additional Help and Information includes a glossary of terms related to cardiovascular disease and a directory of resources offering additional help and support.

Bibliographic Note

This volume contains documents and excerpts from publications issued by the following U.S. government agencies: Centers for Disease Control and Prevention (CDC); Genetic and Rare Diseases Information Center (GARD); Genetics Home Reference (GHR); National Center for Complementary and Integrative Health (NCCIH); National Heart, Lung, and Blood Institute (NHLBI); National Institute of Arthritis and Musculoskeletal and Skin Diseases (NIAMS); National Institute of Diabetes and Digestive and Kidney Diseases (NIDDK); National Institute of Neurological Disorders and Stroke (NINDS); National Institute on Aging (NIA); National Institutes of Health (NIH); *NIH News in Health*; Office of Minority Health (OMH); Office on Women's Health (OWH); and U.S. Food and Drug Administration (FDA).

It may also contain original material produced by Omnigraphics and reviewed by medical consultants.

About the Health Reference Series

The *Health Reference Series* is designed to provide basic medical information for patients, families, caregivers, and the general public. Each volume takes a particular topic and provides comprehensive coverage. This is especially important for people who may be dealing with a newly diagnosed disease or a chronic disorder in themselves or in a family member. People looking for preventive guidance, information about disease warning signs, medical statistics, and risk factors for health problems will also find answers to their questions in the *Health Reference Series*. The *Series*, however, is not intended to serve as a tool for diagnosing illness, in prescribing treatments, or as a substitute for the physician/patient relationship. All people concerned about medical symptoms or the possibility of disease are encouraged to seek professional care from an appropriate healthcare provider.

A Note about Spelling and Style

Health Reference Series editors use *Stedman's Medical Dictionary* as an authority for questions related to the spelling of medical terms and the *Chicago Manual of Style* for questions related to grammatical structures, punctuation, and other editorial concerns. Consistent adherence is not always possible, however, because the individual volumes within the *Series* include many documents from a wide variety of different producers, and the editor's primary goal is to present material from each source as accurately as is possible. This sometimes means that information in different chapters or sections may follow other guidelines and alternate spelling authorities. For example, occasionally a copyright holder may require that eponymous terms be shown in possessive forms (Crohn's disease vs. Crohn disease) or that British spelling norms be retained (leukaemia vs. leukemia).

Medical Review

Omnigraphics contracts with a team of qualified, senior medical professionals who serve as medical consultants for the *Health Reference Series*. As necessary, medical consultants review reprinted and originally written material for currency and accuracy. Citations including the phrase "Reviewed (month, year)" indicate material reviewed by this team. Medical consultation services are provided to the *Health Reference Series* editors by:

Dr. Vijayalakshmi, MBBS, DGO, MD
Dr. Senthil Selvan, MBBS, DCH, MD
Dr. K. Sivanandham, MBBS, DCH, MS (Research), PhD

Our Advisory Board

We would like to thank the following board members for providing initial guidance on the development of this series:

- Dr. Lynda Baker, Associate Professor of Library and Information Science, Wayne State University, Detroit, MI

- Nancy Bulgarelli, William Beaumont Hospital Library, Royal Oak, MI

- Karen Imarisio, Bloomfield Township Public Library, Bloomfield Township, MI

- Karen Morgan, Mardigian Library, University of Michigan-Dearborn, Dearborn, MI

- Rosemary Orlando, St. Clair Shores Public Library, St. Clair Shores, MI

Health Reference Series *Update Policy*

The inaugural book in the *Health Reference Series* was the first edition of *Cancer Sourcebook* published in 1989. Since then, the *Series* has been enthusiastically received by librarians and in the medical community. In order to maintain the standard of providing high-quality health information for the layperson the editorial staff at Omnigraphics felt it was necessary to implement a policy of updating volumes when warranted.

Medical researchers have been making tremendous strides, and it is the purpose of the *Health Reference Series* to stay current with the most recent advances. Each decision to update a volume is made on an individual basis. Some of the considerations include how much new information is available and the feedback we receive from people who use the books. If there is a topic you would like to see added to the update list, or an area of medical concern you feel has not been adequately addressed, please write to:

Managing Editor
Health Reference Series
Omnigraphics
615 Griswold, Ste. 520
Detroit, MI 48226

xvii

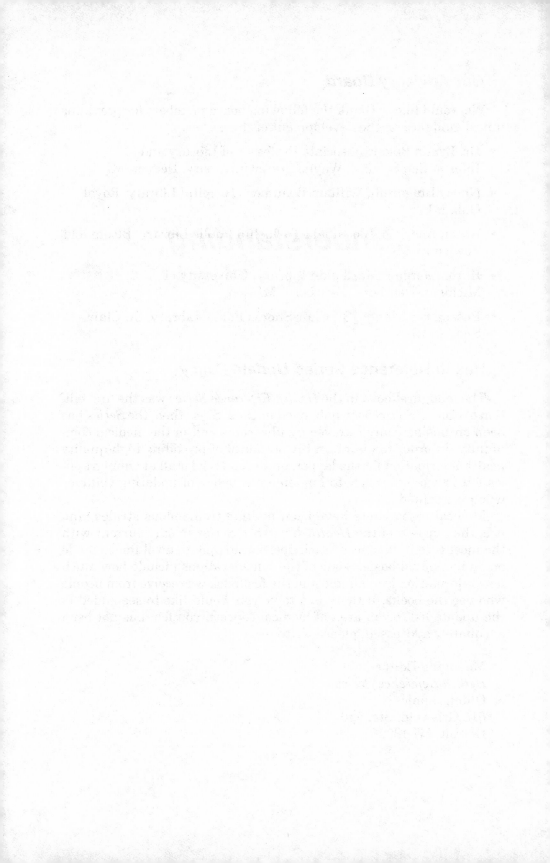

Part One

Understanding Cardiovascular Risks and Emergencies

Chapter 1

How the Heart Works

What Is the Heart?

Your heart is a muscular organ that pumps blood to your body. Your heart is at the center of your circulatory system. This system consists of a network of blood vessels, such as arteries, veins, and capillaries. These blood vessels carry blood to and from all areas of your body.

An electrical system controls your heart and uses electrical signals to contract the heart's walls. When the walls contract, blood is pumped into your circulatory system. Inlet and outlet valves in your heart chambers ensure that blood flows in the right direction.

Your heart is vital to your health and nearly everything that goes on in your body. Without the heart's pumping action, blood cannot move throughout your body.

Your blood carries the oxygen and nutrients that your organs need to work well. Blood also carries carbon dioxide (a waste product) to your lungs so you can breathe it out.

A healthy heart supplies your body with the right amount of blood at the rate needed to work well. If disease or injury weakens your heart, your body's organs will not receive enough blood to work normally.

This chapter includes text excerpted from "How the Heart Works," National Heart, Lung, and Blood Institute (NHLBI), July 29, 2015. Reviewed May 2019.

Anatomy of the Heart

Your heart is located under your ribcage, in the center of your chest, and between your right and left lungs. Its muscular walls beat, or contract, pumping blood to all parts of your body.

The size of your heart can vary depending on your age, size, and the condition of your heart. A normal, healthy, adult heart usually is the size of an average clenched adult fist. Some diseases can cause the heart to enlarge.

The Exterior of the Heart

Below is a picture of the outside of a normal, healthy human heart.

Heart Exterior

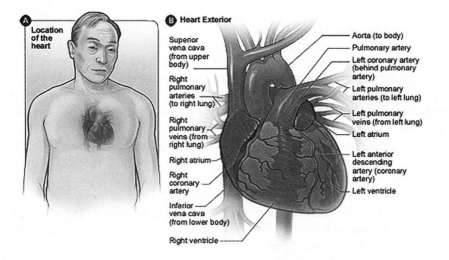

Figure 1.1. *Heart and Its Exterior View*

Figure A shows the location of the heart in the body. Figure B shows the front surface of the heart, including the coronary arteries and major blood vessels.

In figure 1.1. (B), the heart is the muscle in the lower half of the picture. The heart has four chambers. The heart's upper chambers are called the "right atria" and "left atria." The heart's lower chambers are called the "right ventricles" and "left ventricles."

Some of the main blood vessels (arteries and veins) that make up your circulatory system are directly connected to the heart.

The Right Side of Your Heart

In figure 1.1. (B) above, the superior and inferior vena cavae (IVC) are shown to the left of the heart muscle as you look at the picture. These veins are the largest veins in your body.

After your body's organs and tissues have used the oxygen in your blood, the vena cavae carry the oxygen-poor blood back to the right atrium of your heart.

The superior vena cava (SVC) carries oxygen-poor blood from the upper parts of your body, including your head, chest, arms, and neck. The inferior vena cava carries oxygen-poor blood from the lower parts of your body.

The oxygen-poor blood from the vena cava flows into your heart's right atrium and then to the right ventricle. From the right ventricle, the blood is pumped through the pulmonary arteries (shown in the center of figure B) to your lungs.

Once in the lungs, the blood travels through many small, thin blood vessels called "capillaries." There, the blood picks up more oxygen and transfers carbon dioxide to the lungs—a process called "gas exchange."

The oxygen-rich blood passes from your lungs back to your heart through the pulmonary veins (shown to the left of the right atrium in figure 1.1. B).

The Left Side of Your Heart

Oxygen-rich blood from your lungs passes through the pulmonary veins (shown to the right of the left atrium in figure B above). The blood enters the left atrium and is pumped into the left ventricle.

From the left ventricle, the oxygen-rich blood is pumped to the rest of your body through the aorta. The aorta is the main artery that carries oxygen-rich blood to your body.

As with all of your organs, your heart needs oxygen-rich blood. As blood is pumped out of your heart's left ventricle, some of it flows into the coronary arteries.

Your coronary arteries are located on your heart's surface at the beginning of the aorta. They carry oxygen-rich blood to all parts of your heart.

The Interior of the Heart

Below is a picture of the inside of a normal, healthy, human heart.

Heart Interior

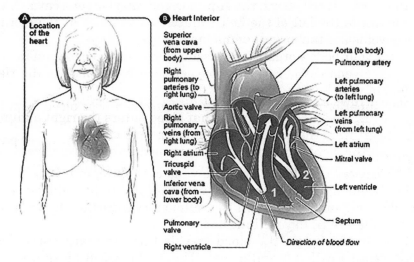

Figure 1.2. *Interior of Heart and Flow of Blood*

Figure A shows the location of the heart in the body. Figure B shows a cross-section of a healthy heart and its inside structures. The blue arrow shows the direction in which oxygen-poor blood flows through the heart to the lungs. The red arrow shows the direction in which oxygen-rich blood flows from the lungs into the heart and then out to the body.

Heart Chambers

Figure B shows the inside of your heart and how it is divided into four chambers. The two upper chambers of your heart are called the "atria." They receive and collect blood.

The two lower chambers of your heart are called "ventricles." The ventricles pump blood out of your heart to other parts of your body.

The Septum

An internal wall of tissue divides the right and left sides of your heart. This wall is called the "septum."

The area of the septum that divides the atria is called the "atrial septum" or "interatrial septum." The area of the septum that divides the ventricles is called the "ventricular septum" or "interventricular septum."

Heart Valves

Figure B shows your heart's four valves. Shown counterclockwise in the picture, the valves include the aortic valve, the tricuspid valve, the pulmonary valve, and the mitral valve.

Blood Flow

The arrows in figure B show the direction that blood flows through your heart. The arrow (1) shows that blood enters the right atrium of your heart from the superior and inferior vena cava.

From the right atrium, blood is pumped into the right ventricle. From the right ventricle, blood is pumped to your lungs through the pulmonary arteries.

The arrow (2) shows oxygen-rich blood coming from your lungs through the pulmonary veins into your heart's left atrium. From the left atrium, the blood is pumped into the left ventricle. The left ventricle pumps the blood to the rest of your body through the aorta.

For the heart to work well, your blood must flow in only one direction. Your heart's valves make this possible. Both of your heart's ventricles have an "in" (inlet) valve from the atria and an "out" (outlet) valve leading to your arteries.

Healthy valves open and close in exact coordination with the pumping action of your heart's atria and ventricles. Each valve has a set of flaps called "leaflets" or "cusps" that seal or open the valve. This allows blood to pass through the chambers and into your arteries without backing up or flowing backward.

Heart Contraction and Blood Flow
Heartbeat

Almost everyone has heard the real or recorded sound of a heartbeat. When your heart beats, it makes a "lub-DUB" sound. Between the time you hear "lub" and "DUB," blood is pumped through your heart and circulatory system.

A heartbeat may seem as if it is a simple, repeated event. However, it is a complex series of very precise and coordinated events. These events take place inside and around your heart.

Each side of your heart uses an inlet valve to help move blood between the atrium and ventricle. The tricuspid valve does this between the right atrium and ventricle. The mitral valve does this between the left atrium and ventricle. The "lub" is the sound of the tricuspid and mitral valves closing.

Each of your heart's ventricles also has an outlet valve. The right ventricle uses the pulmonary valve to help move blood into the pulmonary arteries. The left ventricle uses the aortic valve to do the same for the aorta. The "DUB" is the sound of the aortic and pulmonary valves closing.

Each heartbeat has two basic parts: diastole and systole.

During diastole, the atria and ventricles of your heart relax and begin to fill with blood. At the end of diastole, your heart's atria contract (atrial systole) and pump blood into the ventricles.

The atria then begin to relax. Next, your heart's ventricles contract (ventricular systole) and pump blood out of your heart.

Pumping Action

Your heart uses its four valves to ensure that your blood flows in only one direction. Healthy valves open and close in coordination with the pumping action of your heart's atria and ventricles.

Each valve's leaflets or cusps seal or open the valve. The cusps allow pumped blood to pass through the chambers and into your blood vessels without backing up or flowing backward.

Oxygen-poor blood from the vena cava fills your heart's right atrium. The atrium contracts (atrial systole). The tricuspid valve located between the right atrium and ventricle opens for a short time and then shuts. This allows blood to enter the right ventricle without flowing back into the right atrium.

When your heart's right ventricle fills with blood, it contracts (ventricular systole). The pulmonary valve located between your right ventricle and pulmonary artery opens and closes quickly.

This allows blood to enter into your pulmonary arteries without flowing back into the right ventricle. This is important because the right ventricle begins to refill with more blood through the tricuspid valve. Blood travels through the pulmonary arteries to your lungs to pick up oxygen.

Oxygen-rich blood returns from the lungs to your heart's left atrium through the pulmonary veins. As your heart's left atrium fills with blood, it contracts. This event is called "atrial systole."

The mitral valve located between the left atrium and left ventricle opens and closes quickly. This allows blood to pass from the left atrium into the left ventricle without flowing backward.

As the left ventricle fills with blood, it contracts. The aortic valve, located between the left ventricle and aorta, opens and closes quickly.

This allows blood to flow into the aorta. The aorta is the main artery that carries blood from your heart to the rest of your body.

The aortic valve closes quickly to prevent blood from flowing back into the left ventricle, which already is filling up with new blood.

Taking Your Pulse

When your heart pumps blood through your arteries, it creates a pulse that you can feel on the arteries close to the skin's surface. For example, you can feel the pulse on the artery inside of your wrist, below your thumb.

You can count how many times your heart beats by taking your pulse. You will need a watch with a second hand.

To find your pulse, gently place your index and middle fingers on the artery located on the inner wrist of either arm, below your thumb. You should feel a pulsing or tapping against your fingers.

Watch the second hand and count the number of pulses you feel in 30 seconds. Double that number to find out your heart rate or pulse for 1 minute.

The usual resting pulse for an adult is 60 to 100 beats per minute. To find your resting pulse, count your pulse after you have been sitting or resting quietly for at least 10 minutes.

Circulation and Blood Vessels

Your heart and blood vessels make up your overall blood circulatory system. Your blood circulatory system is made up of four subsystems.

Arterial Circulation

Arterial circulation is the part of your circulatory system that involves arteries, such as the aorta and pulmonary arteries. Arteries are blood vessels that carry blood away from your heart. (The exception is the coronary arteries, which supply your heart muscle with oxygen-rich blood.)

Healthy arteries are strong and elastic (stretchy). They become narrow between heartbeats, and they help keep your blood pressure consistent. This helps blood move through your body.

Arteries branch into smaller blood vessels called "arterioles." Arteries and arterioles have strong, flexible walls that allow them to adjust the amount and rate of blood flowing to parts of your body.

Venous Circulation

Venous circulation is the part of your circulatory system that involves veins, such as the vena cava and pulmonary veins. Veins are blood vessels that carry blood to your heart.

Veins have thinner walls than arteries. Veins can widen as the amount of blood passing through them increases.

Capillary Circulation

Capillary circulation is the part of your circulatory system where oxygen, nutrients, and waste pass between your blood and parts of your body.

Capillaries are very small blood vessels. They connect the arterial and venous circulatory subsystems.

The importance of capillaries lies in their very thin walls. Oxygen and nutrients in your blood can pass through the walls of the capillaries to the parts of your body that need them to work normally.

Capillaries' thin walls also allow waste products, such as carbon dioxide, to pass from your body's organs and tissues into the blood, where it is taken away to your lungs.

Pulmonary Circulation

Pulmonary circulation is the movement of blood from the heart to the lungs and back to the heart again. Pulmonary circulation includes both arterial and venous circulation.

Oxygen-poor blood is pumped to the lungs from the heart (arterial circulation). Oxygen-rich blood moves from the lungs to the heart through the pulmonary veins (venous circulation).

Pulmonary circulation also includes capillary circulation. Oxygen you breathe in from the air passes through your lungs and into your blood through the many capillaries in the lungs. Oxygen-rich blood moves through your pulmonary veins to the left side of your heart and out of the aorta to the rest of your body.

Capillaries in the lungs also remove carbon dioxide from your blood so that your lungs can breathe the carbon dioxide out into the air.

Your Heart's Electrical System

Your heart's electrical system controls all the events that occur when your heart pumps blood. The electrical system also is called the "cardiac conduction system" (CCS). If you have ever seen the heart test called an "electrocardiogram" (EKG), you have seen a graphical picture of the heart's electrical activity.

Your heart's electrical system is made up of three main parts:

- The sinoatrial (SA) node, located in the right atrium of your heart

- The atrioventricular (AV) node, located on the interatrial septum close to the tricuspid valve

- The His-Purkinje system, located along the walls of your heart's ventricles

A heartbeat is a complex series of events. These events take place inside and around your heart. A heartbeat is a single cycle in which your heart's chambers relax and contract to pump blood. This cycle includes the opening and closing of the inlet and outlet valves of the right and left ventricles of your heart.

Each heartbeat has two basic parts: diastole and systole. During diastole, the atria and ventricles of your heart relax and begin to fill with blood.

At the end of diastole, your heart's atria contract (atrial systole) and pump blood into the ventricles. The atria then begin to relax. Your heart's ventricles then contract (ventricular systole), pumping blood out of your heart.

Each beat of your heart is set in motion by an electrical signal from within your heart muscle. In a normal, healthy heart, each beat begins with a signal from the SA node. This is why the SA node sometimes is called your "heart's natural pacemaker." Your pulse, or heart rate, is the number of signals the SA node produces per minute.

The signal is generated as the vena cava fill your heart's right atrium with blood from other parts of your body. The signal spreads across the cells of your heart's right and left atria.

This signal causes the atria to contract. This action pushes blood through the open valves from the atria into both ventricles.

The signal arrives at the AV node near the ventricles. It slows for an instant to allow your heart's right and left ventricles to fill with blood. The signal is released and moves along a pathway called the "Bundle of His," which is located in the walls of your heart's ventricles.

From the bundle of His, the signal fibers divide into left and right bundle branches through the Purkinje fibers. These fibers connect directly to the cells in the walls of your heart's left and right ventricles.

The signal spreads across the cells of your ventricle walls, and both ventricles contract. However, this does not happen at exactly the same moment.

The left ventricle contracts an instant before the right ventricle. This pushes blood through the pulmonary valve (for the right ventricle) to your lungs and through the aortic valve (for the left ventricle) to the rest of your body.

As the signal passes, the walls of the ventricles relax and await the next signal.

This process continues over and over as the atria refill with blood, and more electrical signals come from the SA node.

Heart Disease

Your heart is made up of many parts working together to pump blood. In a healthy heart, all the parts work well so that your heart pumps blood normally. As a result, all parts of your body that depend on the heart to deliver blood also stay healthy.

Heart disease can disrupt a heart's normal electrical system and pumping functions. Diseases and conditions of the heart's muscle make it hard for your heart to properly pump blood.

Damaged or diseased blood vessels make the heart work harder than normal. Problems with the heart's electrical system, called "arrhythmias," can make it hard for the heart to pump blood efficiently.

Chapter 2

Risk Factors for
Cardiovascular Disorders

Chapter Contents

Section 2.1

Coronary Heart Disease Risk Factors

This section includes text excerpted from "Learn More about
Heart Disease," National Heart, Lung, and Blood
Institute (NHLBI), January 20, 2019.

What Is Coronary Heart Disease?

Coronary heart disease (CHD) is a disease in which a waxy substance called "plaque" builds up inside the coronary arteries. These arteries supply oxygen-rich blood to your heart muscle.

When plaque builds up in the arteries, the condition is called "atherosclerosis." The buildup of plaque occurs over many years.

Atherosclerosis

Over time, plaque can harden or rupture (break open). Hardened plaque narrows the coronary arteries and reduces the flow of oxygen-rich blood to the heart.

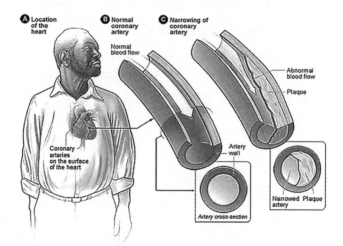

Figure 2.1. *Atherosclerosis*

Figure A shows the location of the heart in the body. Figure B shows a normal coronary artery with normal blood flow. The inset image shows a cross-section of a normal coronary artery. Figure C shows a coronary artery narrowed by plaque. The buildup of plaque limits the flow of oxygen-rich blood through the artery. The inset image shows a cross-section of the plaque-narrowed artery.

If the plaque ruptures, a blood clot can form on its surface. A large blood clot can mostly or completely block blood flow through a coronary artery. Over time, ruptured plaque also hardens and narrows the coronary arteries.

Risk Factors for Coronary Heart Disease
High Blood Cholesterol and Triglyceride Levels
Cholesterol

High blood cholesterol is a condition in which your blood has too much cholesterol—a waxy, fat-like substance. The higher your blood cholesterol level, the greater your risk of CHD and heart attack.

Cholesterol travels through the bloodstream in small packages called "lipoproteins." Two major kinds of lipoproteins carry cholesterol throughout your body:

- **Low-density lipoproteins (LDL).** LDL cholesterol sometimes is called "bad cholesterol." This is because it carries cholesterol to tissues, including to your heart arteries. A high LDL cholesterol level raises your risk of CHD.

- **High-density lipoproteins (HDL).** HDL cholesterol sometimes is called "good cholesterol." This is because it helps remove cholesterol from your arteries. A low HDL cholesterol level raises your risk of CHD.

Many factors affect your cholesterol levels. For example, after menopause, women's LDL cholesterol levels tend to rise, and their HDL cholesterol levels tend to fall. Other factors—such as age, gender, diet, and physical activity—also affect your cholesterol levels.

Healthy levels of both LDL and HDL cholesterol will prevent plaque from building up in your arteries. Routine blood tests can show whether your blood cholesterol levels are healthy. Talk with your doctor about having your cholesterol tested and what the results mean.

Children also can have unhealthy cholesterol levels, especially if they are overweight or their parents have high blood cholesterol. Talk with your child's doctor about testing your child's cholesterol levels.

Triglycerides

Triglycerides are a type of fat found in the blood. Some studies suggest that a high level of triglycerides in the blood may raise the risk of CHD, especially in women.

High Blood Pressure

Blood pressure is the force of blood pushing against the walls of your arteries as your heart pumps blood. If this pressure rises and stays high over time, it can damage your heart and lead to plaque buildup. All levels above 120/80 mmHg raise your risk of CHD. This risk grows as blood pressure levels rise. Only 1 of the 2 blood pressure numbers has to be above normal to put you at a greater risk of CHD and heart attack.

Most adults should have their blood pressure checked at least once a year. If you have high blood pressure, you will likely need to be checked more often. Talk with your doctor about how often you should have your blood pressure checked.

Children also can develop high blood pressure, especially if they are overweight. Your child's doctor should check your child's blood pressure at each routine checkup.

Both children and adults are more likely to develop high blood pressure if they are overweight or have diabetes.

Diabetes and Prediabetes

Diabetes is a disease in which the body's blood sugar level is too high. The two types of diabetes are type 1 and type 2.

In type 1 diabetes, the body's blood sugar level is high because the body does not make enough insulin. Insulin is a hormone that helps move blood sugar into cells, where it is used for energy. In type 2 diabetes, the body's blood sugar level is high mainly because the body does not use its insulin properly.

Over time, a high blood sugar level can lead to increased plaque buildup in your arteries. Having diabetes doubles your risk of CHD.

Prediabetes is a condition in which your blood sugar level is higher than normal but not as high as it is in diabetes. If you have prediabetes and do not take steps to manage it, you will likely develop type 2 diabetes within ten years. You are also at higher risk of CHD.

Being overweight or obese raises your risk of type 2 diabetes. With modest weight loss and moderate physical activity, people who have prediabetes may be able to delay or prevent type 2 diabetes. They also may be able to lower their risk of CHD and heart attack. Weight loss and physical activity also can help control diabetes.

Even children can develop type 2 diabetes. Most children who have type 2 diabetes are overweight.

Type 2 diabetes develops over time and sometimes has no symptoms. Go to your doctor or local clinic to have your blood sugar levels tested regularly to check for diabetes and prediabetes.

Overweight and Obesity

The terms "overweight" and "obesity" refer to body weight that is greater than what is considered healthy for a certain height. More than two-thirds of American adults are overweight, and almost one-third of these adults are obese.

The most useful measure of overweight and obesity is body mass index (BMI). You can use the National Heart, Lung, and Blood Institute's (NHLBI) online BMI calculator to figure out your BMI, or your doctor can help you.

Being overweight is defined differently for children and teens than it is for adults. Children are still growing, and boys and girls mature at different rates. Thus, BMIs for children and teens compare their heights and weights against growth charts that take age and gender into account. This is called the "BMI-for-age percentile."

Being overweight or obese can raise your risk of CHD and heart attack. This is mainly because being overweight or obese is linked to other CHD risk factors, such as high blood cholesterol and triglyceride levels, high blood pressure, and diabetes.

Smoking

Smoking tobacco or long-term exposure to secondhand smoke raises your risk of CHD and heart attack.

Smoking triggers a buildup of plaque in your arteries. Smoking also increases the risk of blood clots forming in your arteries. Blood clots can block plaque-narrowed arteries and cause a heart attack. Some research shows that smoking raises your risk of CHD in part by lowering HDL cholesterol levels.

The more you smoke, the greater your risk of heart attack. The benefits of quitting smoking occur no matter how long or how much you have smoked. Heart disease risk associated with smoking begins to decrease soon after you quit, and, for many people, it continues to decrease over time.

Most people who smoke start when they are teens. Parents can help prevent their children from smoking by not smoking themselves. Talk with your child about the health dangers of smoking and ways to overcome peer pressure to smoke.

17

Lack of Physical Activity

Inactive people are nearly twice as likely to develop CHD as those who are active. A lack of physical activity can worsen other CHD risk factors, such as high blood cholesterol and triglyceride levels, high blood pressure, diabetes and prediabetes, and being overweight or obese.

It is important for children and adults to make physical activity part of their daily routines. One reason many Americans are not active enough is because of hours spent in front of TVs and computers doing work, schoolwork, and leisure activities.

Some experts advise that children and teens should reduce screen time because it limits time for physical activity. They recommend that children two years of age and older should spend no more than two hours a day watching TV or using a computer (except for school work).

Being physically active is one of the most important things you can do to keep your heart healthy. The good news is that even modest amounts of physical activity are good for your health. The more active you are, the more you will benefit.

Unhealthy Diet

An unhealthy diet can raise your risk of CHD. For example, foods that are high in saturated and trans fats and cholesterol raise LDL cholesterol. Thus, you should try to limit these foods.

It is also important to limit foods that are high in sodium (salt) and added sugars. A high-salt diet can raise your risk of high blood pressure.

Added sugars will give you extra calories without nutrients, such as vitamins and minerals. This can cause you to gain weight, which raises your risk of CHD. Added sugars are found in many desserts, canned fruits packed in syrup, fruit drinks, and non-diet sodas.

Stress

Stress and anxiety may play a role in causing CHD. Stress and anxiety also can trigger your arteries to tighten. This can raise your blood pressure and your risk of heart attack.

The most commonly reported trigger for a heart attack is an emotionally upsetting event, especially one involving anger. Stress also may indirectly raise your risk of CHD if it makes you more likely to smoke or overeat foods high in fat and sugar.

Age

In men, the risk for CHD increases starting around 45 years of age. In women, the risk for CHD increases starting around 55 years of age. Most people have some plaque buildup in their heart arteries by the time they are in their seventies. However, only about 25 percent of those people have chest pain, heart attacks, or other signs of CHD.

Gender

Some risk factors may affect CHD risk differently in women than in men. For example, estrogen provides women some protection against CHD, whereas diabetes raises the risk of CHD more in women than in men.

Also, some risk factors for heart disease only affect women, such as preeclampsia, a condition that can develop during pregnancy. Preeclampsia is linked to an increased lifetime risk of heart disease, including CHD, heart attack, heart failure, and high blood pressure. (Likewise, having heart disease risk factors, such as diabetes or being obese, increases a woman's risk of preeclampsia.)

Family History

A family history of early CHD is a risk factor for developing CHD, specifically if a father or brother is diagnosed before the age of 55, or a mother or sister is diagnosed before the age of 65.

Section 2.2

Risk Factors for Stroke

This section includes text excerpted from "About Stroke," Centers for Disease Control and Prevention (CDC), May 3, 2018.

A stroke, sometimes called a "brain attack," occurs when something blocks blood supply to part of the brain or when a blood vessel in the brain bursts. In either case, parts of the brain become damaged or die. A stroke can cause lasting brain damage, long-term disability, or even death.

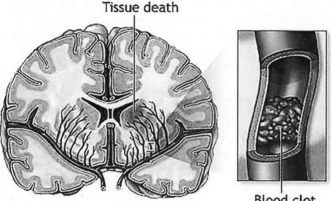

Figure 2.2. *Blood Clot in Brain*

A stroke happens when a blood clot blocks blood flow to the brain. This causes brain tissue to become damaged or die.

Stroke Risk

Anyone can have a stroke at any age. But certain things can increase your chances of having a stroke. The best way to protect yourself and your loved ones from a stroke is to understand your risk and how to control it.

While you cannot control your age or family history, you can take steps to lower your chances of having a stroke.

Conditions That Increase Risk for Stroke

Many common medical conditions can increase your chances of having a stroke. Work with your healthcare team to control your risk.

Previous Stroke or Transient Ischemic Attack

If you have already had a stroke or a transient ischemic attack (TIA), also known as a "mini-stroke," your chances of having another stroke are higher.

High Blood Pressure

High blood pressure is a leading cause of stroke. It occurs when the pressure of the blood in your arteries and other blood vessels is too high.

There are often no symptoms of high blood pressure. Get your blood pressure checked often. If you have high blood pressure, lowering your blood pressure through lifestyle changes or medicine can also lower your risk for stroke.

High Cholesterol

Cholesterol is a waxy, fat-like substance made by the liver or found in certain foods. Your liver makes enough for your body's needs, but we often get more cholesterol from the foods we eat. If we take in more cholesterol than the body can use, the extra cholesterol can build up in the arteries, including those of the brain. This can lead to narrowing of the arteries, stroke, and other problems.

A blood test can tell your doctor if you have high levels of cholesterol and triglycerides (a related kind of fat) in your blood.

Heart Disease

Common heart disorders can increase your risk for stroke. For example, coronary artery disease increases your risk for stroke because plaque builds up in the arteries and blocks the flow of oxygen-rich blood to the brain. Other heart conditions, such as heart valve defects, an irregular heartbeat (including atrial fibrillation (AF)), and enlarged heart chambers, can cause blood clots that may break loose and cause a stroke.

Diabetes

Diabetes increases your risk for stroke. Your body needs glucose (sugar) for energy. Insulin is a hormone made in the pancreas that helps move glucose from the food you eat to your body's cells. If you have diabetes, your body does not make enough insulin, cannot use its own insulin as well as it should, or both.

Diabetes causes sugars to build up in the blood and prevent oxygen and nutrients from getting to the various parts of your body, including your brain. High blood pressure is also common in people with diabetes. High blood pressure is the leading cause of stroke and is the main cause for the increased risk of stroke among people with diabetes.

Talk to your doctor about ways to keep diabetes under control.

Sickle Cell Disease

Sickle cell disease (SCD) is a blood disorder linked to ischemic stroke that affects mainly black and Hispanic children. The disease causes some red blood cells to form an abnormal sickle shape. A stroke can happen if sickle cells get stuck in a blood vessel and block the flow of blood to the brain.

Section 2.3

Targeting Cardiovascular Disease Risk Factors May Be Important across a Lifetime

This section includes text excerpted from "Targeting Cardiovascular Disease Risk Factors May Be Important across a Lifetime," National Institutes of Health (NIH), October 3, 2016.

Findings suggest that all adults, including those over 65, should be mindful of risk factors for cardiovascular disease. The results, published in the Journal of the American Geriatric Society, are part of the Reasons for Geographic and Racial Differences in Stroke (REGARDS) study, which looks at stroke incidence in approximately 30,000 individuals. The REGARDS study is funded by the National Institutes of Health's (NIH) National Institute of Neurological Disorders and Stroke (NINDS).

"As life expectancy continues to increase, we need to improve risk factor prevention and management for stroke and heart disease across the lifespan, including for those adults over the age of 65," said Claudia Moy, Ph.D., Acting Director of the Office of Clinical Research at the National Institute of Neurological Disorders and Stroke (NINDS), and one of the study authors. "The latest findings from the [Reasons for Geographic and Racial Differences in Stroke] REGARDS study reveal that no age group is immune to risk factors related to cardiovascular disease and that prevention efforts should target all adults."

In the current study, led by George Howard, Dr.PH, a biostatistics professor at the University of Alabama at Birmingham, researchers examined individuals over the course of ten years to determine how many developed risk factors known to be associated with stroke and heart disease. The specific risk factors that the researchers focused on in the current study were high blood pressure, diabetes mellitus, high cholesterol, and atrial fibrillation (AF), a type of problem with heart rate and rhythm that is greatly associated with stroke. The authors noted that while smoking is also a risk factor for stroke and heart disease, it is uncommon for individuals to begin smoking after the age of 30.

The REGARDS study is made up of a sample of Black and White Americans, with more than half of the participants living in the Stroke Belt, an area of the southeastern United States, where stroke mortality is higher than in the rest of the country.

Dr. Howard's team discovered that development of cardiovascular disease risk factors remains high among adults older than 65 years of age. The study also confirmed large racial disparities in the incidence of high blood pressure, diabetes mellitus, high cholesterol, and atrial fibrillation.

Overall, nearly half of the participants whose blood pressure was normal at the beginning of the study went on to develop high blood pressure during the 10 years of follow-up. Across all age groups, including participants older than 75 years of age, Black men had a 24 percent greater risk of developing high blood pressure than White men. Black women between the ages of 45 and 54 had a 93 percent higher risk of developing high blood pressure than White women. However, that racial disparity shrank among women older than 75 years of age because in that age group, the incidence of high blood pressure continued to increase in White women while remaining stable among Black women. The findings suggest that efforts to prevent high blood pressure may be beneficial in all subgroups.

As study participants got older, their risk of developing diabetes mellitus decreased, although a large racial disparity was seen across all age groups. Overall, compared to White men, Black men were 52 percent and Black women were 114 percent more likely to develop diabetes mellitus.

The incidence of high cholesterol increased through the age of 74 then decreased slightly among participants older than 75 years of age. Among all age groups, Dr. Howard's team found that there was at least a 20 percent risk of developing high cholesterol and that the incidence for Black participants was greater than among White participants. The researchers also discovered that the risk of atrial fibrillation increased as participants got older, with White participants more likely to develop the condition than Black participants.

"In addition to improving treatment and control of potent risk factors for stroke and heart disease, finding ways to prevent the development of those risk factors may be a potential strategy to lower rates of cardiovascular disease across the age span, but especially in Black Americans," said Dr. Moy.

In 2016, the NINDS launched a stroke prevention campaign called "Mind Your Risks," designed to educate people between the ages of 45 and 65 about the link between uncontrolled high blood pressure and the risk of having a stroke or developing dementia later in life.

This study emphasizes the importance of providing evidence-based clinical preventive services to adults 65 years of age and older. The U.S. Preventive Services Task Force (USPSTF) offers recommendations on healthful diet and physical activity, screening for diabetes and lipid disorders, and the use of aspirin to prevent cardiovascular disease (CVD) in patients who are at an increased risk.

Chapter 3

Conditions That Increase the Risk of Cardiovascular Disorders

Chapter Contents

Section 3.1

Depression and Heart Disease

This section includes text excerpted from "Heart Disease and
Depression: A Two-Way Relationship," National Heart, Lung, and
Blood Institute (NHLBI), April 16, 2017.

Heart Disease and Depression: A Two-Way Relationship

For years, scientists have known about the relationship between
depression and heart disease. At least a quarter of cardiac patients
suffer from depression, and adults with depression often develop
heart disease. What researchers now want to know is why. So far,
they have unearthed a treasure trove of important clues, but a definitive explanation on the curious nature of this relationship has yet
to emerge.

It is a puzzle: Is depression a causal risk factor for heart disease?
Is it a warning sign because depressed people engage in behaviors
that increase the risks for heart disease? Is depression just a secondary event, prompted by the trauma of major medical problems, such
as heart surgery? Experts say the urgent need for answers is clear;
according to the World Health Organization (WHO), 350 million people
suffer from depression worldwide, and 17.3 million die of heart disease
each year, making it the number 1 global cause of death.

The promising news, they say, is that new insights are emerging
because of the data researchers continue to amass, scientific inno-
vation, and heightened public awareness. It was in part because of
better diagnostic tools and an increased recognition of the prevalence
of depression that scientists could establish a connection between
depression and heart disease in the first place.

"30 years of epidemiological data indicate that depression does predict the development of heart disease," said Jesse C. Stewart, Ph.D.,
an associate professor of psychology in the School of Science at Indi-
ana University-Purdue University Indianapolis. Stewart noted that
there is now "an impressive body of evidence" showing that, compared
to people without depression, adults with a depressive disorder or
symptoms have a 64 percent greater risk of developing coronary artery
disease (CAD); and depressed CAD patients are 59 percent more likely
to have a future adverse cardiovascular event, such as a heart attack
or cardiac death.

But, does depression cause heart disease? Is it a risk factor on its own? Many investigators recoil at the use of the word "cause" because almost all evidence connecting heart disease and depression comes from observational studies.

"Those who have elevated depressive symptoms are at increased risk for heart disease, and this association seems to be largely independent of the traditional risk markers for heart disease," said Karina W. Davidson, Ph.D., professor at Columbia University Medical Center. Indeed, she said, the association between depression and heart disease is similar to the association of factors such as high cholesterol, hypertension, diabetes, smoking, obesity, and heart disease.

To establish a true cause-effect link between depression and heart disease, according to Stewart, scientists need evidence from randomized controlled trials showing that treating depression reduces the risk of future heart disease. In other words, what needs to be studied is whether treating depression prevents heart disease in the way that treating high cholesterol and blood pressure does.

A 2014 paper by Stewart and his colleagues suggests that early treatment for depression, before the development of symptomatic cardiovascular disease, could decrease the risk of heart attacks and strokes by almost half. With funding from the National Heart, Lung, and Blood Institute (NHLBI), Stewart is currently conducting a clinical trial which would help answer this cause-effect question.

In the meantime, the existing evidence prompted the American Heart Association (AHA) to issue a statement external link in 2015, warning that teens with depression and bipolar disorder stand at increased risk for developing cardiovascular disease earlier in life and urging doctors to actively monitor these patients and intervene to try to prevent its onset.

Just as concerning, say doctors, is the prognosis for older patients who already have heart disease. Researchers have discovered that depression actually worsens the prognosis—and dramatically. Conversely, people who are diagnosed with heart disease have an increased risk of developing depression. It is a two-way relationship.

The prevalence of depression among cardiac patients ranges from 20 to 30 percent. "Even the lower limit of this range is more than double the prevalence of this treatable condition in the general population," wrote Bruce L. Rollman, M.D., and Stewart in their 2014 study.

A study presented at the American College of Cardiology's (ACC) 66th Annual Scientific Session shows that patients are twice as likely to die if they develop depression after being diagnosed with heart disease. In fact, depression is the strongest predictor of death in the first decade after a heart disease diagnosis.

"We are confident that depression is an independent risk factor for cardiac morbidity and mortality in patients with established heart disease," said Robert Carney, Ph.D., professor of psychiatry at Washington University School of Medicine. "However, depression is also associated with other risk factors, including smoking, so it can be difficult to disentangle its effects from those of other risk factors."

In other words, cardiac patients with depression have worse outcomes, which translate to more deaths and repeated cardiovascular events. But how does depression have such an effect?

Researchers agree that while the pathways are not completely understood, there are many likely explanations. Some point to the biology of depression, such as autonomic nervous system dysfunction, elevated cortisol levels, and elevated markers of inflammation.

"There are also plausible behavioral explanations, such as poor adherence to diet, exercise, and medications, and a higher prevalence of smoking, that have been associated with depression with or without established heart disease," said Ken Freedland, Ph.D., also from Washington University School of Medicine.

"We think that there are likely to be multiple pathways, and this has been one of the foci of our research over the years," he said.

Section 3.2

Diabetes and Cardiovascular Disease

This section includes text excerpted from "Diabetes, Heart Disease, and Stroke," National Institute of Diabetes and Digestive and Kidney Diseases (NIDDK), February 2017.

Having diabetes means that you are more likely to develop heart disease and have a greater chance of a heart attack or a stroke. People with diabetes are also more likely to have certain conditions, or risk factors, that increase the chances of having heart disease or stroke, such as high blood pressure or high cholesterol. If you have diabetes, you can protect your heart and health by managing your blood glucose, also called "blood sugar," as well as your blood pressure and cholesterol. If you smoke, get help to stop.

What Is the Link among Diabetes, Heart Disease, and Stroke?

Over time, high blood glucose from diabetes can damage your blood vessels and the nerves that control your heart and blood vessels. The longer you have diabetes, the higher the chances that you will develop heart disease.

People with diabetes tend to develop heart disease at a younger age than people without diabetes. In adults with diabetes, the most common causes of death are heart disease and stroke. Adults with diabetes are nearly twice as likely to die from heart disease or stroke as people without diabetes. The good news is that the steps you take to manage your diabetes also help to lower your chances of having heart disease or stroke.

What Else Increases Your Chances of Heart Disease or Stroke If You Have Diabetes?

If you have diabetes, other factors add to your chances of developing heart disease or having a stroke.

Smoking

Smoking raises your risk of developing heart disease. If you have diabetes, it is important to stop smoking because smoking and diabetes both narrow blood vessels. Smoking also increases your chances of developing other long-term problems, such as lung disease. Smoking also can damage the blood vessels in your legs and increase the risk of lower leg infections, ulcers, and amputation.

High Blood Pressure

If you have high blood pressure, your heart must work harder to pump blood. High blood pressure can strain your heart, damage blood vessels, and increase your risk of heart attack, stroke, eye problems, and kidney problems.

Abnormal Cholesterol Levels

Cholesterol is a type of fat produced by your liver and found in your blood. You have two kinds of cholesterol in your blood: low-density lipoprotein (LDL) and high-density lipoprotein (HDL).

LDL, often called "bad cholesterol," can build up and clog your blood vessels. High levels of LDL cholesterol raise your risk of developing heart disease.

Another type of blood fat, triglycerides, also can raise your risk of heart disease when the levels are higher than recommended by your healthcare team.

Obesity and Belly Fat

Being overweight or obese can affect your ability to manage your diabetes and increase your risk for many health problems, including heart disease and high blood pressure. If you are overweight, a healthy eating plan with reduced calories often will lower your glucose levels and reduce your need for medications. Excess belly fat around your waist, even if you are not overweight, can raise your chances of developing heart disease.

You have excess belly fat if your waist measures:

- More than 40 inches and you are a man

- More than 35 inches and you are a woman

Family History of Heart Disease

A family history of heart disease may also add to your chances of developing heart disease. If one or more of your family members had a heart attack before the age of 50, you may have an even higher chance of developing heart disease.

You cannot change whether heart disease runs in your family, but if you have diabetes, it is even more important to take steps to protect yourself from heart disease and decrease your chances of having a stroke.

How Can I Lower My Chances of a Heart Attack or Stroke If I Have Diabetes?

Taking care of your diabetes is important to help you take care of your heart. You can lower your chances of having a heart attack or stroke by taking the following steps to manage your diabetes to keep your heart and blood vessels healthy.

Manage Your Diabetes ABCs

Knowing your diabetes ABCs will help you manage your blood glucose, blood pressure, and cholesterol. Stopping smoking if you have diabetes is also important to lower your chances for heart disease.

A is for the A1C test. The A1C test shows your average blood glucose level over the past three months. This is different from the blood glucose checks that you do every day. The higher your A1C number, the higher your blood glucose levels have been during the past three months. High levels of blood glucose can harm your heart, blood vessels, kidneys, feet, and eyes.

The A1C goal for many people with diabetes is below seven percent. Some people may do better with a slightly higher A1C goal. Ask your healthcare team what your goal should be.

B is for blood pressure. Blood pressure is the force of your blood against the wall of your blood vessels. If your blood pressure gets too high, it makes your heart work too hard. High blood pressure can cause a heart attack or stroke and damage your kidneys and eyes.

The blood pressure goal for most people with diabetes is below 140/90 mm Hg. Ask your healthcare team what your goal should be.

C is for cholesterol. You have two kinds of cholesterol in your blood: LDL and HDL. LDL, or "bad cholesterol," can build up and clog your blood vessels. Too much bad cholesterol can cause a heart attack or stroke. HDL, or "good cholesterol," helps remove the bad cholesterol from your blood vessels.

Ask your healthcare team what your cholesterol numbers should be. If you are over 40 years of age, you may need to take medicine, such as a statin, to lower your cholesterol and protect your heart. Some people with very high LDL cholesterol may need to take medicine at a younger age.

S is for stop smoking. Not smoking is especially important for people with diabetes because smoking and diabetes both narrow blood vessels, so your heart has to work harder.

If you quit smoking:

- You will lower your risk for heart attack, stroke, nerve disease, kidney disease, eye disease, and amputation.

- Your blood glucose, blood pressure, and cholesterol levels may improve.

- Your blood circulation will improve.

- You may have an easier time being physically active.

If you smoke or use other tobacco products, stop. Ask for help so you do not have to do it alone. You can start by calling the national quitline at 800-784-8669. For tips on quitting, go to Smokefree.gov.

Ask your healthcare team about your goals for A1C, blood pressure, and cholesterol, and what you can do to reach these goals.

How Do Doctors Diagnose Heart Disease in Diabetes?

Doctors diagnose heart disease in diabetes based on:

- Your symptoms

- Your medical and family history

- How likely you are to have heart disease

- A physical exam

- Results from tests and procedures

Tests used to monitor your diabetes—A1C, blood pressure, and cholesterol—help your doctor decide whether it is important to do other tests to check your heart health.

What Are the Warning Signs of Heart Attack and Stroke?

Warning signs of a heart attack include:

- Pain or pressure in your chest that lasts longer than a few minutes or goes away and comes back

- Pain or discomfort in one or both of your arms or shoulders, your back, your neck, or your jaw

- Shortness of breath

- Sweating or light-headedness

- Indigestion or nausea (feeling sick to your stomach)
- Feeling very tired

Treatment works best when it is given right away. Warning signs can be different in different people. You may not have all of these symptoms. If you have angina, it is important to know how and when to seek medical treatment. Women sometimes have nausea and vomiting; feel very tired (sometimes for days); and have pain in the back, shoulders, or jaw without any chest pain. People with diabetes-related nerve damage may not notice any chest pain.

Warning signs of a stroke include:

- Sudden weakness or numbness of your face, arm, or leg on one side of your body
- Confusion, or trouble talking or understanding
- Dizziness, loss of balance, or trouble walking
- Trouble seeing out of one or both eyes
- Severe headache

If you have any one of these warning signs, call 911. You can help prevent permanent damage by getting to a hospital within an hour of a stroke.

Section 3.3

High Blood Pressure and Heart Disease

This section includes text excerpted from "High Blood Pressure,"
National Heart, Lung, and Blood Institute (NHLBI), May 17, 2018.

High blood pressure is a common disease in which blood flows through blood vessels, or arteries, at higher than normal pressures. Blood pressure is the force of blood pushing against the walls of your arteries as the heart pumps blood. High blood pressure, sometimes called "hypertension," is when this force against the artery walls is too high. Your doctor may diagnose you with high blood pressure if you have consistently high blood pressure readings.

To control or lower high blood pressure, your doctor may recommend that you adopt heart-healthy lifestyle changes, such as heart-healthy eating patterns, like the Dietary Approaches to Stop Hypertension (DASH) eating plan, alone or with medicines. Controlling or lowering blood pressure can also help prevent or delay high blood pressure complications, such as chronic kidney disease, heart attack, heart failure, stroke, and possibly vascular dementia.

Causes of High Blood Pressure

Eating too much sodium and having certain medical conditions can cause high blood pressure. Taking certain medicines, including birth control pills or over-the-counter cold relief medicines, can also make blood pressure rise.

Eating Too Much Sodium

Unhealthy eating patterns, particularly eating too much sodium, are a common cause of high blood pressure in the United States. Healthy lifestyle changes, such as heart-healthy eating, can help prevent or treat high blood pressure.

Do You Know How Sodium Causes Blood Pressure to Rise?

Sodium is a key part of how the body controls blood pressure levels. The kidneys help balance fluid and sodium levels in the body. They use sodium and potassium to remove excess fluid from the blood. The body gets rid of this excess fluid as urine. When sodium levels in the blood are high, blood vessels retain more fluid. This increases blood pressure against the blood vessel walls.

Other Medical Conditions

Other medical conditions change the way your body controls fluids, sodium, and hormones in your blood.

Other medical causes of high blood pressure include:

- Certain tumors
- Chronic kidney disease
- Being overweight or obese
- Sleep apnea
- Thyroid problems

Risk Factors for High Blood Pressure

There are many risk factors for high blood pressure. Some risk factors, such as unhealthy lifestyle habits, can be changed. Other risk factors, such as age, family history and genetics, race and ethnicity, and sex, cannot be changed. Healthy lifestyle changes can decrease your risk for developing high blood pressure.

Age

Blood pressure tends to increase with age. Our blood vessels naturally thicken and stiffen over time. These changes increase the risk for high blood pressure.

However, the risk of high blood pressure is increasing for children and teens, possibly due to the rise in the number of children and teens who are overweight or obese.

As we age, blood vessel structure and function changes in the following ways:

- **Changes in blood vessel function.** The lining of blood vessels sustains more damage over time. This may be caused by oxidative stress or deoxyribonucleic acid (DNA) damage, among other factors. With age, levels of the hormone angiotensin also rise, triggering inflammation in blood vessels. At the same time, vessels slowly lose the ability to release substances that protect or repair the lining. When the blood vessel lining does not work as well, higher diastolic blood pressures can result.

- **Changes in blood vessel structure.** Blood vessels have layers of the proteins elastin and collagen. Elastin is what makes blood vessels flexible. Collagen, which is stiffer, gives vessels structure. With age, elastin breaks down. Even the elastin that remains becomes less elastic. Meanwhile, collagen deposits in the vessels increase. As a result, blood vessels grow thicker and bend less easily over time. These changes may lead to higher systolic blood pressure.

Family History and Genetics

High blood pressure often runs in families. Much of the understanding of the body systems involved in high blood pressure has come from genetic studies. Research has identified many gene variations associated with small increases in the risk of developing high blood pressure. New research suggests that certain DNA changes during fetal development may also lead to the development of high blood pressure later in life. Some people have a high sensitivity to sodium. This can also run in families.

Sodium sensitivity can increase the risk of developing high blood pressure. It is more common in:

- African Americans
- Older adults
- People who have elevated blood pressure, with systolic readings of 120 to 129 millimeters of mercury (mm Hg)
- People with chronic kidney disease, diabetes, or metabolic syndrome

Unhealthy Lifestyle Habits

Unhealthy lifestyle habits can increase the risk of high blood pressure. These habits include:

- Unhealthy eating patterns, such as eating too much sodium
- Drinking too much alcohol
- Being physically inactive

Race or Ethnicity

High blood pressure is more common in African American adults than in White, Hispanic, or Asian adults. Compared with other racial or ethnic groups, African Americans tend to have higher average blood pressure numbers and get high blood pressure earlier in life.

Sex

Before the age of 55, men are more likely than women to develop high blood pressure. After the age of 55, women are more likely than men to develop high blood pressure.

Signs, Symptoms, and Complications of High Blood Pressure

It is important to have regular blood pressure readings taken and to know your numbers because high blood pressure usually does not cause symptoms until serious complications occur. Undiagnosed or uncontrolled high blood pressure can cause the following complications:

- Aneurysms

- Chronic kidney disease

- Eye damage

- Heart attack

- Heart failure

- Peripheral artery disease

- Stroke

- Vascular dementia

Section 3.4

High Cholesterol and Heart Disease

This section includes text excerpted from "High Blood Cholesterol," National Heart, Lung, and Blood Institute (NHLBI) June 30, 2019.

High blood cholesterol is a condition that causes the levels of certain bad fats, or lipids, to be too high in the blood. This condition is usually caused by lifestyle factors, such as diet, in combination with the genes that you inherit from your parents. Less commonly, it is caused by other medical conditions or some medicines.

You may be diagnosed with high blood cholesterol if you consistently have high levels of bad cholesterol in your blood in a routine test called a "lipid panel." To treat high blood cholesterol, your doctor may recommend heart-healthy lifestyle changes, such as following a heart-healthy diet, quitting smoking, or aiming for a healthy weight. Your doctor may also prescribe medicines, such as statins, to lower and control your high blood cholesterol. Untreated high blood cholesterol can lead to the buildup of plaque in the blood vessels, called "atherosclerosis." Plaque buildup increases your risk for heart attack, stroke, and peripheral artery disease.

Causes of High Cholesterol

The most common cause of high blood cholesterol is an unhealthy lifestyle. However, the genes that you inherit from your parents, other medical conditions, and some medicines may also cause high blood cholesterol.

Unhealthy Lifestyle Habits

Unhealthy eating patterns, lack of physical activity, and smoking can cause high blood cholesterol.

- Unhealthy eating patterns, such as consuming high amounts of saturated fats or trans fats, can increase bad low-density lipoprotein cholesterol (LDL cholesterol).

- Lack of physical activity, such as spending a lot of time during the day sitting and watching TV or using the computer, is linked with lower levels of good high-density lipoprotein cholesterol (HDL cholesterol).

- Smoking lowers HDL cholesterol, particularly in women, and increases LDL cholesterol.

Genes

Some people may develop high blood cholesterol because of mutations, or changes, in their genes. These mutations make it harder for the body to clear LDL cholesterol from the blood or break it down in the liver. Familial hypercholesterolemia is one inherited form of high blood cholesterol.

Other Medical Conditions

The following medical conditions may cause high blood cholesterol:

- Chronic kidney disease (CKD)

- Diabetes

- Human immunodeficiency virus (HIV)

- Hypothyroidism

- Overweight or obese

- Polycystic ovary syndrome (PCOS)

- Inflammatory diseases, such as psoriasis, lichen planus, pemphigus, histiocytosis, lupus erythematosus, and rheumatoid arthritis (RA)

Medicines

Some medicines that you take for other medical conditions can increase your cholesterol levels. Examples of these medicines include the following:

- Diuretics, such as thiazide that are used for high blood pressure

- Immunosuppressive drugs, such as cyclosporine that are used to treat inflammatory diseases, such as psoriasis or to prevent rejection after a transplant

- Steroids, such as prednisone that are used to treat inflammatory diseases, such as lupus and psoriasis

- Retinoids, such as retinol that are used to treat acne

- Antiretroviral medicines used to treat HIV

- Antiarrhythmic medicines, such as amiodarone that are used in treatment for irregular rhythm of the heart

Risk Factors for High Cholesterol

You may have an increased risk for high blood cholesterol because of your age, your family history and genetics, and your race.

Age

Your body's metabolism and chemistry change as you age. For example, your liver does not remove LDL cholesterol as efficiently as when you were young. These normal age-related changes may increase your risk of developing high blood cholesterol.

Family History and Genetics

Genetic studies have found that related family members tend to have similar levels of LDL cholesterol, known as "bad cholesterol," or HDL cholesterol, known as "good cholesterol." Depending on the genes in your family, you may have an increased risk for high blood cholesterol. Learn more about current research to better understand how genetic differences may affect how our bodies absorb cholesterol from the foods that we eat, how much cholesterol the liver produces and removes, and how we respond to high blood cholesterol treatments.

Race

Your race may also increase your risk for high blood cholesterol. Compared to White individuals, Black individuals have higher HDL and LDL cholesterol levels.

Levels of one type of blood fat can signal your risk of developing heart disease separately from the others. It is called "lipoprotein-a," or "Lp(a)." Lipoproteins, including HDL and LDL, carry cholesterol in your blood. Unlike HDL and LDL, Lp(a) is not part of standard lipid panels, but your doctor can request a test for it in special cases. Genes determine how much Lp(a) you have. This level is unlikely to change much from childhood to old age. If other cholesterol measurements on your lipid panel are low, high Lp(a) could explain other signs of heart disease, especially in children, or suggest a particular treatment approach.

Signs, Symptoms, and Complications of High Cholesterol

High blood cholesterol does not cause specific symptoms. But people who have very high blood cholesterol may show signs, such as xanthomas and corneal arcus. Undiagnosed or untreated high blood cholesterol can lead to serious complications, such as heart attack and stroke.

Complications

High blood cholesterol levels lead to atherosclerosis, or the buildup of plaque deposits in blood vessels throughout the body. Over time, chronic or uncontrolled high blood cholesterol can cause serious complications including the following:

- Carotid artery disease
- Coronary heart disease (CHD), including angina or heart attack
- Peripheral artery disease (PAD)
- Stroke

Do You Know Why High Blood Cholesterol Can Cause These Complications?

Cells are not able to destroy cholesterol, so they transfer excess cholesterol to the HDL to transport it back to the liver for elimination. In this way, HDL protects your heart from atherosclerotic disease, so HDL cholesterol is sometimes called "good cholesterol." LDL is a lipoprotein that carries 75 percent of the cholesterol in blood to the peripheral tissues. LDL is removed from the blood by the liver to be eliminated or reused. When the amount of LDL is too high, the liver is not able to remove all of it. It is deposited in the blood vessels, contributing to the development of atherosclerosis, so LDL cholesterol is sometimes called "bad cholesterol."

Section 3.5

Metabolic Syndrome and Cardiovascular Disease

This section includes text excerpted from "Metabolic Syndrome," National Heart, Lung, and Blood Institute (NHLBI) January 30, 2019.

What Is Metabolic Syndrome?

Metabolic syndrome is the name for a group of risk factors that raises your risk for heart disease and other health problems, such as diabetes and stroke.

The term "metabolic" refers to the biochemical processes involved in the body's normal functioning. Risk factors are traits, conditions, or habits that increase your chance of developing a disease.

In this section, "heart disease" refers to ischemic heart disease, a condition in which a waxy substance called "plaque" builds up inside the arteries that supply blood to the heart.

Plaque hardens and narrows the arteries, reducing blood flow to your heart muscle. This can lead to chest pain, a heart attack, heart damage, or even death.

Metabolic Risk Factors

The five conditions described below are metabolic risk factors. You can have any one of these risk factors by itself, but they tend to occur together. You must have at least three metabolic risk factors to be diagnosed with metabolic syndrome.

- A large waistline. This also is called "abdominal obesity" or "having an apple shape." Excess fat in the stomach area is a greater risk factor for heart disease than excess fat in other parts of the body, such as on the hips.

- A high triglyceride level (or you are on medicine to treat high triglycerides). Triglycerides are a type of fat found in the blood.

- A low HDL cholesterol level (or you are on medicine to treat low HDL cholesterol). HDL sometimes is called "good cholesterol." This is because it helps remove cholesterol from your arteries. A low HDL cholesterol level raises your risk for heart disease.

- High blood pressure (or you are on medicine to treat high blood pressure). Blood pressure is the force of blood pushing against the walls of your arteries as your heart pumps blood. If this pressure rises and stays high over time, it can damage your heart and lead to plaque buildup.

High fasting blood sugar (or you are on medicine to treat high blood sugar). Mildly high blood sugar may be an early sign of diabetes.

Causes of Metabolic Syndrome

Metabolic syndrome has several causes that act together. You can control some of the causes, such as being overweight or obese, an inactive lifestyle, and insulin resistance.

You cannot control other factors that may play a role in causing metabolic syndrome, such as growing older. Your risk for metabolic syndrome increases with age.

You also cannot control genetics (ethnicity and family history), which may play a role in causing the condition. For example, genetics can increase your risk for insulin resistance, which can lead to metabolic syndrome.

People who have metabolic syndrome often have two other conditions: excessive blood clotting and constant, low-grade inflammation throughout the body. Researchers do not know whether these conditions cause metabolic syndrome or worsen it.

Researchers continue to study conditions that may play a role in metabolic syndrome, such as:

- A fatty liver (excess triglycerides and other fats in the liver)

- Polycystic ovarian syndrome (PCOS), a tendency to develop cysts on the ovaries

- Gallstones

- Breathing problems during sleep (such as sleep apnea)

Risk Factors for Metabolic Syndrome

People at greatest risk for metabolic syndrome have these underlying causes:

- Abdominal obesity (a large waistline)

- An inactive lifestyle

- Insulin resistance

Some people are at risk for metabolic syndrome because they take medicines that cause weight gain or changes in blood pressure, blood cholesterol, and blood sugar levels. These medicines most often are used to treat inflammation, allergies, human immunodeficiency virus (HIV), and depression and other types of mental illness.

Populations Affected

Some racial and ethnic groups in the United States are at higher risk for metabolic syndrome than others. Mexican Americans have the highest rate of metabolic syndrome, followed by Whites and Blacks.

Other groups at increased risk for metabolic syndrome include:

- People who have a personal history of diabetes

- People who have a sibling or parent who has diabetes

- Women, when compared with men

- Women who have a personal history of PCOS, a tendency to develop cysts on the ovaries

Heart Disease Risk

Metabolic syndrome increases your risk for ischemic heart disease. Other risk factors, besides metabolic syndrome, also increase your risk for heart disease. For example, a high LDL cholesterol ("bad cholesterol") level and smoking are major risk factors for heart disease.

Even if you do not have metabolic syndrome, you should find out your short-term risk for heart disease. The National Cholesterol Education Program (NCEP) divides short-term heart disease risk into four categories. Your risk category depends on which risk factors you have and how many you have.

Your risk factors are used to calculate your ten-year risk of developing heart disease. The NCEP has an online calculator (www.nhlbi. nih.gov/health-topics/assessing-cardiovascular-risk) that you can use to estimate your ten-year risk of having a heart attack.

- **High risk.** You are in this category if you already have heart disease or diabetes, or if your 10-year risk score is more than 20 percent.

- **Moderately high risk.** You are in this category if you have 2 or more risk factors and your 10-year risk score is 10 percent to 20 percent.

- **Moderate risk.** You are in this category if you have 2 or more risk factors and your 10-year risk score is less than 10 percent.

- **Lower risk.** You are in this category if you have 0 or 1 risk factor.

Even if your 10-year risk score is not high, metabolic syndrome will increase your risk for coronary heart disease over time.

Signs, Symptoms, and Complications of Metabolic Syndrome

Metabolic syndrome is a group of risk factors that raises your risk for heart disease and other health problems, such as diabetes and stroke. These risk factors can increase your risk for health problems even if they are only moderately raised (borderline-high risk factors).

Most of the metabolic risk factors have no signs or symptoms, although a large waistline is a visible sign.

Some people may have symptoms of high blood sugar if diabetes—especially type 2 diabetes—is present. Symptoms of high blood sugar often include increased thirst; increased urination, especially at night; fatigue (tiredness); and blurred vision.

High blood pressure usually has no signs or symptoms. However, some people in the early stages of high blood pressure may have dull headaches, dizzy spells, or more nosebleeds than usual.

Section 3.6

Sleep Apnea and Cardiovascular Disease

This section includes text excerpted from "Sleep Apnea Information Page," National Institute of Neurological Disorders and Stroke (NINDS) July 30, 2018.

Sleep apnea is a common sleep disorder characterized by brief interruptions of breathing during sleep. These episodes usually last 10 seconds or more and occur repeatedly throughout the night. People with sleep apnea will partially awaken as they struggle to breathe, but in the morning, they will not be aware of the disturbances in their sleep. The most common type of sleep apnea is obstructive sleep apnea (OSA), which is caused by relaxation of soft tissue in the back of the throat that blocks the passage of air. Central sleep apnea (CSA) is caused by irregularities in the brain's normal signals to breathe. Most people with sleep apnea will have a combination of both types. The hallmark symptom of the disorder is excessive daytime sleepiness. Additional symptoms of sleep apnea include restless sleep, loud snoring (with periods of silence followed by gasps), falling asleep during the day, morning headaches, trouble concentrating, irritability, forgetfulness, mood or behavior changes, anxiety, and depression. Not everyone who has these symptoms will have sleep apnea, but it is recommended that people who are experiencing even a few of these symptoms visit their doctor for evaluation. Sleep apnea is more likely to occur in men than women, and in people who are overweight or obese.

Treatment of Sleep Apnea

There are a variety of treatments for sleep apnea, depending on an individual's medical history and the severity of the disorder. Most treatment regimens begin with lifestyle changes, such as avoiding alcohol and medications that relax the central nervous system (for example, sedatives and muscle relaxants), losing weight, and quitting smoking. Some people are helped by special pillows or devices that keep them from sleeping on their backs, or oral appliances to keep the airway open during sleep. If these conservative methods are inadequate, doctors often recommend continuous positive airway pressure (CPAP), in which a face mask is attached to a tube and a machine that blows pressurized air into the mask and through the airway to keep it open. Also available are machines that offer variable positive airway pressure (VPAP) and automatic positive airway pressure (APAP). There are also surgical procedures that can be used to remove tissue and widen the airway. The U.S. Food and Drug Administration (FDA) has approved a surgically implantable device placed in the upper chest that monitors a person's respiratory signals during sleep and stimulates a nerve to send signals to a muscle to stimulate and restore normal breathing. Some individuals may need a combination of therapies to successfully treat their sleep apnea.

Prognosis for Sleep Apnea

Untreated sleep apnea can be life-threatening. Excessive daytime sleepiness can cause people to fall asleep at inappropriate times, such as while driving. Sleep apnea also appears to put individuals at risk for stroke and transient ischemic attacks (TIAs), also known as "mini-strokes"), and is associated with coronary heart disease, heart failure, irregular heartbeat, heart attack, and high blood pressure. Although there is no cure for sleep apnea, recent studies show that successful treatment can reduce the risk of heart and blood pressure problems.

Section 3.7

Stress and Cardiovascular Disease

This section includes text excerpted from "Your Guide to Living Well with Heart Disease," National Heart, Lung, and Blood Institute (NHLBI), November 2005. Reviewed May 2019.

A number of other factors also contribute to heart disease, including certain health conditions, medicines, and other substances. Stress is one among them.

Stress is linked to heart disease in a number of ways. Research shows that the most commonly reported trigger for a heart attack is an emotionally upsetting event, particularly one involving anger. In addition, some common ways of coping with stress, such as overeating, heavy drinking, and smoking, are clearly bad for your heart.

The good news is that sensible health habits can have a protective effect. For people with heart disease, regular physical activity not only relieves stress but also can directly lower the risk of heart disease complications. Participating in a stress management program can help to prevent recurrent heart attacks and repeat heart procedures. Good relationships count too; developing strong personal ties can help to improve recovery after a heart attack.

Much remains to be learned about the connections between stress and heart disease, but a few things are clear. Staying physically active, developing a wide circle of supportive people in your life, and sharing your feelings and concerns with them can help you to be happier and live longer.

Chapter 4

Aging and Cardiovascular Risk Factors

How Does Your Heart Change with Age?

People 65 years of age and older are much more likely than younger people to suffer a heart attack, have a stroke, or develop coronary heart disease (CHD) (commonly called "heart disease") and heart failure. Heart disease is also a major cause of disability, limiting the activity and eroding the quality of life (QOL) of millions of older people.

Aging can cause changes in the heart and blood vessels. For example, as you get older, your heart cannot beat as fast during physical activity or times of stress as it did when you were younger. However, the number of heartbeats per minute (heart rate) at rest does not change significantly with normal aging.

Changes that happen with age may increase a person's risk of heart disease. A major cause of heart disease is the buildup of fatty deposits in the walls of arteries over many years. The good news is there are things you can do to delay, lower, or possibly avoid or reverse your risk.

The most common aging change is increased stiffness of the large arteries, called "arteriosclerosis," or hardening of the arteries. This causes high blood pressure, or hypertension, which becomes more common as we age.

This chapter includes text excerpted from "Heart Health and Aging," National Institute on Aging (NIA), National Institutes of Health (NIH), June 1, 2018.

High blood pressure and other risk factors, including advancing age, increase the risk of developing atherosclerosis. Because there are several modifiable risk factors for atherosclerosis, it is not necessarily a normal part of aging. Plaque builds up inside the walls of your arteries and, over time, hardens, and narrows your arteries, which limits the flow of oxygen-rich blood to your organs and other parts of your body. Oxygen and blood nutrients are supplied to the heart muscle through the coronary arteries. Heart disease develops when plaque builds up in the coronary arteries, reducing blood flow to your heart muscle. Over time, the heart muscle can become weakened and/or damaged, resulting in heart failure. Heart damage can be caused by heart attacks, long-standing hypertension and diabetes, and chronic heavy alcohol use.

Age can cause other changes to the heart. For example:

- There are age-related changes in the electrical system that can lead to arrhythmias—a rapid, slowed, or irregular heartbeat—and/or the need for a pacemaker. Valves—the one-way, door-like parts that open and close to control blood flow between the chambers of your heart—may become thicker and stiffer. Stiffer valves can limit the flow of blood out of the heart and become leaky, both of which can cause fluid to build up in the lungs or in the body (legs, feet, and abdomen.)

- The chambers of your heart may increase in size. The heart wall thickens, so the amount of blood that a chamber can hold may decrease despite the increased overall heart size. The heart may fill more slowly. Long-standing hypertension is the main cause of increased thickness of the heart wall, which can increase the risk of atrial fibrillation (AF), a common heart rhythm problem in older people.

- With increasing age, people become more sensitive to salt, which may cause an increase in blood pressure and/or ankle or foot swelling (edema).

Other factors, such as thyroid disease or chemotherapy, may also weaken the heart muscle. Things you cannot control, such as your family history, might increase your risk of heart disease. But, leading a heart-healthy lifestyle might help you avoid or delay serious illness.

What Is Heart Disease?

Heart disease is caused by atherosclerosis, which is the buildup of fatty deposits, or plaques, in the walls of the coronary arteries over many years. The coronary arteries surround the outside of the heart and supply blood nutrients and oxygen to the heart muscle. When plaque builds up inside the arteries, there is less space for blood to flow normally and deliver oxygen to the heart. If the flow of blood to your heart is reduced by plaque buildup or is blocked if plaque suddenly ruptures, it can cause angina (chest pain or discomfort) or a heart attack. When the heart muscle does not get enough oxygen and blood nutrients, the heart muscle cells will die (heart attack) and weaken the heart, diminishing its ability to pump blood to the rest of the body.

Signs of Heart Disease

Early heart disease often does not have symptoms, or the symptoms may be barely noticeable. That is why regular checkups with your doctor are important.

Contact your doctor right away if you feel any chest pain, pressure, or discomfort. However, chest pain is a less common sign of heart disease as it progresses, so be aware of other symptoms. Tell your doctor if you have:

- Pain, numbness, and/or tingling in the shoulders, arms, neck, jaw, or back

- Shortness of breath when active, at rest, or while lying flat

- Chest pain during physical activity that gets better when you rest

- Light-headedness

- Dizziness

- Confusion

- Headaches

- Cold sweats

- Nausea/vomiting

- Tiredness or fatigue

- Swelling in the ankles, feet, legs, stomach, and/or neck

- Reduced ability to exercise or be physically active

- Problems doing your normal activities

Problems with arrhythmia are much more common in older adults than younger people. Arrhythmia needs to be treated. See a doctor if you feel a fluttering in your chest or have the feeling that your heart is skipping a beat or beating too hard, especially if you are weaker than usual, dizzy, tired, or get short of breath when active.

If you have any signs of heart disease, your doctor may send you to a cardiologist, a doctor who specializes in the heart.

What Can You Do to Prevent Heart Disease?

There are many steps you can take to keep your heart healthy.

Try to be more physically active. Talk to your doctor about the type of activities that would be best for you. If possible, aim to get at least 150 minutes of physical activity each week. Every day is best. It does not have to be done all at once.

Start by doing activities you enjoy—brisk walking, dancing, bowling, bicycling, or gardening, for example. Avoid spending hours every day sitting.

If you smoke, quit. Smoking is the leading cause of preventable death. Smoking adds to the damage to the artery walls. It is never too late to get some benefit from quitting smoking. Quitting, even in later life, can lower your risk of heart disease, stroke, and cancer over time.

Follow a heart-healthy diet. Choose foods that are low in trans and saturated fats, added sugars, and salt. As we get older, we become more sensitive to salt, which can cause swelling in the legs and feet. Eat plenty of fruits, vegetables, and foods high in fiber, such as those made from whole grains.

Keep a healthy weight. Balancing the calories, you eat and drink with the calories burned by being physically active helps to maintain a healthy weight. Some ways you can maintain a healthy weight include limiting portion size and being physically active.

Keep your diabetes, high blood pressure, and/or high cholesterol under control. Follow your doctor's advice to manage these conditions, and take medications as directed.

Do not drink a lot of alcohol. Men should not have more than 2 drinks a day and women only 1. One drink is equal to:

- One 12-ounce can or bottle of regular beer, ale, or wine cooler

- One 8- or 9-ounce can or bottle of malt liquor

- One 5-ounce glass of red or white wine

- One 1.5-ounce shot glass of distilled spirits, such as gin, rum, tequila, vodka, or whiskey

Manage stress. Learn how to manage stress, relax, and cope with problems to improve physical and emotional health. Consider activities, such as a stress management program, meditation, physical activity, and talking things out with friends or family.

Cholesterol

High blood cholesterol levels can lead to plaque buildup in your arteries. Your doctor can check the level of cholesterol in your blood with a blood test. You must be fasting overnight or for eight hours before this blood test. This will tell you your overall or total cholesterol level, as well as low-density lipoprotein or "bad cholesterol" (LDL), High-density lipoprotein or "healthy cholesterol" (HDL), and triglycerides (another type of fat in the blood that puts you at risk for heart problems).

Questions to Ask Your Doctor

Ask your doctor questions to learn more about your risk for heart disease and what to do about it. Learn what you can do if you are at increased risk or already have a heart problem.

- What is my risk for heart disease?

- What is my blood pressure?

- What are my cholesterol numbers? (These include total cholesterol, LDL, HDL, and triglycerides.) Make sure your doctor has checked a fasting blood sample to determine your cholesterol levels.

- Do I need to lose weight for my health?

- What is my blood sugar level, and does it mean that I am at risk for diabetes?

- What other screening tests do I need to tell me if I am at risk for heart disease and how to lower my risk?

- What can you do to help me quit smoking?

- How much physical activity do I need to help protect my heart?

- What is a heart-healthy eating plan for me?

- How can I tell if I am having a heart attack? If I think I am having one, what should I do?

The Future of Research on Aging and the Heart

Adults 65 years of age and older are more likely than younger people to suffer from cardiovascular disease (CVD), which is problems with the heart, blood vessels, or both. Aging can cause changes in the heart and blood vessels that may increase a person's risk of developing cardiovascular disease.

To understand how aging is linked to cardiovascular disease so that we can ultimately develop cures for this group of diseases, we need to first understand what is happening in the healthy, but aging heart and blood vessels. This understanding has advanced dramatically in the past 30 years.

Nowadays, more than ever, scientists understand what causes your blood vessels and heart to age and how your aging cardiovascular system leads to cardiovascular disease. In addition, they have pinpointed risk factors that increase the odds a person will develop cardiovascular disease. They are learning much more about how physical activity, diet, and other lifestyle factors that influence the "rate of aging" in the healthy heart and arteries. The aging of other organ systems, including the muscles, kidneys, and lungs, also likely contributes to heart disease. Research is ongoing to unravel how these aging systems influence each other, which may reveal new targets for treatments.

In the future, interventions or treatments that slow accelerated aging of the heart and arteries in young and middle-aged people who seem to be healthy could prevent or delay the onset of heart disease, stroke, and other cardiovascular disorders in later life. Some interventions that we already know slow the rate of aging in the heart and arteries include healthy eating, exercise, reducing stress, and quitting smoking. The more we understand the changes that take place in cells and molecules during aging, for example, the closer we get to the possibility of designing drugs that target those changes. Gene therapies can also target specific cellular changes and could potentially be a way to intervene in the aging process. While waiting for these new therapies to be developed, you can still enjoy activities, such as exercise and a healthy diet, that can benefit your heart.

Chapter 5

Smoking and Cardiovascular Disease

Smoking is a major cause of cardiovascular disease (CVD) and causes approximately 1 of every 4 deaths from CVD, according to the 2014 Surgeon General's *The Health Consequences of Smoking—50 Years of Progress.* CVD is the single largest cause of death in the United States, killing more than 800,000 people a year. More than 16 million Americans have heart disease. Almost 8 million have had a heart attack, and 7 million have had a stroke.

Even people who smoke fewer than five cigarettes a day may show signs of early CVD. The risk of CVD increases with the number of cigarettes smoked per day and when smoking continues for many years. Smoking cigarettes with lower levels of tar or nicotine does not reduce the risk for cardiovascular disease.

Exposure to secondhand smoke causes heart disease in nonsmokers. More than 33,000 nonsmokers die every year in the United States from coronary heart disease (CHD) caused by exposure to secondhand smoke. Exposure to secondhand smoke can also cause heart attacks and strokes in nonsmokers.

This chapter includes text excerpted from "Smoking and Cardiovascular Disease," Centers for Disease Control and Prevention (CDC), October 15, 2014. Reviewed May 2019.

How Smoking Harms the Cardiovascular System

Chemicals in cigarette smoke cause the cells that line blood vessels to become swollen and inflamed. This can narrow the blood vessels and lead to many cardiovascular conditions.

- **Atherosclerosis,** in which arteries narrow and become less flexible, occurs when fat, cholesterol, and other substances in the blood form plaque that builds up in the walls of arteries. The opening inside the arteries narrows as plaque builds up, and blood can no longer flow properly to various parts of the body. Smoking increases the formation of plaque in blood vessels.

- **Coronary heart disease (CHD)** occurs when arteries that carry blood to the heart muscle are narrowed by plaque or blocked by clots. Chemicals in cigarette smoke cause the blood to thicken and form clots inside veins and arteries. Blockage from a clot can lead to a heart attack and sudden death.

- **Stroke** is a loss of brain function caused when blood flow within the brain is interrupted.

Strokes can cause permanent brain damage and death. Smoking increases the risk of strokes. Deaths from strokes are more likely among smokers than among former smokers or people who have never smoked.

- **Peripheral arterial disease (PAD)** and peripheral vascular disease occur when blood vessels become narrower and the flow of blood to arms, legs, hands, and feet is reduced. Cells and tissue are deprived of needed oxygen when blood flow is reduced. In extreme cases, an infected limb must be removed. Smoking is the most common preventable cause of PAD.

- **Abdominal aortic aneurysm (AAA)** is a bulge or weakened area that occurs in the portion of the aorta that is in the abdomen. The aorta is the main artery that carries oxygen-rich blood throughout the body. Smoking is a known cause of early damage to the abdominal aorta, which can lead to an aneurysm. A ruptured abdominal aortic aneurysm is life-threatening; almost all deaths from abdominal aortic aneurysms are caused by smoking. Women smokers have a higher risk of dying from an aortic aneurysm than men who smoke. Autopsies have shown early narrowing of the abdominal aorta in young adults who smoked as adolescents.

Quitting Smoking Cuts Cardiovascular Disease Risks

Even though we do not know exactly which smokers will develop cardiovascular disease risks from smoking, the best thing all smokers can do for their hearts is to quit. Smokers who quit start to improve their heart health and reduce their risk for CVD immediately. Within a year, the risk of heart attack drops dramatically, and even people who have already had a heart attack can cut their risk of having another if they quit smoking. Within five years of quitting, smokers lower their risk of stroke to about that of a person who has never smoked.

Save Your Heart: Avoid the Smoke

Smoking damages the heart and blood vessels very quickly, but the damage is repaired quickly for most smokers who stop smoking. Even long-time smokers can see rapid health improvements when they quit. Within a year, heart attack risk drops dramatically. Within five years, most smokers cut their risk of stroke to nearly that of a nonsmoker. Even a few cigarettes now and then damage the heart, so the only proven strategy to keep your heart safe from the effects of smoking is to quit.

Chapter 6

Recent Research Regarding Cardiovascular Disease Risks

Chapter Contents

Section 6.1

Disrupted Sleep May Lead to Heart Disease

This section includes text excerpted from "How Disrupted
Sleep May Lead to Heart Disease," National
Institutes of Health (NIH), March 5, 2019.

Heart disease is the leading cause of death among women and men
in the United States. The most common cause of heart disease is when
fatty deposits called "plaque" build up inside your arteries, the blood
vessels that carry oxygen-rich blood around your body. This is called
"atherosclerosis." White blood cells (WBCs) from the immune system
collect at the plaque and cause inflammation.

Over time, the plaque hardens and narrows your arteries. This
limits the flow of oxygen-rich blood to your heart and other organs.
Atherosclerosis can lead to serious problems, including heart attack,
stroke, or even death.

Research has linked sleep deficiency and certain sleep disorders,
such as sleep apnea, to an increased risk of heart disease and other
health conditions. But the molecular mechanisms underlying the link
between sleep and heart disease has been unclear.

To learn more about the impact of sleep deficiency on heart disease, a team led by Dr. Filip Swirski at Harvard Medical School and
Massachusetts General Hospital studied a group of mice that were
genetically engineered to develop atherosclerosis. The research was
supported in part by the National Institutes of Health's (NIH) National
Heart, Lung, and Blood Institute (NHLBI).

The researchers repeatedly disrupted the sleep cycles of half
the mice, and the other half slept normally. After 16 weeks, the
sleep-disrupted mice developed larger arterial plaques than the mice
with normal sleep patterns.

The sleep-disrupted mice also had twice the level of certain WBCs
in their circulation than the control mice. And they had lower amounts
of hypocretin, a hormone made by the brain that plays a key role in
regulating sleep and wake states (also known as "orexin"). Further
experiments showed that hypocretin suppressed the production of stem
cells that make the white blood cells in their bone marrow.

Sleep-deficient mice that received hypocretin supplementation
tended to produce fewer immune cells and develop smaller artery wall
plaques than mice that were not given the supplementation. These

results suggest that hypocretin loss during disrupted sleep contributes to inflammation and atherosclerosis.

"We have identified a mechanism by which a brain hormone controls the production of inflammatory cells in the bone marrow in a way that helps protect the blood vessels from damage," Swirski explains. "This anti-inflammatory mechanism is regulated by sleep, and it breaks down when you frequently disrupt sleep or experience poor sleep quality. It is a small piece of a larger puzzle."

"This appears to be the most direct demonstration yet of the molecular connections linking blood and cardiovascular risk factors to sleep health," says Dr. Michael Twery, director of NHLBI's National Center on Sleep Disorders Research (NCSDR).

If disrupted sleep proves to have similar effects in people, these findings could open new avenues for developing ways to treat heart disease.

Section 6.2

Eating Red Meat Daily Triples Heart Disease-Related Chemical

This section includes text excerpted from "Eating Red Meat Daily Triples Heart Disease-Related Chemical," National Institutes of Health (NIH), January 8, 2019.

Trimethylamine N-oxide (TMAO) is a dietary byproduct that is formed by gut bacteria during digestion. The chemical is derived in part from nutrients that are abundant in red meat. High saturated fat levels in red meat have long been known to contribute to heart disease, the leading cause of death in the United States. A growing number of studies have identified TMAO as another culprit.

The exact mechanisms by which TMAO may affect heart disease is complex. Prior research has shown that TMAO enhances cholesterol deposits in the artery wall. Studies also suggest that the chemical interacts with platelets—blood cells that are responsible for normal clotting responses—to increase the risk for clot-related events such as heart attack and stroke.

To investigate the effects of dietary protein on TMAO production, a research team led by Dr. Stanley L. Hazen at the Cleveland Clinic enrolled 113 healthy men and women in a clinical trial. The participants were given 3 diets for a month in random order. All meals were prepared for them, with 25 percent of calories from protein. The dietary proteins came from either red meat, white meat, or nonmeat sources. The research was largely supported by the National Institutes of Health's (NIH) National Heart, Lung, and Blood Institute (NHLBI).

When on the red meat diet, the participants consumed roughly the equivalent of 8 ounces of steak daily, or 2 quarter-pound beef patties. After 1 month on this diet, blood levels of TMAO were 3 times higher than when participants were on the diets based on either white meat or nonmeat protein sources.

Half of the participants were also placed on high-saturated fat versions of the three diets. The diets all had equal amounts of calories. The researchers found that saturated fat had no additional effect on TMAO levels.

Importantly, the TMAO increases were reversible. When the participants discontinued the red meat diet and ate either the white meat or nonmeat diet for another month, their TMAO levels decreased significantly.

"This study shows for the first time what a dramatic effect changing your diet has on levels of TMAO, which is increasingly linked to heart disease," Hazen says.

"These findings reinforce current dietary recommendations that encourage all ages to follow a heart-healthy eating plan that limits red meat," says nutrition researcher Dr. Charlotte Pratt, the NHLBI project officer for the study. "This means eating a variety of foods, including more vegetables, fruits, whole grains, low-fat dairy foods, and plant-based protein sources, such as beans and peas."

Section 6.3

Risk Factors for Heart Disease Linked to Dementia

This section includes text excerpted from "Risk Factors
for Heart Disease Linked to Dementia," National Institutes
of Health (NIH), August 15, 2017.

People with dementia have problems thinking, remembering, and communicating. They may repeat the same question over and over, get lost in familiar places, or have other problems managing everyday life.

Dementia can be caused by a number of disorders, such as strokes, brain tumors, Alzheimer disease (AD), and late-stage Parkinson disease (PD). Most forms of dementia slowly worsen. Risk factors include aging, diabetes, high blood pressure (hypertension), smoking cigarettes, and a family history of dementia.

Past studies suggest that problems in the vascular system—the heart and blood vessels that supply blood to the brain—can contribute to the development of dementia. To explore the effect of vascular risk factors on dementia, a research team led by Dr. Rebecca Gottesman at Johns Hopkins University studied nearly 16,000 middle-aged people who participated in the Atherosclerosis Risk in Communities (ARIC) study. ARIC was funded by the National Institutes of Health's (NIH) National Heart, Lung, and Blood Institute (NHLBI). The study was also supported by NIH's National Institute of Neurological Disorders and Stroke (NINDS).

The people enrolled in the study were between 44 and 66 years of age in 1987-1989 and located in 4 states. Over a 25-year period, the researchers examined the participants 5 times with a variety of medical tests. Cognitive tests of memory and thinking were given during the second, fourth, and fifth exams. In addition to in-person visits, the researchers collected health data from telephone interviews, caregiver interviews, hospitalization records, and death certificates.

More than 1,500 of the participants were diagnosed with dementia over the 25-year period. The analysis confirmed prior findings that those with vascular risk factors in midlife, such as diabetes or hypertension, had a greater chance of developing dementia as they aged. Also confirming other studies, smoking cigarettes increased the risk of dementia (although this effect was seen only in White people). In addition, the researchers detected a higher risk of dementia among

63

people with prehypertension, in which blood pressure levels are higher than normal but lower than hypertension.

The team reanalyzed the data to determine whether having had a stroke influenced these associations. They found that diabetes, hypertension, prehypertension, and smoking during midlife increased the risk of developing dementia whether or not the person had a stroke.

"With an aging population, dementia is becoming a greater health concern. This study supports the importance of controlling vascular risk factors like high blood pressure early in life in an effort to prevent dementia as we age," says NINDS Director Dr. Walter J. Koroshetz. "What is good for the heart is good for the brain."

Section 6.4

Too Little Potassium May Contribute to Cardiovascular Disease

This section includes text excerpted from "How Too Little Potassium May Contribute to Cardiovascular Disease," National Institutes of Health (NIH), October 24, 2017.

Potassium is a mineral that is essential for health. A healthy diet usually provides enough potassium, but problems sometimes develop because too much sodium in the diet or certain medicines can increase the need for it. Previous studies have shown that increasing potassium intake can reduce the risk of cardiovascular diseases, such as high blood pressure, heart disease, and stroke. However, the mechanism is not known.

One explanation is that potassium might prevent vascular calcification, the buildup of calcium in the smooth muscle cells within arteries. Vascular calcification contributes to atherosclerosis, also known as "hardening of the arteries." This is a serious disease in which plaques of fat, cholesterol, calcium, and other substances can diminish blood flow.

A research team led by Dr. Yabing Chen at the University of Alabama at Birmingham and the Birmingham VA Medical Center set out to discover how dietary potassium affects the vascular calcification process. The study was supported in part by the National Institutes of Health's (NIH) National Heart, Lung, and Blood Institute (NHLBI) and the National Institute of Diabetes and Digestive and Kidney Diseases (NIDDK).

For 30 weeks, the researchers fed three groups of atherosclerosis-prone male mice a high-fat, high-cholesterol diet that contained normal, low, or high levels of potassium. Using tissue staining and ultrasound imaging methods, the team showed that mice fed a low-potassium diet had increased vascular calcification and artery stiffness. Conversely, a high-potassium diet reduced calcification and stiffness. Using smooth muscle cell cultures, the team confirmed that low potassium enhanced vascular calcification, and high potassium inhibited it.

Next, the research team analyzed changes in proteins made by vascular smooth muscle cells when the potassium level was low. They found large increases in proteins often associated with bone cells and decreases in those associated with smooth muscle cells. This rise in bone-associated proteins suggests that low potassium directly affects the calcification of smooth muscle cells.

The team also showed that low potassium increased the calcium level within smooth muscle cells. Higher levels of calcium led to activation of a protein called "CREB" (cAMP response element-binding protein). Smooth muscle cell calcification could be blocked by inhibiting the activity of CREB. This suggested that CREB is a critical part of the calcification process when the potassium level is low. CREB activation was linked to increased autophagy, the process by which waste within the cell is broken down and recycled. Further work will be needed to define the role of autophagy in vascular calcification and artery stiffness.

"The findings have important translational potential," says co-author Dr. Paul W. Sanders of the University of Alabama at Birmingham, "since they demonstrate the benefit of adequate potassium supplementation on prevention of vascular calcification in atherosclerosis-prone mice, and the adverse effect of low potassium intake."

Section 6.5

Consumers Missing Out on Health Benefits of Seafood Consumption

This section includes text excerpted from "Consumers Missing Out on Health Benefits of Seafood Consumption," National Institutes of Health (NIH), August 22, 2017.

While most U.S. consumers eat some seafood, the amounts are inadequate to meet federal dietary guidelines, according to studies conducted by the U.S. Department of Agriculture (USDA) scientists. Both fish and shellfish, referred to as "seafood," are nutrient-rich protein foods, and consumption has been associated with reduced heart disease risk.

Seafood contains healthful natural compounds known as "omega-3 fatty acids." *The Dietary Guidelines for Americans, 2010*, recommends eating 2 servings of seafood (about 8 ounces) weekly to get at least 1,750 milligrams of 2 omega-3s known as "eicosapentaenoic acid" (EPA) and "docosahexaenoic acid" (DHA) weekly.

Agricultural Research Service (ARS) nutritionist Lisa Jahns led a study with colleagues based on an evaluation of food-intake data collected from a representative sampling of the U.S. population. The data were collected during the national survey known as "What We Eat in America/The National Health and Nutrition Examination Survey (NHANES)." Overall, about 80 to 90 percent of U.S. consumers did not meet their seafood recommendations. Jahns is with the ARS Grand Forks Human Nutrition Research Center (GFHNRC) in Grand Forks, North Dakota.

Additionally, a review of published studies that explored fish consumption's link to heart health pointed to consistent evidence supporting a reduced risk of heart disease due particularly to eating oily fish. The review was led by GFHNRC nutritionist Susan Raatz. EPA and DHA are abundant in oily fish such as salmon, mackerel, herring, sardines, anchovies, trout, and tuna.

In the published study, Raatz and colleagues concluded that getting the message of the benefits of fish consumption to consumers is key and suggested a public-health education program on the health benefits of eating fish.

Both studies were published in the journal *Nutrients*. Data on the nutrient content of seafood can be found in the United States

Department of Agriculture-Agricultural Research Service (USDA-ARS) National Nutrient Database for Standard Reference.

Section 6.6

When High-Density Lipoprotein Cholesterol Does Not Protect against Heart Disease

This section includes text excerpted from "When HDL Cholesterol Doesn't Protect against Heart Disease," National Institutes of Health (NIH), March 22, 2016.

Cholesterol has many important functions. It is carried through the bloodstream in several forms, including attached to low-density lipoproteins (LDL) and high-density lipoproteins (HDL). When there is too much cholesterol in your blood, the LDL-cholesterol can combine with other substances to form plaque that coats artery walls, causing them to narrow. This condition, called "atherosclerosis," increases your risk for cardiovascular diseases, such as heart attack and stroke.

High-density lipoprotein, in contrast, is thought to remove cholesterol from arteries and carry it to the liver for removal from the body. Higher levels of HDL have been associated with a lower risk of cardiovascular disease. However, pharmaceutical approaches to reduce heart disease risk by raising HDL levels have had disappointing results.

An international research team led by Dr. Daniel J. Rader at the University of Pennsylvania aimed to gain further insights into the relationship between HDL-cholesterol (HDL-C) and cardiovascular disease. They examined 328 people with very high HDL-C (average of 107 mg/dl) and 398 people with low HDL-C (average of 30 mg/dl). The scientists sequenced nearly a thousand genes near genetic regions previously associated with plasma lipid levels. Their work was funded in part by National Institutes of Health's (NIH) National Center for Research Resources (NCRR) and National Center for Advancing Translational Sciences (NCATS).

In five people with high HDL-C, the researchers found a genetic variant within the gene SCARB1, which codes for the major HDL receptor on liver cells, scavenger receptor class BI (SR-BI). One of the individuals had two mutant copies of the variant. In mice, genetic manipulations of this gene had effects opposite from those expected if HDL-C were protective. Overexpression of the gene lowered HDL-C levels but reduced atherosclerosis. Deletion raised HDL-C levels but increased atherosclerosis.

Genetic analyses of well over 300,000 people confirmed that the variant, called "*SCARB1* P376L," was associated with elevated HDL-C levels. The researchers found that people with the variant had unusually high levels of large HDL-C particles in their blood.

To see whether *SCARB1* P376L was associated with heart disease, the team acquired data from nearly 50,000 people with coronary heart disease and about 88,000 controls. They found that those with the variant had a significantly higher risk of heart disease.

Experiments in cell cultures and mice revealed that the P376L SR-BI protein was not processed properly by the cell and often failed to reach the cell surface. As a result, liver cells became incapable of taking up HDL cholesterol from the blood.

"The work demonstrates that the protective effects of HDL are more dependent upon how it functions than merely how much of it is present," Rader says. "We still have a lot to learn about the relationship between HDL function and heart disease risk."

The team plans to study how other SCARB1 mutations affect HDL levels and heart disease. Other genes, they suggest, may also have similar effects.

Chapter 7

Warning Signs of Cardiovascular Emergencies

Chapter Contents

Section 7.1

Signs and Symptoms of a Heart Attack

This section includes text excerpted from "Heart Attack Symptoms,"
Office on Women's Health (OWH), U.S. Department of Health and
Human Services (HHS), March 14, 2019.

Many people think that the warning signs of a heart attack are sudden, such as a movie heart attack, where someone clutches their chest and falls over. A real heart attack may look and feel very different for women. Women are more likely to have nontraditional symptoms of heart attack than men. And women are also more likely to have silent heart attacks.

How Do You Know If You Are Having a Heart Attack?

For both women and men, the most common heart attack symptom is pain or discomfort in the center of the chest. The pain or discomfort can be mild or strong. It can last more than a few minutes, or it can go away and come back.

The more heart attack symptoms that you have, the more likely it is that you are having a heart attack. Also, if you have already had a heart attack, your symptoms may not be the same for another one. Even if you are not totally sure you are having a heart attack, call 911 right away.

What Should You Do If You Have Heart Attack Symptoms?

If you think you or someone else may be having a heart attack, call 911 right away. Do not drive yourself to the hospital, and do not let a friend drive you. You may need medical help on the way to the hospital. Ambulance workers are trained to treat you on the way to the emergency room.

Getting to the hospital quickly is important. Treatments for opening clogged arteries work best within the first hour after a heart attack starts.

If you think you are having a heart attack, get emergency help right away. Do not let anyone tell you that you are overreacting or to wait and see. Get tips on how best to describe your symptoms and how to ask for tests that can show whether you are having a heart attack.

Section 7.2

Signs and Symptoms of Cardiac Arrest

This section includes text excerpted from "Cardiac Arrest,"
MedlinePlus, National Institutes of Health (NIH), May 3, 2018.

The heart has an internal electrical system that controls the rhythm of the heartbeat. Problems can cause abnormal heart rhythms, called "arrhythmias." There are many types of arrhythmia. During an arrhythmia, the heart can beat too fast, too slow, or it can stop beating. Sudden cardiac arrest (SCA) occurs when the heart develops an arrhythmia that causes it to stop beating. This is different than a heart attack, where the heart usually continues to beat but blood flow to the heart is blocked.

There are many possible causes of SCA. They include coronary heart disease (CHD), physical stress, and some inherited disorders. Sometimes there is no known cause for the SCA.

Without medical attention, the person will die within a few minutes. People are less likely to die if they have early defibrillation. Defibrillation sends an electric shock to restore the heart rhythm to normal. You should give cardiopulmonary resuscitation (CPR) to a person having SCA until defibrillation can be done.

If you have had an SCA, an implantable cardiac defibrillator (ICD) reduces the chance of dying from a second SCA.

Section 7.3

Warning Signs of a Stroke

This section includes text excerpted from "About Stroke," Centers for
Disease Control and Prevention (CDC), March 5, 2019.

A stroke, sometimes called a "brain attack," occurs when something blocks blood supply to part of the brain or when a blood vessel in the brain bursts. In either case, parts of the brain become damaged or die. A stroke can cause lasting brain damage, long-term disability, or even death.

Stroke Signs and Symptoms

During a stroke, every minute counts. Fast treatment can lessen the brain damage that stroke can cause.

By knowing the signs and symptoms of stroke, you can take quick action and perhaps save a life—maybe even your own.

Signs of Stroke in Men and Women

- Sudden numbness or weakness in the face, arm, or leg, especially on one side of the body

- Sudden confusion, trouble speaking, or difficulty understanding speech

- Sudden trouble seeing in one or both eyes

- Sudden trouble walking, dizziness, loss of balance, or lack of coordination

- Sudden severe headache with no known cause

Call 911 right away if you or someone else has any of these symptoms.

Acting F.A.S.T. Is Key for Stroke

Acting F.A.S.T. can help stroke patients get the treatments they desperately need. The stroke treatments that work best are available only if the stroke is recognized and diagnosed within three hours of the first symptoms. Stroke patients may not be eligible for these if they do not arrive at the hospital in time.

If you think someone may be having a stroke, act F.A.S.T. and do the following simple test:

F—Face: Ask the person to smile. Does one side of the face droop?

A—Arms: Ask the person to raise both arms. Does one arm drift downward?

S—Speech: Ask the person to repeat a simple phrase. Is the speech slurred or strange?

T—Time: If you see any of these signs, call 911 right away.

Note the time when any symptoms first appear. This information helps healthcare providers determine the best treatment for each person. Do not drive to the hospital or let someone else drive you. Call an ambulance so that medical personnel can begin life-saving treatment on the way to the emergency room.

Treating a Transient Ischemic Attack

If your symptoms go away after a few minutes, you may have had a transient ischemic attack (TIA). Although brief, a TIA is a sign of a serious condition that will not go away without medical help.

Unfortunately, because TIAs clear up, many people ignore them. But paying attention to a TIA can save your life. Tell your healthcare team about your symptoms right away.

Chapter 8

What to Do in a Cardiac Emergency

Chapter Contents

Section 8.1

What to Do during a Heart Attack

This section includes text excerpted from "Heart Attack Know the Symptoms. Take Action." National Heart, Lung, and Blood Institute (NHLBI), December 2011. Reviewed May 2019.

Heart Attacks Do Not Always Cause Common Symptoms

Not all heart attacks begin with the sudden, crushing chest pain often seen on TV or in the movies or include other common symptoms, such as chest discomfort. The symptoms of a heart attack can vary from person to person. Some people can have few symptoms and are surprised to learn that they have had a heart attack. If you have already had a heart attack, your symptoms may not be the same for another one. It is important for you to know the most common symptoms of a heart attack and also remember these facts:

- Heart attacks can start slowly and cause only mild pain or discomfort. Symptoms can be mild or more intense and sudden. Symptoms also may come and go over several hours.

- People who have high blood sugar (diabetes) may have no symptoms or very mild ones.

- The most common symptom, in both women and men, is chest pain or discomfort. But women also are somewhat more likely to have shortness of breath; nausea and vomiting; unusual tiredness (sometimes lasting for days); and pain in the back, shoulders, and jaw.

- There will be excessive sweating, especially over the forehead.

- Some may have coughing or wheezing.

- Some may experience an overwhelming feeling of anxiety, such as a panic attack.

Quick Action Can Save Your Life

Any time you think you might be having heart attack symptoms or a heart attack, do not ignore it or feel embarrassed to call for help. Call 911 for emergency medical care, even if you are not sure whether you are having a heart attack. Here is why:

- Acting fast can save your life.

- An ambulance is the best and safest way to get to the hospital. Emergency medical services (EMS) personnel can check how you are doing and start life-saving medicines and other treatments right away. People who arrive by ambulance often receive faster treatment at the hospital.

- The 911 operator or EMS technician can give you advice. You might be told to crush or chew an aspirin if you are not allergic, unless there is a medical reason for you not to take one. Aspirin taken during a heart attack can limit the damage to your heart and save your life.

- Every minute matters. Never delay calling 911 to take aspirin or do anything else you think might help.

- Your heart may stop beating during a heart attack. EMS technicians have the training and equipment needed to treat you if this happens.

- If you are unable to reach 911, have someone else drive you to the hospital right away. Do not drive yourself to the hospital. You can cause a car accident if your symptoms worsen.

- When given quickly, medicines and other treatments can stop a heart attack.

Action Steps to Take Now—Before a Heart Attack Happens

Talk about an emergency heart attack action plan with your spouse or someone else close to you, so you will know what to do if a heart attack occurs. This is especially important if you are at high risk for a heart attack or have already had one. Steps you can take now include:

- During a routine office visit, talk to your doctor or healthcare provider about your risk for a heart attack. Find out now whether you can take aspirin if you have heart attack symptoms in the future.

- Write down important information to share with EMS and hospital staff in case of a medical emergency.

- Put your written information in a handy place, and tell someone else where it is. Share it with family, coworkers, and neighbors, and always keep it with you.

- Consider taking part in a research study (clinical trial) if you have had or are at risk for a heart attack. Research supported by the National Heart, Lung, and Blood Institute (NHLBI) has uncovered some of the causes of heart diseases and conditions, as well as ways to prevent or treat them.

Write down and keep in a handy place:

- Medicines you are taking and medicines you cannot take because you are allergic

- Important phone numbers, including those of your healthcare provider and the person who should be contacted if you go to the hospital

Section 8.2

Emergency Treatment of Cardiac Arrest

This section includes text excerpted from "Three Things You May Not Know about CPR," Centers for Disease Control and Prevention (CDC), October 9, 2018.

How Can You Tell Whether Someone Is in Cardiac Arrest?

A person might be in cardiac arrest in case:

- The person is unresponsive, even if you shake or shout at them

- The person is not breathing or is only gasping

If you see someone in cardiac arrest, call 911 right away and then start cardiopulmonary resuscitation (CPR). Keep doing CPR until medical professionals arrive. Most cardiac arrests happen outside of the hospital, either at home or in public places. If CPR is performed within the first few minutes of cardiac arrest, it can double or triple a person's chance of survival.

What Is Cardiopulmonary Resuscitation and When Should You Use It?

Cardiopulmonary resuscitation is an emergency procedure that can help save a person's life if their breathing or heart stops. When a person's heart stops beating, they are in cardiac arrest. During cardiac arrest, the heart cannot pump blood to the rest of the body, including the brain and lungs. Death can happen in minutes without treatment. CPR uses chest compressions to mimic how the heart pumps. These compressions help keep blood flowing throughout the body.

Cardiac arrest is not the same as a heart attack. A heart attack happens when blood flow to the heart is blocked. A person having a heart attack is still talking and breathing. This person does not need CPR, but they do need to get to the hospital right away. Heart attack increases the risk for going into cardiac arrest.

Cardiopulmonary Resuscitation Saves Lives

Currently, about 9 in 10 people who have cardiac arrest outside the hospital die. But, CPR can help improve those odds. If it is performed within the first few minutes of cardiac arrest, CPR can double or triple a person's chance of survival.

Certain people, including people in low-income, Black, and Hispanic neighborhoods, are less likely to receive CPR from bystanders than people in high-income, White neighborhoods. Women may also be less likely to receive CPR if they experience cardiac arrest in a public place.

Cardiac Arrests Often Happen at Home

About 350,000 cardiac arrests happen outside of hospitals each year—and about 7 in 10 of those happen at home. Unfortunately, about half of the people who experience cardiac arrests at home do not get the help they need from bystanders before an ambulance arrives.

If you see cardiac arrest happen, call 911 right away and then do CPR until medical professionals arrive.

You Do Not Need Formal Training to Perform Cardiopulmonary Resuscitation

You do not need a special certification or formal training to perform CPR, but you do need education. If cardiac arrest happens to someone near you, do not be afraid; just be prepared. Follow these steps if you see someone in cardiac arrest:

- Call 911 right away. If another bystander is nearby, save time by asking that person to call 911 and look for an automated external defibrillator (AED) while you begin CPR. AEDs are portable machines that can electrically shock the heart and cause it to start beating again.

- Give CPR. Push down hard and fast in the center of the chest at a rate of 100 to 120 pushes a minute. Let the chest come back up to its normal position after each push. The American Heart Association (AHA) recommends timing your pushes to the beat of the song "Stayin' Alive." This method of CPR is called "hands-only" and does not involve breathing into the person's mouth.

- Continue giving CPR until medical professionals arrive or until a person with formal CPR training can take over.

Chapter 9

Role of Automated External Defibrillator (AED) in Cardiac Emergencies

Defibrillators are devices that restore a normal heartbeat by sending an electric pulse or shock to the heart. They are used to prevent or correct an arrhythmia, a heartbeat that is uneven or that is too slow or too fast. Defibrillators can also restore the heart's beating if the heart suddenly stops.

Different types of defibrillators work in different ways. Automated external defibrillators (AEDs), which are in many public spaces, were developed to save the lives of people experiencing sudden cardiac arrest (SCA). Even untrained bystanders can use these devices in an emergency.

Other defibrillators can prevent sudden death among people who have a high risk of a life-threatening arrhythmia. They include implantable cardioverter defibrillators (ICDs), which are surgically placed inside your body, and wearable cardioverter defibrillators (WCDs), which rest on the body. It can take time and effort to get used to living with a defibrillator, and it is important to be aware of possible risks and complications.

This chapter includes text excerpted from "Defibrillators," National Heart, Lung, and Blood Institute (NHLBI), June 30, 2018.

How They Work

There are three types of defibrillators: AEDs, ICDs, and WCDs. Each type works by checking for arrhythmias. Once detected, each defibrillator will send a shock to restore a normal rhythm.

It may also help to understand how the heart works.

How Do Automated External Defibrillators Work?

An automated external defibrillator is a lightweight, battery-operated, portable device that checks the heart's rhythm and sends a shock to the heart to restore a normal rhythm. The device is used to help people having sudden cardiac arrest.

Sticky pads with sensors, called "electrodes," are attached to the chest of someone who is having cardiac arrest. The electrodes send information about the person's heart rhythm to a computer in the AED. The computer analyzes the heart rhythm to find out whether an electric shock is needed. If needed, the electrodes deliver the shock.

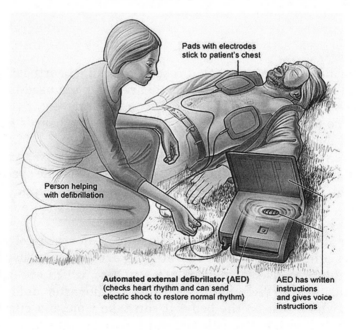

Figure 9.1. *Automated External Defibrillator in Use*

The image shows a typical setup using an automated external defibrillator (AED). The AED has step-by-step instructions and voice prompts that enable an untrained bystander to use the machine correctly.

How Do Implantable Cardioverter Defibrillators Work?

Implantable cardioverter defibrillators are placed surgically in the chest or abdomen, where it checks for arrhythmias. Arrhythmias can interrupt the flow of blood from your heart to the rest of your body or cause your heart to stop. The ICD sends a shock to correct the arrhythmia.

An implantable cardioverter defibrillator can give off a low-energy shock to speed up or slow down an abnormal heart rate or a high-energy shock, which can correct a fast or irregular heartbeat. If the low-energy shocks do not restore your normal heart rhythm, the device will switch to high-energy shocks for defibrillation. The device also will switch to high-energy shocks if your ventricles start to quiver rather than contract strongly. ICDs are similar to pacemakers, but pacemakers deliver only low-energy electrical shocks.

Implantable cardioverter defibrillators have a generator connected to wires to detect your heart's pulses and deliver a shock when needed. Some models have wires that rest in one or two chambers of the heart. Others do not have wires threaded into the heart chambers but rest on the heart to monitor its rhythm.

The implantable cardioverter defibrillator can also record the heart's electrical activity and heart rhythms. The recordings can help your doctor fine-tune the programming of your device so it works better to correct irregular heartbeats. Your device will be programmed to respond to the type of arrhythmia you are most likely to have.

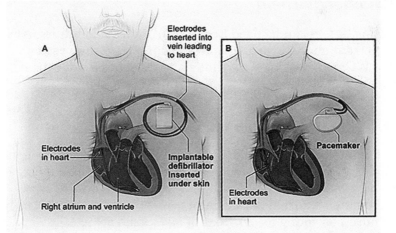

Figure 9.2. *Comparison of an Implantable Cardioverter Defibrillator and a Pacemaker*

The image compares an ICD with a pacemaker. Figure A shows the location and general size of an ICD in the upper chest. The wires with electrodes on the ends are inserted into the heart through a vein in the upper chest. Figure B shows the location and general size of a pacemaker in the upper chest. The wires with electrodes on the ends are inserted into the heart through a vein in the upper chest.

How Do Wearable Cardioverter Defibrillators Work?

Wearable cardioverter defibrillators have sensors that attach to the skin. They are connected by wires to a unit that checks your heart's rhythm and delivers shocks when needed. As with an ICD, the WCD can deliver low- and high-energy shocks. The device has a belt attached to a vest and is worn under your clothes. Your doctor will fit the device to your size. The device is programmed to detect a particular heart rhythm.

The sensors detect when an arrhythmia occurs and notifies you with an alert. You can turn off the alert to prevent a shock if not needed, but if you do not respond, the device will administer a shock to correct the rhythm. Typically, this happens within one minute. The device can deliver repeated shocks during an episode. After each episode, the sensors must be replaced.

The device can also send a record of your heart's activity to your doctors.

Who Needs Them

Defibrillators can be used in children, teens, and adults. AEDs are used to treat sudden cardiac arrest. Your doctor may recommend an ICD or WCD to treat an arrhythmia and prevent new or repeat sudden cardiac arrests.

Who Needs an Automated External Defibrillator

Automated external defibrillators can save the life of someone having sudden cardiac arrest, when the heart suddenly and unexpectedly stops beating.

Automated external defibrillators can be used for adults, as well as for children as young as one year of age. Some devices have pads and cables designed especially for children.

Doing cardiopulmonary resuscitation, or CPR, on someone having sudden cardiac arrest also can improve her or his chance of survival.

Who Needs an Implantable Cardioverter Defibrillator

Implantable cardioverter defibrillators can correct a dangerous arrhythmia or keep an irregular heartbeat from triggering sudden cardiac arrest. Life-threatening arrhythmias can develop for many reasons and can affect people of any age, from newborns to older adults. Your doctor may recommend an ICD if you have a type of arrhythmia that causes your heart's ventricles to quiver instead of pumping blood. This type of arrhythmia is most likely to cause sudden cardiac arrest.

If you have the following conditions, you may be at risk for a life-threatening arrhythmia and your doctor may recommend an ICD:

- You survived sudden cardiac arrest.

- You developed an arrhythmia during or after treatment for a heart attack.

- You have a genetic condition that causes arrhythmia. This includes having congenital heart disease or an inherited conduction disorder.

- You have a neuromuscular disorder. For example, the progression of muscular dystrophy can damage the heart and cause unpredictable heart rhythms. This can lead to unexplained fainting and a high risk of death.

- You have an abnormally slow heart rate or other problem with the heart's electrical signals.

- You have cardiac sarcoidosis.

- You have poor heart function following a procedure to improve blood flow.

- Your doctor detected an arrhythmia during an electrocardiogram (EKG) or stress test. If this happened several times, you may be at an increased risk.

Who Needs a Wearable Cardioverter Defibrillator

Wearable cardioverter defibrillators are used to protect against sudden cardiac arrest in certain circumstances, such as if you are at risk of arrhythmia for just a short time. This might occur under these conditions:

- You are recovering from a heart attack.

- You are waiting for a heart transplant.

- You are fighting an infection.

- You are removing or waiting to replace your ICD.

Using an Automated External Defibrillators in an Emergency

Automated external defibrillators are found in many public spaces. They may be used in an emergency to help someone who is experiencing sudden cardiac arrest. Learn how to recognize sudden cardiac arrest emergencies—when you might use an AED, how to find an AED if you need one, and how to use an AED until help arrives.

When to Use an Automated External Defibrillators

A person whose heart stops from sudden cardiac arrest must get help within 10 minutes to survive. Fainting is usually the first sign of sudden cardiac arrest. If you think someone may be in cardiac arrest, try the following steps:

- If you see a person faint or if you find a person already unconscious, first confirm that the person cannot respond. The person may not move, or her or his movements may be reminiscent of a seizure.

- You can shout at or gently shake the person to make sure she or he is not sleeping, but never shake an infant or young child. Instead, you can gently pinch the child to try to wake her or him up.

- Check the person's breathing and pulse. If the person is not breathing and has no pulse or has an irregular heartbeat, prepare to use the AED as soon as possible.

Where to Find an Automated External Defibrillators

You often can find AEDs in places with large numbers of people, such as shopping malls, golf courses, gyms and swimming pools, businesses, airports, hotels, sports venues, and schools. You can also purchase a home-use AED.

The automated external defibrillator is in a case about the size of a large first-aid kit. Many AEDs have a heart logo in red or green. Large letters on the case or the wall where it is stored might spell out A–E–D.

How to Use an Automated External Defibrillators

Even someone without special training can respond in an emergency by following the instructions relayed by the device. If someone is having sudden cardiac arrest, using an AED and giving CPR can save that person's life. When using an AED:

- Call 911 or have someone else call 911. If two rescuers are present, one can provide CPR while the other calls 911 and gets the AED.

- Make sure the area around the person is clear; touching the person could interfere with the AED's reading of the person's heart.

- If an electric pulse or shock is needed to restore a normal rhythm, the AED uses voice prompts to tell you when and how to give the shock, and electrodes deliver it. Some AEDs can deliver more than one shock with increasing energy.

- The device may instruct you to start CPR again after delivering the shock.

Part Two

Heart Disorders

Chapter 10

Coronary Artery Disease

Coronary artery disease (CAD) is the most common type of heart disease in the United States. For some people, the first sign of CAD is a heart attack. You and your healthcare team may be able to help you reduce your risk for CAD.

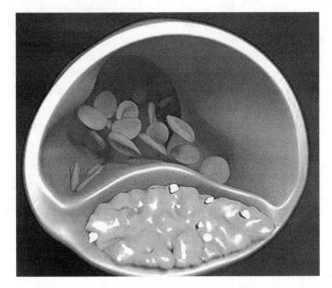

Figure 10.1. *Plaque Buildup in the Wall of the Arteries*

This chapter includes text excerpted from "Coronary Artery Disease (CAD)," Centers for Disease Control and Prevention (CDC), August 10, 2015. Reviewed May 2019.

Causes of Coronary Artery Disease

Coronary artery disease is caused by plaque buildup in the walls of the arteries that supply blood to the heart (called the "coronary arteries") and to other parts of the body. Plaque is made up of deposits of cholesterol and other substances in the artery. Plaque buildup causes the inside of the arteries to narrow over time, which could partially or totally block the blood flow. This process is called "atherosclerosis."

Too much plaque buildup and narrowed artery walls can make it harder for blood to flow through your body. When your heart muscle does not get enough blood, you may have chest pain or discomfort, called "angina." Angina is the most common symptom of CAD.

Over time, CAD can weaken the heart muscle. This may lead to heart failure, a serious condition where the heart cannot pump blood the way that it should. An irregular heartbeat, or arrhythmia, also can develop.

Diagnosing Coronary Artery Disease

To find out your risk for CAD, your healthcare team may measure your blood pressure, cholesterol, and sugar levels. Being overweight, physical inactivity, unhealthy eating, and smoking tobacco are risk factors for CAD. A family history of heart disease also increases your risk for CAD. If you are at high risk for heart disease or already have symptoms, your doctor can use several tests to diagnose CAD.

Table 10.1. Tests to Diagnose Coronary Artery Disease

Electrocardiogram (ECG or EKG)	Measures the electrical activity, rate, and regularity of your heartbeat.
Echocardiogram	Uses ultrasound (special sound wave) to create a picture of the heart.
Exercise stress test	Measures your heart rate while you walk on a treadmill. This helps to determine how well your heart is working when it has to pump more blood.
Chest X-ray	Uses X-rays to create a picture of the heart, lungs, and other organs in the chest.

Table 10.1. Continued

Cardiac catheterization	Checks the inside of your arteries for blockage by inserting a thin, flexible tube through an artery in the groin, arm, or neck to reach the heart. Healthcare professionals can measure blood pressure within the heart and the strength of blood flow through the heart's chambers as well as collect blood samples from the heart or inject dye into the arteries of the heart (coronary arteries).
Coronary angiogram	Monitors blockage and flow of blood through the coronary arteries. Uses X-rays to detect dye injected via cardiac catheterization.

Reducing Your Risk for Coronary Artery Disease

If you have CAD, your healthcare team may suggest the following steps to help lower your risk for heart attack or worsening heart disease:

- Lifestyle changes, such as eating a healthier (lower sodium, lower fat) diet, increasing physical activity, and quitting smoking

- Medications to treat the risk factors for CAD, such as high cholesterol, high blood pressure (HBP), an irregular heartbeat, and low blood flow

- Surgical procedures to help restore blood flow to the heart

Chapter 11

Angina

Angina is chest pain or discomfort that occurs if an area of your heart muscle does not get enough oxygen-rich blood. It is a common symptom of ischemic heart disease, which limits or cuts off blood flow to the heart.

There are several types of angina, and the signs and symptoms depend on which type you have. Angina chest pain, called an "angina event," can happen when your heart is working hard. It can go away when you stop to rest again, or it can happen at rest. This pain can feel like pressure or squeezing in your chest. It also can spread to your shoulders, arms, neck, jaw, or back, as with a heart attack. Angina pain can even feel like an upset stomach. Symptoms can be different for women and men.

Angina can be a warning sign that you are at an increased risk of a heart attack. If you have chest pain that does not go away, call 911 immediately.

To diagnose angina, your doctor will ask you about your signs and symptoms and may run blood tests, take an X-ray, or order tests, such as an electrocardiogram (EKG), an exercise stress test, or cardiac catheterization, to determine how well your heart is working. With some types of angina, you may need emergency medical treatment to try to prevent a heart attack. To control your condition, your doctor may recommend heart-healthy lifestyle changes, medicines, medical procedures, and cardiac rehabilitation.

This chapter includes text excerpted from "Angina," National Heart, Lung, and Blood Institute (NHLBI), December 10, 2018.

Types of Angina

The types of angina are stable, unstable, microvascular, and variant. The types vary based on their severity or cause.

Stable Angina

Stable angina follows a pattern that has been consistent for at least two months. That means the following factors have not changed:

- How long your angina events last
- How often your angina events occur
- How well the angina responds to rest or medicines
- The causes or triggers of your angina

If you have stable angina, you can learn its pattern and predict when an event will occur, such as during physical exertion or mental stress. The pain usually goes away a few minutes after you rest or take your angina medicine. If the condition causing your angina gets worse, stable angina can become unstable angina.

Unstable Angina

Unstable angina does not follow a pattern. It may be new or occur more often and be more severe than stable angina. Unstable angina can also occur with or without physical exertion. Rest or medicine may not relieve the pain.

Unstable angina is a medical emergency, as it can progress to a heart attack. Medical attention may be needed right away to restore blood flow to the heart muscle.

Microvascular Angina

Microvascular angina is a sign of ischemic heart disease and affects the tiny arteries of the heart. Microvascular angina events can be stable or unstable. They can be more painful and last longer than other types of angina, and symptoms can occur during exercise or at rest. Medicine may not relieve symptoms of this type of angina.

Variant Angina

Variant angina, also known as "Prinzmetal's angina," is rare. It occurs when a spasm—a sudden tightening of the muscles within the arteries of your heart—causes the angina rather than a blockage. This type of angina usually occurs while you are at rest, and the pain can be severe. It usually happens between midnight and early morning and in a pattern. Medicine can ease symptoms of variant angina.

Causes of Angina

Angina happens when your heart muscle does not get enough oxygen-rich blood. Medical conditions, particularly ischemic heart disease, or lifestyle habits can cause angina. To understand the causes of angina, it helps to understand how the heart works.

Ischemic Heart Disease

Two types of ischemic heart disease can cause angina.

- **Coronary artery disease (CAD)** happens when plaque builds up inside the large arteries that supply blood to the heart. This is called "atherosclerosis." Plaque narrows or blocks the arteries, reducing blood flow to the heart muscle. Sometimes, plaque breaks open and causes blood clots to form. Blood clots can partially or totally block the coronary arteries.

- **Coronary microvascular disease (MVD)** affects the tiny arteries that branch off the larger coronary arteries. Reduced blood flow in these arteries causes microvascular angina. The arteries may be damaged and unable to expand as usual when the heart needs more oxygen-rich blood.

Spasm of the Coronary Arteries

A spasm that tightens your coronary arteries can cause angina. Spasms can occur whether or not you have ischemic heart disease and can affect large or small coronary arteries. Damage to your heart's arteries may cause them to narrow instead of widen when the heart needs more oxygen-rich blood.

What Happens in the Heart during an Angina Event

In one day, your heart beats about 100,000 times and pumps about 2,400 gallons of blood throughout your body. To meet this demand, your heart's cells need a great deal of oxygen, which is supplied by the large coronary arteries and the tiny arteries that branch off the large arteries. When your heart is working hard, such as during physical activity or emotional stress, its demand for oxygen increases. Angina occurs when there is an imbalance between the heart's need for oxygen-rich blood and the ability of the arteries to deliver blood to all areas of the heart.

Risk Factors for Angina

You may have an increased risk for angina because of your age, environment or occupation, family history, and genetics, lifestyle, other medical conditions, race, or sex.

Age

Genetic or lifestyle factors can cause plaque to build up in your arteries as you age. This means that your risk for ischemic heart disease and angina increases as you get older.

Variant angina is rare, but people who have variant angina often are younger than those who have other types of angina.

Environment or Occupation

Angina may be linked to a type of air pollution called "particle pollution." Particle pollution can include dust from roads, farms, dry riverbeds, construction sites, and mines.

Your work life can increase your risk of angina. Examples include work that limits your time available for sleep; involves high stress; requires long periods of sitting or standing; is noisy; or exposes you to potential hazards, such as radiation.

Family History and Genetics

Ischemic heart disease often runs in families. Also, people who have no lifestyle-related risk factors can develop ischemic heart disease. These factors suggest that genes are involved in ischemic heart disease and can influence a person's risk of developing angina.

Variant angina has also been linked to specific deoxyribonucleic acid (DNA) changes.

Lifestyle Habits

The more heart disease risk factors you have, the greater your risk of developing angina. The main lifestyle risk factors for angina include:

- Alcohol use, for variant angina

- Illegal-drug use

- Lack of physical activity

- Smoking tobacco or long-term exposure to secondhand smoke

- Stress

- Unhealthy eating patterns

Other Medical Conditions

Medical conditions in which your heart needs more oxygen-rich blood than your body can supply increase your risk for angina. They include:

- Anemia

- A racing heart rate or blood vessel damage due to cocaine or methamphetamine use

- Cardiomyopathy, or disease of the heart muscle

- Damage to the heart caused by injury

- Heart failure

- Heart valve disease

- High blood pressure

- Inflammation

- Insulin resistance or diabetes

- Low blood pressure

- Metabolic syndrome

- Being overweight or obese

- Unhealthy cholesterol levels

Medical Procedures

Heart procedures, such as stent placement, percutaneous coronary intervention (PCI), or coronary artery bypass grafting (CABG), can trigger coronary spasms and angina. Although rare, noncardiac surgery can also trigger unstable angina or variant angina.

Race or Ethnicity

Some groups of people are at higher risk of developing ischemic heart disease and one of its main symptoms, angina. African Americans who have already had a heart attack are more likely to develop angina when compared to White individuals.

Variant angina is more common among people living in Japan, especially men, than among people living in Western countries.

Sex

Angina affects both men and women but at different ages and is based on men and women's risk of developing ischemic heart disease. In men, ischemic heart disease risk starts to increase at 45 years of age. Before the age of 55, women have a lower risk for heart disease than men. After the age of 55, the risk rises in both women and men. Women who have already had a heart attack are more likely to develop angina when compared to men.

Microvascular angina most often begins in women around the time of menopause.

Screening and Prevention of Angina

Typically, doctors screen for angina only when you have symptoms. However, your doctor may assess your risk factors for ischemic heart disease every few years as part of your regular office visits. If you have 2 or more risk factors, then your doctor may estimate the chance that you will develop ischemic heart disease, which may include angina, over the next 10 years.

Prevention Strategies

To prevent angina, your doctor may recommend that you adopt heart-healthy lifestyle changes to lower your risk of ischemic heart disease, the most common cause of angina. Heart-healthy lifestyle changes include choosing a heart-healthy eating pattern, such as the dietary approaches to stop hypertension (DASH) eating plan; being physically active; aiming for a healthy weight; quitting smoking; and managing stress. You should also avoid using illegal drugs.

Signs, Symptoms, and Complications of Angina

Signs and symptoms vary based on the type of angina you have and on whether you are a man or a woman. Angina symptoms can differ in severity, location in the body, timing, and how much relief you may feel with rest or medicines. Since symptoms of angina and a heart attack can be the same, call 911 if you feel chest discomfort that does not go away with rest or medicine. Angina can also lead to a heart attack and other complications that can be life-threatening.

Signs and Symptoms

Pain and discomfort are the main symptoms of angina. Angina is often described as pressure, squeezing, burning, indigestion, or tightness in the chest. The pain or discomfort usually starts behind the breastbone. Some people say that angina pain is hard to describe or that they cannot tell exactly where the pain is coming from.

Other symptoms include:

- Fatigue
- Light-headedness or fainting
- Nausea, or feeling sick in the stomach
- Shortness of breath
- Sweating
- Weakness

Symptoms of angina can be different for women and men. Instead of chest pain, or in addition to it, women may feel pain in the neck, jaw, throat, abdomen, or back. Sometimes, this pain is not recognized as a symptom of a heart condition. As a result, treatment for women can be delayed.

Because angina has so many possible symptoms and causes, all chest pain should be checked by a doctor.

Each type of angina has certain typical symptoms. Learn more about the symptoms that are characteristic of each type.

Stable Angina

- Discomfort that feels like gas or indigestion
- Pain during physical exertion or mental stress
- Pain that spreads from your breastbone to your arms or back
- Pain that is relieved by medicines
- Pattern of symptoms that has not changed in the last two months

- Symptoms that go away within five minutes

Unstable Angina

- Changes in your stable angina symptoms
- Pain that grows worse
- Pain that is not relieved by rest or medicines
- Pain that lasts longer than 20 minutes or goes away and then comes back
- Pain while you are resting or sleeping
- Severe pain
- Shortness of breath

Microvascular Angina

- Pain after physical or emotional stress
- Pain that is not immediately relieved by medicines
- Pain that lasts a long time
- Pain that you feel while doing regular daily activities
- Severe pain
- Shortness of breath

Variant Angina

- Cold sweats
- Fainting
- Numbness or weakness of the left shoulder and upper arm
- Pain that is relieved by medicines
- Pain that occurs during rest or while sleeping
- Pain that starts in the early morning hours
- Severe pain
- Vague pain with a feeling of pressure in the lower chest, perhaps spreading to the neck, jaw, or left shoulder

Complications

Angina is not a heart attack, but it suggests that a heart attack or other life-threatening complications are more likely to happen in the future.

The following are other possible complications of angina:

- Arrhythmia

- Cardiomyopathy

- Sudden cardiac arrest (SCA)

Diagnosis of Angina

Your doctor may diagnose angina based on your medical history, a physical exam, and diagnostic tests and procedures. These tests can help assess whether you need immediate treatment for a heart attack. Some of these tests may help rule out other conditions.

Medical History

Your doctor will want to learn about your signs and symptoms, risk factors, personal health history, and family health history to determine whether your chest pain is angina or is caused by something else. Other heart and blood vessel problems or problems with your chest muscles, lungs, or digestive system can cause chest pain.

Tell your doctor if you notice a pattern to your symptoms. Ask yourself these questions:

- How long does the pain or discomfort last?

- How often does the pain occur?

- How severe is the pain or discomfort?

- What brings on the pain or discomfort, and what makes it better?

- Where do you feel the pain or discomfort?

- What does the pain or discomfort feel like?

Your doctor will also need information about ischemic heart disease risk factors and other medical conditions you might have, including diabetes and kidney disease. Even if your chest pain is not angina, it can still be a symptom of a serious medical problem. Your doctor can recommend steps you need to take to get medical care.

Physical Examination

As part of a physical examination, your doctor will measure your blood pressure and heart rate, feel your chest and belly, take your temperature, listen to your heart and lungs, and feel your pulse.

Diagnostic Tests and Procedures

Your doctor may have you undergo some of the following tests and procedures.

- **Blood tests** to check the level of cardiac troponins. Troponin levels can help doctors differentiate unstable angina from heart attacks. Your doctor may also check levels of certain fats, cholesterol, sugar, and proteins in your blood.

- **Chest X-ray** to look for lung disorders and other causes of chest pain not related to ischemic heart disease. A chest X-ray alone is not enough to diagnose angina or ischemic heart disease, but it can help rule out other causes.

- **Computed tomography (CT) angiography** to examine blood flow through the coronary arteries. This test can rapidly diagnose ischemic heart disease as the source of your chest pain and help your doctor decide whether a procedure to improve blood flow will benefit your future health.

- **Coronary angiography** with cardiac catheterization to see if ischemic heart disease is the cause of your chest pain. This test lets your doctor study the flow of blood through your heart and blood vessels to confirm whether plaque buildup is the problem. The results of the scan can also help your doctor assess whether unstable angina might be relieved by surgery or other procedures.

- **Echocardiogram** to assess the strength of your heart beating to help the doctor determine your risk of future heart problems.

- **Electrocardiogram** to check for the possibility of a heart attack. Certain EKG patterns are associated with variant angina and unstable angina. These patterns may indicate serious ischemic heart disease or prior heart damage as a cause of angina. However, some people who have angina have normal EKGs.

- **Hyperventilation testing** to diagnose variant angina. Rapid breathing under controlled conditions with careful medical monitoring may bring on EKG changes that help your doctor diagnose variant angina.

- **Magnetic resonance imaging (MRI)** or other noninvasive tests to check for problems with the heart's movement or with blood flow in the heart's small blood vessels.

- **Provocation tests** to diagnose variant angina. Your doctor may give you a medicine, such as acetylcholine, during coronary angiography to see if the coronary arteries start to spasm.

- **Stress testing** to assess your heart's function during exercise. A stress test can show possible signs and symptoms of ischemic heart disease causing your angina. Stress testing in the early morning can help diagnose variant angina. Stress echocardiography tests can help your doctor diagnose the cause of your angina.

Treatment of Angina

Your doctor will decide on a treatment approach based on the type of angina you have, your symptoms, test results, and risk of complications. Unstable angina is a medical emergency that requires immediate treatment in a hospital. If your angina is stable and your symptoms are not getting worse, you may be able to control your angina with heart-healthy lifestyle changes and medicines. If lifestyle changes and medicines cannot control your angina, you may need a medical procedure to improve blood flow and relieve your angina.

Medicines

If you are diagnosed with angina, your doctor will prescribe fast-acting medicines you can take to control angina events and relieve pain. Often, other medicines are also prescribed to help control angina long-term. The choice of medicines may depend on what type of angina you have.

- **Anticoagulant medicines,** or blood thinners, such as heparin, to prevent dangerous blood clots and future complications, such as a heart attack or another angina event.

- **Antiplatelet medicines** to prevent blood clots from forming. If you have stable or unstable angina, your doctor may recommend aspirin to treat angina and reduce the risk of complications of ischemic heart disease. Other platelet inhibitors, such as clopidogrel, may also be prescribed.

- **Beta-blockers** to help your heart beat slower and with less force. These drugs are often prescribed to help relieve angina. If you cannot take beta-blockers for some reason, long-acting nitrates are the preferred alternative.

- **Calcium channel blockers** to keep calcium from entering the muscle cells of your heart and blood vessels. This allows blood vessels to relax. Calcium channel blockers may be an alternative medicine if you are unable to take beta-blockers or nitrates. For variant angina, your doctor is likely to order calcium channel blockers and avoid giving you beta-blockers.

- **Nitrates** to widen and relax blood vessels, which allows more blood to flow to the heart while reducing the heart's workload. Nitrate pills or sprays, including nitroglycerin, act quickly and can relieve pain during an event. Long-acting nitrates are available as pills or skin patches. If you are hospitalized for chest pain, your doctor may order intravenous (IV) nitrates to relieve your angina pain.

- **Statins** to prevent plaque from forming and to relieve blood vessel spasms or inflammation, reducing the risk of a heart attack or other complications after emergency treatment

If you still have symptoms or experience side effects, your doctor may prescribe other medicines, including:

- **Morphine** to relieve pain and help relax the blood vessels. Your doctor may suggest it if other medicines have not helped.

- **Ranolazine** to help you have angina symptoms less often. When given with other anti-angina medicines, ranolazine can also increase the length of time you can be physically active without pain. This medicine may work for coronary microvascular disease, which causes microvascular angina. Ranolazine may be a substitute for nitrates for men with stable angina who take drugs for erectile dysfunction (ED).

Procedures

If lifestyle changes and medicines do not control angina, you may need a medical procedure to treat the underlying heart disease.

- **CABG** to treat ischemic heart disease and relieve angina. CABG can improve blood flow to your heart, relieve chest pain, and possibly prevent a heart attack.

- **Percutaneous coronary intervention (PCI)**, also known as "coronary angioplasty," to open narrowed or blocked blood vessels that supply blood to the heart. This procedure requires cardiac catheterization. If PCI includes certain medicines to expand coronary arteries, the procedure may be helpful for some people who have variant angina.

Living with Angina

Angina is not a heart attack, but it is a signal that you are at greater risk of having a heart attack. The risk is higher if you have unstable angina. For this reason, it is important that you receive follow-up care, monitor your condition, and understand your condition so you know when to get medical help. Your doctor may recommend heart-healthy lifestyle changes and cardiac rehabilitation to help manage angina.

Receive Routine Follow-Up Care

You may need follow-up visits every 4 to 6 months for the first year after diagnosis of angina and every 6 to 12 months as long as your condition is stable. Your care plan may be changed if your angina worsens or if stable angina becomes unstable. Unstable angina is a medical emergency.

- Your doctor may recommend cholesterol-lowering statins as part of your long-term treatment, especially if you have had a heart attack.

- Ask your doctor about when you can resume normal physical activity, such as climbing stairs.

- Ask your doctor whether sexual activity is safe for you. People who have unstable angina or angina that does not respond well to treatment should not engage in sexual activity until their heart condition and angina are stable and well managed.

- Talk to your medical team about vaccinations to prevent the flu and pneumonia.

Monitor Your Condition

To monitor your condition, your doctor may recommend the following tests or procedures:

- **Blood pressure** checks to ensure that your blood pressure is in a healthy range. Keeping your blood pressure under control can help your angina.

- **EKGs** to detect changes in heart health after treatment or for monitoring the heart during exercise as part of cardiac rehabilitation.

- **Repeat lipid panels** to see if blood cholesterol levels are at healthy levels. A lipid panel should be done every year and also two to three months after any change in treatment.

- **Stress testing** to assess your risk for complications either before or after starting angina medicines. Stress tests can also make sure your heart is strong enough for physical and sexual activity.

Adopt Heart-Healthy Lifestyle Changes

Angina is a symptom of ischemic heart disease. Your doctor may recommend the following heart-healthy lifestyle changes to help you manage angina:

- **Heart-healthy eating.** Following a healthy eating plan, including limiting alcohol, can prevent or reduce high blood pressure and high blood cholesterol, helping you reduce angina symptoms and maintain a healthy weight. You should avoid large meals and rich foods if heavy meals trigger your angina. If you have variant angina, drinking alcohol can also be a trigger.

- **Aiming for a healthy weight.** If you are overweight or obese, work with your doctor to create a reasonable weight-loss plan. Controlling your weight helps you manage the risk factors for angina.

- **Being physically active.** Before starting any exercise program, ask your doctor about what level of physical activity is right for you. Slow down or take rest breaks if physical exertion triggers angina.

- **Managing stress.** If emotional stress triggers your angina, try to avoid situations that make you upset or stressed.

- **Quitting smoking.** Smoking can damage and tighten blood vessels, make angina worse, and raise the risk of life-threatening complications. For free help and support to quit smoking, you may call the National Cancer Institute's (NCI) Smoking Quitline at 877-448-7848.

Your doctor may recommend these heart-healthy lifestyle changes as part of a larger cardiac rehabilitation program that your healthcare team oversees.

Prevent Repeat Angina Events

Stable angina usually occurs in a pattern. After several events, you will learn what causes the pain to occur, what the pain feels like, and how long the pain usually lasts. To help learn your angina's pattern and triggers, keep a log of when you feel pain. The log helps your doctor regulate your medicines and evaluate your need for future treatments. When you know what triggers your angina, you can take steps to prevent or lessen the severity of events.

- **Know the limits of your physical activity.** Most people who have stable angina can continue their normal activities. This includes work, hobbies, and sexual relations. Learn how much exertion triggers your angina so you can try to stop and rest before the chest pain starts.

- **Learn how to reduce and manage stress.** Try to avoid or limit situations that cause anger, arguments, and worry. Exercise and relaxation can help relieve stress. Alcohol and drug use play a part in causing stress and do not relieve it. If stress is a problem for you, talk with your doctor about getting help.

- **Avoid exposure to very hot or cold conditions** because temperature extremes strain the heart.

- **Eat smaller meals** if large meals lead to chest pain.

Tell your doctor right away if your pattern changes. Pattern changes may include angina that occurs more often, lasts longer, is more severe, occurs without physical exertion, or does not go away with rest or medicines. These changes may be a sign that your symptoms are getting worse or becoming unstable.

Seek Help for Angina That Does Not Improve

Not all angina improves with medicines or medical procedures. If your symptoms continue, your doctor may change your medicines or therapies to help relieve your chest pain. Additional treatments for hard-to-treat angina include:

- **Enhanced external counterpulsation therapy (EECP)** to improve the flow of oxygen-rich blood to your heart muscle, which may help relieve angina. EECP uses large cuffs, similar to blood pressure cuffs, on your legs. The cuffs inflate and deflate in sync with your heartbeat. You typically get five one-hour treatments per week for seven weeks. Side effects may include back or neck pain and skin abrasions.

- **Spinal cord stimulators** to block the sensation of pain. Emerging research suggests that this technology can help people be more physically active, feel angina less often, and have a better quality of life.

- **Transmyocardial laser therapy** to stimulate growth of new blood vessels or improve blood flow in the heart muscle. It can relieve angina pain and increase your ability to exercise without discomfort. This laser-based treatment is done during open-heart surgery or through cardiac catheterization. Rarely, your doctor may recommend this treatment in combination with CABG.

Know Your Medicines

You should know what medicines you are taking, the purpose of each, how and when to take them, and possible side effects. Learn exactly when and how to take nitroglycerin or other short-acting nitrates to relieve chest pain. Then talk to your doctor about the following:

- **Any other medicines you are taking, including vitamins and nutritional supplements.** Some medicines can cause serious or life-threatening problems if they are taken with nitrates or other angina medicines. For example, men who take nitrates, including nitroglycerin, for their angina should not take medicines for erectile dysfunction without checking with their doctor first.

- **Any side effects you may experience.** Do not stop taking your medicines without talking to your doctor first.

- **Storing and replacing.** How to store your medicines correctly and when to replace them.

- **Safe and effective use.** What is the safest and most effective way to use short-acting nitrates, such as nitroglycerin, to treat stable angina events?

Here are some tips for taking short-acting nitrates.

- Use the short-acting nitrate immediately before any planned exercise or physical exertion.
- Watch for side effects, such as flushing, headache, or dizziness. Find a place to sit down or something to hold on to if you feel dizzy.
- After five minutes, if the pain has not gone away, take another dose.

Call 911 if the pain continues after taking a second dose. This could be a symptom of unstable angina, which is a medical emergency.

Learn the Warning Signs of Serious Complications and Have a Plan

Sometimes it is hard to tell the difference between unstable angina and a heart attack. Angina can be a sign of increased risk of stroke. Angina can also trigger sudden cardiac arrest. These are medical emergencies.

If you think that you or someone else is having the following symptoms, call 911 immediately. Every minute matters.

Heart Attack

Signs of heart attack include mild or severe chest pain or discomfort in the center of the chest or upper abdomen that lasts for more than a few minutes, or goes away and comes back. It can feel like pressure, squeezing, fullness, heartburn, or indigestion. There may also be pain down the left arm. Women may also have chest pain and pain down the left arm, but they are more likely to have symptoms such as shortness of breath, nausea, vomiting, unusual tiredness, and pain in the back, shoulders, or jaw.

Stroke

If you think someone may be having a stroke, act F.A.S.T. and do the following simple test.

F—Face: Ask the person to smile. Does one side of the face droop?

A—Arms: Ask the person to raise both arms. Does one arm drift downward?

S—Speech: Ask the person to repeat a simple phrase. Is his or her speech slurred or strange?

T—Time: If you observe any of these signs, **call 911 immediately. Early treatment is essential.**

Sudden Cardiac Arrest

It is possible for a spasm causing angina to trigger arrhythmia. This can lead to sudden cardiac arrest. Fainting is usually the first sign of sudden cardiac arrest. If you think someone may be in cardiac arrest, try the following steps.

- If you see a person faint or if you find a person already unconscious, first confirm that the person cannot respond. The person may not move, or her or his movements may look similar to a seizure.

- You can shout at or gently shake the person to make sure she or he is not sleeping, but never shake an infant or young child. Instead, you can gently pinch the child to try to wake her or him up.

- Check the person's breathing and pulse. If the person is not breathing and has no pulse or has an irregular heartbeat, prepare to use an automated external defibrillator as soon as possible.

Chapter 12

Heart Attack (Myocardial Infarction)

What Is a Heart Attack?

A heart attack happens when the flow of oxygen-rich blood to a section of heart muscle suddenly becomes blocked, and the heart cannot receive oxygen. If blood flow is not restored quickly, the section of heart muscle begins to die.

Heart attack treatment works best when it is given right after symptoms occur. If you think you or someone else is having a heart attack, even if you are not sure, call 911 right away.

Heart with Muscle Damage and a Blocked Artery

A less common cause of heart attack is a severe spasm (tightening) of a coronary artery. The spasm cuts off blood flow through the artery. Spasms can occur in coronary arteries that are not affected by atherosclerosis.

Heart attacks can be associated with or lead to severe health problems, such as heart failure and life-threatening arrhythmias.

Heart failure is a condition in which the heart cannot pump enough blood to meet the body's needs. Arrhythmias are irregular heartbeats.

This chapter includes text excerpted from "Heart Attack," National Heart, Lung, and Blood Institute (NHLBI), June 12, 2017.

Ventricular fibrillation (VF) is a life-threatening arrhythmia that can cause death if not treated right away.

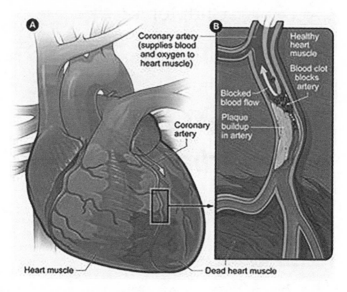

Figure 12.1. *Overview of a Heart*

Figure A is an overview of a heart and coronary artery showing damage (dead heart muscle) caused by a heart attack. Figure B is a cross-section of the coronary artery with plaque buildup and a blood clot.

Causes of Heart Attack
Coronary Heart Disease

A heart attack happens if the flow of oxygen-rich blood to a section of heart muscle suddenly becomes blocked, and the heart cannot get oxygen. Most heart attacks occur as a result of ischemic heart disease.

Ischemic heart disease is a condition in which a waxy substance, called "plaque," builds up inside of the coronary arteries. These arteries supply oxygen-rich blood to your heart.

When plaque builds up in the arteries, the condition is called "atherosclerosis." The buildup of plaque occurs over many years.

Eventually, an area of plaque can rupture (break open) inside of an artery. This causes a blood clot to form on the plaque's surface. If the clot becomes large enough, it can mostly or completely block blood flow through a coronary artery.

If the blockage is not treated quickly, the portion of heart muscle fed by the artery begins to die. Healthy heart tissue is replaced with scar tissue. This heart damage may not be obvious, or it may cause severe or long-lasting problems.

Coronary Artery Spasm

A less common cause of heart attack is a severe spasm (tightening) of a coronary artery. The spasm cuts off blood flow through the artery. Spasms can occur in coronary arteries that are not affected by atherosclerosis.

What causes a coronary artery to spasm is not always clear. A spasm may be related to:

- Taking certain drugs, such as cocaine

- Emotional stress or pain

- Exposure to extreme cold

- Cigarette smoking

Risk Factors for Heart Attack

Certain risk factors make it more likely that you will develop ischemic heart disease and have a heart attack. You can control many of these risk factors.

Risk Factors You Can Control

The major risk factors for a heart attack that you can control include:

- Smoking

- High blood pressure (HBP)

- High blood cholesterol

- Overweight and obesity

- An unhealthy diet (for example, a diet high in saturated fat, trans fat, cholesterol, and sodium)

- Lack of routine physical activity

- High blood sugar due to insulin resistance or diabetes

Some of these risk factors—such as obesity, high blood pressure, and high blood sugar—tend to occur together. When they do, it is called "metabolic syndrome."

In general, a person who has metabolic syndrome is twice as likely to develop heart disease and five times as likely to develop diabetes when compared to someone who does not have metabolic syndrome.

Risk Factors You Cannot Control

Risk factors that you cannot control include:

- **Age.** The risk of heart disease increases for men after the age of 45 and for women after the age of 55 (or after menopause).

- **Family history of early heart disease.** Your risk increases if your father or a brother was diagnosed with heart disease before 55 years of age, or if your mother or a sister was diagnosed with heart disease before 65 years of age.

- **Preeclampsia.** This condition can develop during pregnancy. The two main signs of preeclampsia are a rise in blood pressure and excess protein in the urine. Preeclampsia is linked to an increased lifetime risk of heart disease, including CHD, heart attack, heart failure, and high blood pressure.

Screening and Prevention of Heart Attack

Lowering your risk factors for ischemic heart disease can help you prevent a heart attack. Even if you already have heart disease, you still can take steps to lower your risk for a heart attack. These steps involve making heart-healthy lifestyle changes and getting ongoing medical care for related conditions that make a heart attack more likely. Talk to your doctor about whether you may benefit from aspirin primary prevention or from using aspirin to help prevent your first heart attack.

Heart-Healthy Lifestyle Changes

A heart-healthy lifestyle can help prevent a heart attack and includes heart-healthy eating, being physically active, quitting smoking, managing stress, and managing your weight.

Ongoing Care
Treat Related Conditions

Treating conditions that make a heart attack more likely also can help lower your risk for a heart attack. These conditions may include:

- **Diabetes (high blood sugar).** If you have diabetes, try to control your blood sugar level through diet and physical activity (as your doctor recommends). If needed, take medicine as prescribed.

- **High blood cholesterol.** Your doctor may prescribe a statin medicine to lower your cholesterol if diet and exercise are not enough.

- **High blood pressure.** Your doctor may prescribe medicine to keep your blood pressure under control.

- **Chronic kidney disease (CKD).** Your doctor may prescribe medicines to control your high blood pressure or high blood sugar levels.

- **Peripheral artery disease (PAD).** Your doctor may recommend surgery or procedures to unblock the affected arteries.

Have an Emergency Action Plan

Make sure that you have an emergency action plan in case you or someone in your family has a heart attack. This is very important if you are at high risk for, or have already had, a heart attack.

Write down a list of medicines you are taking, medicines you are allergic to, your healthcare provider's phone numbers (both during and after office hours), and contact information for a friend or relative. Keep the list in a handy place to share in a medical emergency.

Talk with your doctor about the signs and symptoms of a heart attack, when you should call 911, and steps you can take while waiting for medical help to arrive.

Signs, Symptoms, and Complications of Heart Attack

Not all heart attacks begin with the sudden, crushing chest pain that often is shown on TV or in the movies. In one study, for example, one-third of the patients who had heart attacks had no chest pain. These patients were more likely to be older, female, or diabetic.

The symptoms of a heart attack can vary from person to person. Some people can have few symptoms and are surprised to learn that they have had a heart attack. If you have already had a heart attack, your symptoms may not be the same for another one. It is important for you to know the most common symptoms of a heart attack and also remember these facts:

- Heart attacks can start slowly and cause only mild pain or discomfort. Symptoms can be mild or more intense and sudden. Symptoms also may come and go over several hours.

- People who have high blood sugar (diabetes) may have no symptoms or very mild ones.

- The most common symptom, in both men and women, is chest pain or discomfort.

- Women are somewhat more likely to have shortness of breath, nausea, and vomiting, unusual tiredness (sometimes for days), and pain in the back, shoulders, and jaw.

Some people do not have symptoms at all. Heart attacks that occur without any symptoms or with very mild symptoms are called "silent heart attacks."

Most Common Symptoms

The most common warning symptoms of a heart attack for both men and women are:

- **Chest pain or discomfort.** Most heart attacks involve discomfort in the center or left side of the chest. The discomfort usually lasts for more than a few minutes or goes away and comes back. It can feel like pressure, squeezing, fullness, or pain. It also can feel like heartburn or indigestion. The feeling can be mild or severe.

- **Upper body discomfort.** You may feel pain or discomfort in one or both arms, the back, shoulders, neck, jaw, or upper part of the stomach (above the belly button).

- **Shortness of breath.** This may be your only symptom, or it may occur before or along with chest pain or discomfort. It can occur when you are resting or doing a little bit of physical activity.

The symptoms of angina can be similar to the symptoms of a heart attack. Angina is chest pain that occurs in people who have ischemic heart disease, usually when they are active. Angina pain usually lasts for only a few minutes and goes away with rest.

Chest pain or discomfort that does not go away or changes from its usual pattern (for example, occurs more often or while you are resting) can be a sign of a heart attack.

All chest pain should be checked by a doctor.

Other Common Signs and Symptoms

Pay attention to these other possible symptoms of a heart attack:

- Breaking out in a cold sweat
- Feeling unusually tired for no reason, sometimes for days (especially if you are a woman)
- Nausea (feeling sick to the stomach) and vomiting
- Light-headedness or sudden dizziness
- Any sudden, new symptoms or a change in the pattern of symptoms you already have (for example, if your symptoms become stronger or last longer than usual)

Not everyone having a heart attack has typical symptoms. If you have already had a heart attack, your symptoms may not be the same for another one. However, some people may have a pattern of symptoms that recur.

The more signs and symptoms you have, the more likely it is that you are having a heart attack.

Quick Action Can Save Your Life: Call 911

The signs and symptoms of a heart attack can develop suddenly. However, they also can develop slowly—sometimes within hours, days, or weeks of a heart attack.

Any time you think you might be having heart attack symptoms or a heart attack, do not ignore it or feel embarrassed to call for help. Call 911 for emergency medical care, even if you are not sure whether you are having a heart attack. Here is why:

- Acting fast can save your life.
- An ambulance is the best and safest way to get to the hospital. Emergency medical services (EMS) personnel can check how you are doing and start life-saving medicines and other treatments right away. People who arrive by ambulance often receive faster treatment at the hospital.
- The 911 operator or EMS technician can give you advice. You might be told to crush or chew an aspirin if you are not allergic, unless there is a medical reason for you not to take one. Aspirin

taken during a heart attack can limit the damage to your heart and save your life.

Every minute matters. Never delay calling 911 to take aspirin or do anything else you think might help.

Diagnosis of Heart Attack

Your doctor will diagnose a heart attack based on your signs and symptoms, your medical and family histories, and test results.

Diagnostic Tests
Electrocardiogram (EKG)

An electrocardiogram (EKG) is a simple, painless test that detects and records the heart's electrical activity. The test shows how fast the heart is beating and its rhythm (steady or irregular). An EKG also records the strength and timing of electrical signals as they pass through each part of the heart.

An EKG can show signs of heart damage due to ischemic heart disease and signs of a previous or current heart attack.

Blood Tests

During a heart attack, heart muscle cells die and release proteins into the bloodstream. Blood tests can measure the amount of these proteins in the bloodstream. Higher than normal levels of these proteins suggest a heart attack.

Commonly used blood tests include troponin tests, creatine kinase (CK) or creatine kinase-MB (CK-MB) tests, and serum myoglobin tests. Blood tests often are repeated to check for changes over time.

Chapter 13

Sudden Cardiac Arrest

What Is Sudden Cardiac Arrest?

Sudden cardiac arrest (SCA) is a condition in which the heart suddenly and unexpectedly stops beating. If this happens, blood stops flowing to the brain and other vital organs.

If it is not treated within minutes, SCA usually results in death.

To understand sudden cardiac arrest, it helps to understand how the heart works. The heart has an electrical system that controls the rate and rhythm of the heartbeat. Problems with the heart's electrical system can cause irregular heartbeats called "arrhythmias."

There are many types of arrhythmias. During an arrhythmia, the heart can beat too fast, too slow, or with an irregular rhythm. Some arrhythmias can cause the heart to stop pumping blood to the body—these arrhythmias cause SCA.

Sudden cardiac arrest is not the same as a heart attack. A heart attack occurs if blood flow to part of the heart muscle is blocked. During a heart attack, the heart usually does not suddenly stop beating. SCA, however, may happen after or during recovery from a heart attack.

People who have heart disease are at a higher risk for SCA. However, SCA can happen in people who appear healthy and have no known heart disease or other risk factors for SCA.

Most people who have SCA die from it—often within minutes. Rapid treatment of SCA with a defibrillator can be lifesaving. A defibrillator

---

This chapter includes text excerpted from "Sudden Cardiac Arrest," National Heart, Lung, and Blood Institute (NHLBI), August 28, 2018.

is a device that sends an electric shock to the heart to try to restore its normal rhythm.

Automated external defibrillators (AEDs) can be used by bystanders to save the lives of people who are experiencing SCA. These portable devices often are found in public places, such as shopping malls, golf courses, businesses, airports, airplanes, casinos, convention centers, hotels, sports venues, and schools.

Causes of Sudden Cardiac Arrest

Ventricular fibrillation (v-fib) causes most SCAs. V-fib is a type of arrhythmia.

During v-fib, the ventricles (the heart's lower chambers) do not beat normally. Instead, they quiver very rapidly and irregularly. When this happens, the heart pumps little or no blood to the body. V-fib is fatal if not treated within a few minutes.

Other problems with the heart's electrical system also can cause SCA. For example, SCA can occur if the rate of the heart's electrical signals becomes very slow and stops. SCA also can occur if the heart muscle does not respond to the heart's electrical signals.

Certain diseases and conditions can cause the electrical problems that lead to SCA. Examples include ischemic heart disease, also called "coronary heart disease" or "coronary artery disease;" "severe physical stress;" "certain inherited disorders;" and "structural changes in the heart."

Several research studies are underway to try to find the exact causes of SCA and how to prevent them.

Ischemic Heart Disease

Ischemic heart disease is a disease in which a waxy substance called "plaque" builds up in the coronary arteries. These arteries supply oxygen-rich blood to your heart muscle.

Plaque narrows the arteries and reduces blood flow to your heart muscle. Eventually, an area of plaque can rupture (break open). This may cause a blood clot to form on the plaque's surface.

A blood clot can partly or fully block the flow of oxygen-rich blood to the portion of heart muscle fed by the artery. This causes a heart attack.

During a heart attack, some heart muscle cells die and are replaced with scar tissue. The scar tissue damages the heart's electrical system. As a result, electrical signals may spread abnormally throughout the heart. These changes to the heart increase the risk of dangerous arrhythmias and SCA.

Ischemic heart disease seems to cause most cases of SCA in adults. Many of these adults, however, have no signs or symptoms of heart disease before experiencing SCA.

Physical Stress

Certain types of physical stress can cause your heart's electrical system to fail. Examples include:

- Intense physical activity. The hormone adrenaline is released during intense physical activity. This hormone can trigger SCA in people who have heart problems.

- Very low blood levels of potassium or magnesium. These minerals play an important role in your heart's electrical signaling.

- Major blood loss

- Severe lack of oxygen

Inherited Disorders

A tendency to have arrhythmias runs in some families. This tendency is inherited, which means it is passed from parents to children through their genes. Members of these families may be at a higher risk for SCA.

An example of an inherited disorder that makes you more likely to have arrhythmias is long QT syndrome (LQTS). LQTS is a disorder of the heart's electrical activity. Problems with tiny pores on the surface of heart muscle cells cause the disorder. LQTS can cause sudden, uncontrollable, dangerous heart rhythms.

People who inherit structural heart problems also may be at higher risk for SCA. These types of problems often are the cause of SCA in children.

Structural Changes in the Heart

Changes in the heart's normal size or structure may affect its electrical system. Examples of such changes include an enlarged heart due to high blood pressure or advanced heart disease. Heart infections also may cause structural changes in the heart.

Risk Factors for Sudden Cardiac Arrest

The risk of SCA increases:

- With age

- If you are a man. Men are more likely to go into SCA than women.

- Some studies show that Black individuals—particularly those with underlying conditions, diabetes, high blood pressure, heart failure, and chronic kidney disease or those with certain cardiac findings on tests such as an electrocardiogram—have a higher risk for SCA.

Major Risk Factor

The major risk factor for SCA is ischemic heart disease. Most people who have SCA have some degree of ischemic heart disease; however, many people may not know that they have heart disease until SCA occurs. Usually, their heart disease is "silent"—that is, it has no signs or symptoms. Because of this, doctors and nurses have not detected it.

Many people who have SCA also have silent, or undiagnosed, heart attacks before SCA happens. These people have no clear signs of heart attack, and they do not even realize that they have had one.

Other Risk Factors

Other risk factors for SCA include:

- A personal history of arrhythmias

- A personal or family history of SCA or inherited disorders that make you prone to arrhythmias

- Drug or alcohol abuse

- Heart attack

- Heart failure

Screening and Prevention of Sudden Cardiac Arrest

Ways to prevent death due to SCA differ depending on whether:

- You have already had SCA.

- You have never had SCA but are at high risk for the condition.

- You have never had SCA and have no known risk factors for the condition.

For People Who Have Survived Sudden Cardiac Arrest

If you have already had SCA, you are at a high risk of having it again. Research shows that an implantable cardioverter defibrillator (ICD) reduces the chances of dying from a second SCA. An ICD is surgically placed under the skin in your chest or abdomen. The device has wires with electrodes on the ends that connect to your heart's chambers. The ICD monitors your heartbeat.

If the ICD detects a dangerous heart rhythm, it gives an electric shock to restore the heart's normal rhythm. Your doctor may give you medicine to limit irregular heartbeats that can trigger the ICD.

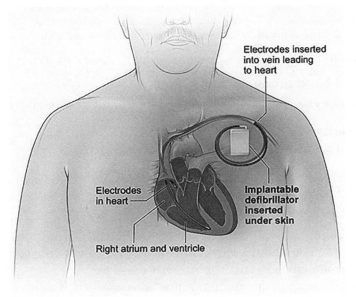

Figure 13.1. *Implantable Cardioverter Defibrillator*

The illustration shows the location of an implantable cardioverter defibrillator in the upper chest. The electrodes are inserted into the heart through a vein.

An ICD is not the same as a pacemaker. The devices are similar, but they have some differences. Pacemakers give off low-energy electrical pulses. They are often used to treat less dangerous heart rhythms, such as those that occur in the upper chambers of the heart. Most new ICDs work as both pacemakers and ICDs.

For People at High Risk for a First Sudden Cardiac Arrest

If you have severe ischemic heart disease, you are at an increased risk for SCA. This is especially true if you have recently had a heart attack.

Your doctor may prescribe a type of medicine called a "beta-blocker" to help lower your risk for SCA. Your doctor also may discuss beginning statin treatment if you have an elevated risk for developing heart disease or having a stroke. Doctors usually prescribe statins for people who have:

- Diabetes

- Heart disease or had a prior stroke

- High low-density lipoprotein (LDL) cholesterol levels

Your doctor also may prescribe other medications to:

- Decrease your chance of having a heart attack or dying suddenly

- Lower blood pressure

- Prevent blood clots, which can lead to heart attack or stroke

- Prevent or delay the need for a procedure or surgery, such as angioplasty or coronary artery bypass grafting

- Reduce your heart's workload and relieve heart disease symptoms

Take all medicines regularly, as your doctor prescribes. Do not change the amount of your medicine or skip a dose unless your doctor tells you to. You should still follow a heart-healthy lifestyle, even if you take medicines to treat your heart disease.

Other treatments for coronary heart disease—such as percutaneous coronary intervention, also known as "coronary angioplasty" or "coronary artery bypass grafting"—also may lower your risk for SCA. Your doctor also may recommend an ICD if you are at high risk for SCA.

For People Who Have No Known Risk Factors for Sudden Cardiac Arrest

Ischemic heart disease seems to be the cause of most SCAs in adults. Heart disease also is a major risk factor for angina (chest pain or discomfort) and heart attack, and it contributes to other heart problems.

Following a heart-healthy lifestyle can help you lower your risk for heart disease, SCA, and other heart problems. A heart-healthy lifestyle includes:

- Heart-healthy eating
- Aiming for a healthy weight
- Managing stress
- Physical activity
- Quitting smoking

Signs, Symptoms, and Complications of Sudden Cardiac Arrest

Usually, the first sign of SCA is loss of consciousness (fainting). At the same time, no heartbeat (or pulse) can be felt.

Some people may have a racing heartbeat or feel dizzy or light-headed just before they faint. Within an hour before SCA, some people may experience chest pain, shortness of breath, nausea (feeling sick to the stomach), or vomiting.

Diagnosis of Sudden Cardiac Arrest

Sudden cardiac arrest happens without warning and requires emergency treatment. Doctors rarely diagnose SCA with medical tests as it is happening. Instead, SCA often is diagnosed after it happens. Doctors do this by ruling out other causes of a person's sudden collapse.

Specialists Involved

If you are at high risk for SCA, your doctor may refer you to a cardiologist. This is a doctor who specializes in diagnosing and treating heart diseases and conditions. Your cardiologist will work with you to decide whether you need treatment to prevent SCA.

Some cardiologists specialize in problems with the heart's electrical system. These specialists are called "cardiac electrophysiologists."

Diagnostic Tests and Procedures

Doctors use several tests to help detect the factors that put people at risk for SCA.

Electrocardiogram

An electrocardiogram (EKG) is a simple, painless test that detects and records the heart's electrical activity. The test shows how fast the heart is beating and its rhythm (steady or irregular). An EKG also records the strength and timing of electrical signals as they pass through each part of the heart.

An EKG can show evidence of heart damage due to ischemic heart disease. The test also can show signs of a previous or current heart attack.

Echocardiography

An echocardiography, or echo, is a painless test that uses sound waves to create pictures of your heart. The test shows the size and shape of your heart and how well your heart chambers and valves are working.

An echo also can identify areas of poor blood flow to the heart, areas of heart muscle that are not contracting normally, and previous injury to the heart muscle caused by poor blood flow.

There are several types of an echo, including a stress echo. This test is done both before and after a cardiac stress test. During this test, you exercise (or are given medicine if you are unable to exercise) to make your heart work hard and beat fast.

A stress echo shows whether you have decreased blood flow to your heart (a sign of coronary heart disease (CHD)).

Multiple Gated Acquisition Test or Cardiac Magnetic Resonance Imaging

A multiple gated acquisition (MUGA) test shows how well your heart is pumping blood. For this test, a small amount of radioactive substance is injected into a vein and travels to your heart.

The substance releases energy, which special cameras outside of your body can detect. The cameras use the energy to create pictures of many parts of your heart.

Cardiac magnetic resonance imaging (MRI) is a safe procedure that uses radio waves and magnets to create detailed pictures of your heart. The test creates still and moving pictures of your heart and major blood vessels.

Doctors use cardiac MRI to get pictures of the beating heart and to look at the structure and function of the heart.

Cardiac Catheterization

Cardiac catheterization is a procedure used to diagnose and treat certain heart conditions. A long, thin, flexible tube called a "catheter" is put into a blood vessel in your arm, groin (upper thigh), or neck and threaded to your heart. Through the catheter, your doctor can do diagnostic tests and treatments on your heart.

Sometimes, dye is put into the catheter. The dye will flow through your bloodstream to your heart. The dye makes your coronary (heart) arteries visible on X-ray pictures. The dye can show whether plaque has narrowed or blocked any of your coronary arteries.

Electrophysiology Study

For an electrophysiology study, doctors use cardiac catheterization to record how your heart's electrical system responds to certain medicines and electrical stimulation. This helps your doctor find where the heart's electrical system is damaged.

Blood Tests

Your doctor may recommend blood tests to check the levels of potassium, magnesium, and other chemicals in your blood. These chemicals play an important role in your heart's electrical signaling.

Treatment of Sudden Cardiac Arrest
Emergency Treatment

Sudden cardiac arrest is an emergency. A person having SCA needs to be treated with a defibrillator right away. This device sends an electric shock to the heart. The electric shock can restore a normal rhythm to a heart that is stopped beating.

To work well, defibrillation must be done within minutes of the SCA. With every minute that passes, the chances of surviving SCA drop rapidly.

Police, emergency medical technicians, and other first responders usually are trained and equipped to use a defibrillator. Call 911 right away if someone has signs or symptoms of SCA. The sooner you call for help, the sooner lifesaving treatment can begin.

Automated External Defibrillators

Automated external defibrillators (AEDs) are special defibrillators that untrained bystanders can use. These portable devices often are found in public places, such as shopping malls, golf courses, businesses, airports, airplanes, casinos, convention centers, hotels, sports venues, and schools.

Automated external defibrillators are programmed to give an electric shock if they detect a dangerous arrhythmia, such as ventricular fibrillation. This prevents giving a shock to someone who may have fainted but is not having SCA.

You should give cardiopulmonary resuscitation (CPR) to a person having SCA until defibrillation can be done.

People who are at risk for SCA may want to consider having an AED at home. A 2008 study by the National Heart, Lung, and Blood Institute (NHLBI) and the National Institutes of Health (NIH) found that AEDs in the home are safe and effective.

Some people feel that placing these devices in homes will save many lives because many SCAs occur at home. Others note that no evidence supports the idea that home-use AEDs save more lives. These people fear that people who have AEDs in their homes will delay calling for help during an emergency. They are also concerned that people who have home-use AEDs will not properly maintain the devices or forget where they are.

When considering a home-use AED, talk with your doctor. She or he can help you decide whether having an AED in your home will benefit you.

Treatment in a Hospital

If you survive SCA, you will likely be admitted to a hospital for ongoing care and treatment. In the hospital, your medical team will closely watch your heart. They may give you medicines to try to reduce the risk of another SCA.

While in the hospital, your medical team will try to find out what caused your SCA. If you are diagnosed with ischemic heart disease, you may have percutaneous coronary intervention. This procedure helps to restore blood flow through narrowed or blocked coronary arteries.

Often, people who have SCA get an ICD. This small device is surgically placed under the skin in your chest or abdomen. An ICD uses electric pulses or shocks to help control dangerous arrhythmias.

Chapter 14

Cardiogenic Shock

What Is Cardiogenic Shock?

Cardiogenic shock is a condition in which a suddenly weakened heart is not able to pump enough blood to meet the body's needs. The condition is a medical emergency and is fatal if not treated right away.

The most common cause of cardiogenic shock is damage to the heart muscle from a severe heart attack. However, not everyone who has a heart attack has cardiogenic shock. In fact, on average, only about seven percent of people who have heart attacks develop the condition.

If cardiogenic shock does occur, it is very dangerous. When people die from heart attacks in hospitals, cardiogenic shock is the most common cause of death.

What Is Shock?

The medical term "shock" refers to a state in which not enough blood and oxygen reach important organs in the body, such as the brain and kidneys. Shock causes very low blood pressure and may be life-threatening.

Shock can have many causes. Cardiogenic shock is only one type of shock. Other types of shock include hypovolemic shock and vasodilatory shock.

This chapter includes text excerpted from "Cardiogenic Shock," National Heart, Lung, and Blood Institute (NHLBI), January 28, 2019.

Hypovolemic shock is a condition in which the heart cannot pump enough blood to the body because of severe blood loss.

In vasodilatory shock, the blood vessels suddenly relax. When the blood vessels are too relaxed, blood pressure drops and blood flow becomes very low. Without enough blood pressure, blood and oxygen do not reach the body's organs.

A bacterial infection in the bloodstream, a severe allergic reaction, or damage to the nervous system (brain and nerves) may cause vasodilatory shock.

When a person is in shock (from any cause), not enough blood and oxygen are reaching the body's organs. If shock lasts more than a few minutes, the lack of oxygen starts to damage the body's organs. If shock is not treated quickly, it can cause permanent organ damage or death.

If you think that you or someone else is in shock, call 911 right away for emergency treatment. Prompt medical care can save your life and prevent or limit damage to your body's organs.

In the past, almost no one survived cardiogenic shock. Now, about half of the people who go into cardiogenic shock survive. This is because of prompt recognition of symptoms and improved treatments, such as medicines and devices. These treatments can restore blood flow to the heart and help the heart pump better.

In some cases, devices that take over the pumping function of the heart are used. Implanting these devices requires major surgery.

Causes of Cardiogenic Shock
Immediate Causes

Cardiogenic shock occurs if the heart suddenly cannot pump enough oxygen-rich blood to the body. The most common cause of cardiogenic shock is damage to the heart muscle from a severe heart attack.

This damage prevents the heart's main pumping chamber, the left ventricle, from working well. As a result, the heart cannot pump enough oxygen-rich blood to the rest of the body.

In about three percent of cardiogenic shock cases, the heart's lower right chamber, the right ventricle, does not work well. This means that the heart cannot properly pump blood to the lungs, where it picks up oxygen to bring back to the heart and the rest of the body.

Without enough oxygen-rich blood reaching the body's major organs, many problems can occur. For example:

- Cardiogenic shock can cause death if the flow of oxygen-rich blood to the organs is not restored quickly. This is why emergency medical treatment is required.

- If organs do not get enough oxygen-rich blood, they will not work well. Cells in the organs die, and the organs may never work well again.

- As some organs stop working, they may cause problems with other bodily functions. This, in turn, can worsen shock. For example:

  - If the kidneys are not working well, the levels of important chemicals in the body change. This may cause the heart and other muscles to become even weaker, limiting blood flow even more.

  - If the liver is not working well, the body stops making proteins that help the blood clot. This can lead to more bleeding if the shock is due to blood loss.

How well the brain, kidneys, and other organs recover will depend on how long a person is in shock. The less time a person is in shock, the less damage will occur to the organs. This is another reason why emergency treatment is so important.

Underlying Causes

The underlying causes of cardiogenic shock are conditions that weaken the heart and prevent it from pumping enough oxygen-rich blood to the body.

Heart Attack

Most heart attacks occur as a result of ischemic heart disease. Ischemic heart disease is a condition in which a waxy substance called "plaque" narrows or blocks the coronary arteries, which supply blood to the heart.

Plaque reduces blood flow to your heart muscle. It also makes it more likely that blood clots will form in your arteries. Blood clots can partially or completely block blood flow.

Conditions Caused by Heart Attack

Heart attacks can cause some serious heart conditions that can lead to cardiogenic shock. One example is a ventricular septal rupture. This condition occurs if the wall that separates the ventricles (the heart's two lower chambers) breaks down.

The breakdown happens because cells in the wall have died due to a heart attack. Without the wall to separate them, the ventricles cannot pump properly.

Heart attacks also can cause papillary muscle infarction or rupture. This condition occurs if the muscles that help anchor the heart valves stop working or break because a heart attack cuts off their blood supply. If this happens, blood does not flow correctly between the heart's chambers. This prevents the heart from pumping properly.

Other Heart Conditions

Serious heart conditions that may occur with or without a heart attack can cause cardiogenic shock. Examples include:

- **Myocarditis.** This is inflammation of the heart muscle.

- **Endocarditis.** This is an infection of the inner lining of the heart chambers and valves.

- **Life-threatening arrhythmias.** These are problems with the rate or rhythm of the heartbeat.

- **Pericardial tamponade.** This is when there is too much fluid or blood around the heart. The fluid squeezes the heart muscle, so it cannot pump properly.

Pulmonary Embolism

Pulmonary embolism (PE) is a sudden blockage in a lung artery. This condition usually is caused by a blood clot that travels to the lung from a vein in the leg. PE can damage your heart and other organs in your body.

Risk Factors for Cardiogenic Shock

The most common risk factor for cardiogenic shock is having a heart attack. If you have had a heart attack, the following factors can further increase your risk for cardiogenic shock:

- Older age

- A history of heart attacks or heart failure

- Ischemic heart disease that affects all of the heart's major blood vessels

- High blood pressure

- Diabetes

Women who have heart attacks are at higher risk for cardiogenic shock than men who have heart attacks.

Screening and Prevention of Cardiogenic Shock

The best way to prevent cardiogenic shock is to lower your risk for ischemic heart disease and heart attack.

If you already have heart disease, it is important to get ongoing treatment from a doctor who has experience with treating heart problems.

If you have a heart attack, you should get treatment right away to try to prevent cardiogenic shock and other possible complications.

- Act timely. Know the warning signs of a heart attack so you can act fast to get treatment. Many heart attack victims wait two hours or more after their symptoms begin before they seek medical help. Delays in treatment increase the risk of complications and death.

- If you think you are having a heart attack, call 911 for help. Do not drive yourself or have friends or family drive you to the hospital. Call an ambulance so that medical personnel can begin life-saving treatment on the way to the emergency room.

Signs, Symptoms, and Complications of Cardiogenic Shock

A lack of oxygen-rich blood reaching the brain, kidneys, skin, and other parts of the body causes the signs and symptoms of cardiogenic shock.

Some of the typical signs and symptoms of shock usually include at least two or more of the following:

- Confusion or lack of alertness

- Loss of consciousness

- A sudden and ongoing rapid heartbeat

- Sweating

- Pale skin

- A weak pulse

- Rapid breathing

- Decreased or no urine output

- Cool hands and feet

Any of these alone is unlikely to be a sign or symptom of shock.

If you or someone else is having these signs and symptoms, call 911 right away for emergency treatment. Prompt medical care can save your life and prevent or limit organ damage.

Diagnosis of Cardiogenic Shock

The first step in diagnosing cardiogenic shock is to identify that a person is in shock. At that point, emergency treatment should begin.

Once emergency treatment starts, doctors can look for the specific cause of the shock. If the reason for the shock is that the heart is not pumping strongly enough, then the diagnosis is cardiogenic shock.

Tests and Procedures to Diagnose Shock and Its Underlying Causes
Blood Pressure Test

Medical personnel can use a simple blood pressure cuff and stethoscope to check whether a person has very low blood pressure. This is the most common sign of shock. A blood pressure test can be done before the person goes to a hospital.

Less serious conditions also can cause low blood pressure, such as fainting or taking certain medicines, such as those used to treat high blood pressure.

Electrocardiogram

An electrocardiogram (EKG) is a simple test that detects and records the heart's electrical activity. The test shows how fast the heart is beating and its rhythm (steady or irregular).

An EKG also records the strength and timing of electrical signals as they pass through each part of the heart. Doctors use EKGs to diagnose severe heart attacks and monitor the heart's condition.

Echocardiography

An echocardiography (echo) uses sound waves to create a moving picture of the heart. The test provides information about the size and shape of the heart and how well the heart chambers and valves are working.

An echo also can identify areas of poor blood flow to the heart, areas of heart muscle that are not contracting normally, and previous injury to the heart muscle caused by poor blood flow.

Chest X-Ray

A chest X-ray takes pictures of organs and structures in the chest, including the heart, lungs, and blood vessels. This test shows whether the heart is enlarged or whether fluid is present in the lungs. These can be signs of cardiogenic shock.

Cardiac Enzyme Test

When cells in the heart die, they release enzymes into the blood. These enzymes are called "markers" or "biomarkers." Measuring these markers can show whether the heart is damaged and the extent of the damage.

Coronary Angiography

Coronary angiography is an X-ray exam of the heart and blood vessels. The doctor passes a catheter (a thin, flexible tube) through an artery in the leg or arm to the heart. The catheter can measure the pressure inside the heart chambers.

Dye that can be seen on an X-ray image is injected into the bloodstream through the tip of the catheter. The dye lets the doctor study the flow of blood through the heart and blood vessels and see any blockages.

Pulmonary Artery Catheterization

For this procedure, a catheter is inserted into a vein in the arm or neck or near the collarbone. Then, the catheter is moved into the pulmonary artery. This artery connects the right side of the heart to the lungs.

The catheter is used to check blood pressure in the pulmonary artery. If the blood pressure is too high or too low, treatment may be needed.

Blood Tests

Some blood tests also are used to help diagnose cardiogenic shock, including:

- **Arterial blood gas measurement.** For this test, a blood sample is taken from an artery. The sample is used to measure oxygen, carbon dioxide, and pH (acidity) levels in the blood. Certain levels of these substances are associated with shock.

- **Tests that measure the function of various organs, such as the kidneys and liver.** If these organs are not working well, they may not be getting enough oxygen-rich blood. This could be a sign of cardiogenic shock.

Treatment of Cardiogenic Shock

Cardiogenic shock is life-threatening and requires emergency medical treatment. The condition usually is diagnosed after a person has been admitted to a hospital for a heart attack. If the person is not already in a hospital, emergency treatment can start as soon as medical personnel arrive.

The first goal of emergency treatment for cardiogenic shock is to improve the flow of blood and oxygen to the body's organs.

Sometimes, both the shock and its cause are treated at the same time. For example, doctors may quickly open a blocked blood vessel that is damaging the heart. Often, this can get the patient out of shock with little or no additional treatment.

Emergency Life Support

Emergency life support treatment is needed for any type of shock. This treatment helps get oxygen-rich blood flowing to the brain, kidneys, and other organs.

Restoring blood flow to the organs keeps the patient alive and may prevent long-term damage to the organs. Emergency life support treatment includes:

- Giving the patient extra oxygen to breathe so that more oxygen reaches the lungs, the heart, and the rest of the body.

- Providing breathing support if needed. A ventilator might be used to protect the airway and provide the patient with extra oxygen. A ventilator is a machine that supports breathing.

- Giving the patient fluids, including blood and blood products, through a needle inserted in a vein (when the shock is due to blood loss). This can help get more blood to major organs and the rest of the body. This treatment usually is not used for cardiogenic shock because the heart cannot pump the blood that is already in the body. Also, too much fluid is in the lungs, making it hard to breathe.

Medicines

During and after emergency life support treatment, doctors will try to find out what is causing the shock. If the reason for the shock is that the heart is not pumping strongly enough, then the diagnosis is cardiogenic shock.

Treatment for cardiogenic shock will depend on its cause. Doctors may prescribe medicines to:

- Prevent blood clots from forming

- Increase the force with which the heart muscle contracts

- Treat a heart attack

Medical Devices

Medical devices can help the heart pump and improve blood flow. Devices used to treat cardiogenic shock may include:

- **An intra-aortic balloon pump.** This device is placed in the aorta, the main blood vessel that carries blood from the heart to the body. A balloon at the tip of the device is inflated and deflated in a rhythm that matches the heart's pumping rhythm. This allows the weakened heart muscle to pump as much blood as it can, which helps get more blood to vital organs, such as the brain and kidneys.

- **A left ventricular assist device (LVAD).** This device is a battery-operated pump that takes over part of the heart's pumping action. An LVAD helps the heart pump blood to the body. This device may be used if damage to the left ventricle, the heart's main pumping chamber, is causing shock.

Medical Procedures and Surgery

Sometimes, medicines and medical devices are not enough to treat cardiogenic shock.

Medical procedures and surgery can restore blood flow to the heart and the rest of the body, repair heart damage, and help keep a patient alive while she or he recovers from shock.

Surgery also can improve the chances of long-term survival. Surgery done within six hours of the onset of shock symptoms has the greatest chance of improving survival.

The types of procedures and surgery used to treat underlying causes of cardiogenic shock include:

- **Percutaneous coronary intervention (PCI) and stents.** PCI, also known as "coronary angioplasty," is a procedure used to open narrowed or blocked coronary (heart) arteries and to treat an ongoing heart attack. A stent is a small mesh tube that is placed in a coronary artery during PCI to help keep it open.

- **Coronary artery bypass grafting.** For this surgery, arteries or veins from other parts of the body are used to bypass (that is, go around) narrowed coronary arteries. This creates a new passage for oxygen-rich blood to reach the heart.

- Surgery to repair damaged heart valves

- Surgery to repair a break in the wall that separates the heart's chambers. This break is called a "septal rupture."

- **Heart transplant.** This type of surgery rarely is done during an emergency situation as with cardiogenic shock because of other available options. Also, doctors need to do very careful testing to make sure a patient will benefit from a heart transplant and to find a matching heart from a donor. Still, in some cases, doctors may recommend a transplant if they feel it is the best way to improve a patient's chances of long-term survival.

Chapter 15

Cardiomyopathy

Cardiomyopathy represents a collection of diverse conditions of the heart muscle. These diseases have many causes, symptoms, and treatments, and they can affect people of all ages and races.

When cardiomyopathy occurs, the normal muscle in the heart can thicken, stiffen, thin out, or fill with substances the body produces that do not belong in the heart muscle. As a result, the heart muscle's ability to pump blood is reduced, which can lead to irregular heartbeats, the backup of blood into the lungs or rest of the body, and heart failure.

Cardiomyopathy can be acquired—developed because of another disease, condition, or factor—or inherited. The cause is not always known.

The main types of cardiomyopathy include the following:

- Dilated is where one of the pumping chambers (ventricles) of the heart is enlarged. This is more common in males and is the most common form of cardiomyopathy in children. It can occur at any age and may or may not be inherited.

- Hypertrophic is where the heart muscle is thickened. This is often present in childhood or early adulthood and can cause sudden death in adolescents and young adult athletes. It is often an inherited condition, and a person may not have any

This chapter includes text excerpted from "Other Related Conditions—Cardiomyopathy," Centers for Disease Control and Prevention (CDC), September 2, 2015. Reviewed May 2019.

symptoms. If there is a family history of this, other family members can be tested and adjust their activities to reduce the risk of sudden death.

- Arrhythmogenic is where the disease causes irregular heartbeats or rhythms. This is often inherited and is more common in males.

- Restrictive is where heart muscle is stiff or scarred, or both. It can occur with amyloidosis or hemochromatosis, and other conditions. This is the least common type.

How Common Is Cardiomyopathy?

Cardiomyopathy often goes undiagnosed, so the numbers can vary. As many as 1 of 500 adults may have this condition. Males and females of all ages and races can have cardiomyopathy. Dilated cardiomyopathy is more common in Blacks than in Whites and in males than in females.

Hypertrophic cardiomyopathy is thought to be the most common inherited or genetic heart disease. While this type of cardiomyopathy occurs at many ages, children and young adults with this condition may have no symptoms, yet they are still at high risk of sudden cardiac death.

What Causes Cardiomyopathy

Although the cause of cardiomyopathy is sometimes unknown, certain diseases or conditions can lead to cardiomyopathy. These include the following:

- A family history of cardiomyopathy, heart failure, or sudden cardiac arrest

- Connective tissue disease and other types of autoimmune disease

- Coronary heart disease or a heart attack

- Diseases that can damage the heart, such as hemochromatosis, sarcoidosis or amyloidosis

- Endocrine diseases, including thyroid conditions and diabetes

- Infections in the heart muscle

- Long-term alcoholism or cocaine abuse

- Muscle conditions, such as muscular dystrophy

- Pregnancy

Symptoms of Cardiomyopathy

Some people who have cardiomyopathy never have symptoms, while others may show signs as the disease progresses. These might include the following:

- Shortness of breath or trouble breathing

- Fatigue

- Swelling in the ankles and legs

- Irregular heartbeat or palpitations

- Syncope, the medical term for fainting or briefly passing out

Treatment and Prevention of Cardiomyopathy

The goal of treatment is to slow down the disease, control symptoms, and prevent sudden death. If you are diagnosed with cardiomyopathy, your doctor may tell you to change your diet and physical activity, reduce stress, avoid alcohol and other drugs, and take medicines. Your doctor may also treat you for the conditions that led to cardiomyopathy, if they exist, or recommend surgery. Treatment also depends on which type of cardiomyopathy you have.

Genetic or inherited types of cardiomyopathy cannot be prevented, but adopting or following a healthier lifestyle can help control symptoms and complications. If you have an underlying disease or condition that can cause cardiomyopathy, early treatment of that condition can help prevent the disease from developing.

Pediatric Cardiomyopathy

Cardiomyopathy can occur in children regardless of age, race, and gender. Pediatric cardiomyopathy can be inherited or acquired through a viral infection, and sometimes, the cause is unknown. It is a frequent cause of sudden cardiac arrest in the young population, according to the National Heart, Lung and Blood Institute (NHLBI). Treatment may include medications, changes to physical activity, or surgery.

In many cases, early detection and intervention can help to improve outcomes for children.

Chapter 16

Heart Failure

What Is Heart Failure?

Heart failure is a condition in which the heart cannot pump enough blood to meet the body's needs. In some cases, the heart cannot fill with enough blood. In other cases, the heart cannot pump blood to the rest of the body with enough force. Some people have both problems.

The term "heart failure" does not mean that your heart has stopped or is about to stop working. However, heart failure is a serious condition that requires medical care.

What Causes Heart Failure

Conditions that damage or overwork the heart muscle can cause heart failure. Over time, the heart weakens. It is not able to fill with and/or pump blood as well as it should. As the heart weakens, certain proteins and substances might be released into the blood. These substances have a toxic effect on the heart and blood flow, and they worsen heart failure.

Causes of heart failure include:

Ischemic Heart Disease

Ischemic heart disease is a condition in which a waxy substance called "plaque" builds up inside the coronary arteries. These arteries supply oxygen-rich blood to your heart muscle.

This chapter includes text excerpted from "Heart Failure," National Heart, Lung, and Blood Institute (NHLBI), October 9, 2018.

Plaque narrows the arteries and reduces blood flow to your heart muscle. The buildup of plaque also makes it more likely that blood clots will form in your arteries. Blood clots can partially or completely block blood flow. Ischemic heart disease can lead to chest pain or discomfort called "angina," a heart attack, and heart damage.

Diabetes

Diabetes is a disease in which the body's blood glucose (sugar) level is too high. The body normally breaks down food into glucose and then carries it to cells throughout the body. The cells use a hormone called "insulin" to turn the glucose into energy.

In diabetes, the body does not make enough insulin or does not use its insulin properly. Over time, high blood sugar levels can damage and weaken the heart muscle and the blood vessels around the heart, leading to heart failure.

High Blood Pressure

Blood pressure is the force of blood pushing against the walls of the arteries. If this pressure rises and stays high over time, it can weaken your heart and lead to plaque buildup.

Blood pressure is considered high if it stays at or above 140/90 mmHg over time. (The mmHg is millimeters of mercury—the units used to measure blood pressure.) If you have diabetes or chronic kidney disease (CKD), high blood pressure is defined as 130/80 mmHg or higher.

Other Heart Conditions or Diseases

Other conditions and diseases also can lead to heart failure, such as:

- Arrhythmia happens when a problem occurs with the rate or rhythm of the heartbeat.

- Cardiomyopathy happens when the heart muscle becomes enlarged, thick, or rigid.

- Congenital heart defects (CHD) are problems with the heart's structure that are present at birth.

- Heart valve disease occurs if one or more of your heart valves does not work properly, which can be present at birth or caused by infection, other heart conditions, and age.

Other Factors

Other factors also can injure the heart muscle and lead to heart failure. Examples include:

- Alcohol abuse or cocaine and other illegal-drug use
- Human immunodeficiency virus (HIV)/acquired immunodeficiency syndrome (AIDS)
- Thyroid disorders (having either too much or too little thyroid hormone in the body)
- Too much vitamin E
- Treatments for cancer, such as radiation and chemotherapy

Risk Factors of Heart Failure

About 5.7 million people in the United States have heart failure. The number of people who have this condition is growing.

Heart failure is more common in:

- People who are 65 years of age or older. Aging can weaken the heart muscle. Older people also may have had diseases for many years that led to heart failure. Heart failure is a leading cause of hospital stays among people on Medicare.

- Blacks are more likely to have heart failure than people of other races. They are also more likely to have symptoms at a younger age, have more hospital visits due to heart failure, and die from heart failure.

- People who are overweight. Excess weight puts strain on the heart. Being overweight also increases your risk of heart disease and type 2 diabetes. These diseases can lead to heart failure.

- People who have had a heart attack. Damage to the heart muscle from a heart attack and can weaken the heart muscle.

Children who have congenital heart defects also can develop heart failure. These defects occur if the heart, heart valves, or blood vessels near the heart did not form correctly in the womb. Congenital heart defects can make the heart work harder. This weakens the heart muscle, which can lead to heart failure. Children do not have the same symptoms of heart failure or get the same treatments as adults.

Screening and Prevention of Heart Failure

You can take steps to prevent heart failure. The sooner you start, the better your chances of preventing or delaying the condition.

For People Who Have Healthy Hearts

If you have a healthy heart, you can take action to prevent heart disease and heart failure. To reduce your risk of heart disease:

- Avoid using illegal drugs

- Adopt heart-healthy lifestyle habits

For People Who Are at High Risk for Heart Failure

Even if you are at high risk for heart failure, you can take steps to reduce your risk. People at high risk include those who have ischemic heart disease, high blood pressure, or diabetes.

- Follow all of the steps listed above. Talk to your doctor about what types and amounts of physical activity are safe for you.

- Treat and control any conditions that can cause heart failure. Take medicines as your doctor prescribes.

- Avoid drinking alcohol.

- See your doctor for ongoing care.

For People Who Have Heart Damage But No Signs of Heart Failure

If you have heart damage but show no signs of heart failure, you can still reduce your risk of developing the condition. In addition to the steps above, take your medicines as prescribed to reduce your heart's workload.

Signs, Symptoms, and Complications of Heart Failure

The most common signs and symptoms of heart failure are:

- Shortness of breath or trouble breathing

- Fatigue (tiredness)

- Swelling in the ankles, feet, legs, abdomen, and veins in the neck

All of these symptoms are the result of fluid buildup in your body. When symptoms start, you may feel tired and short of breath after routine physical effort, such as after climbing stairs.

As your heart grows weaker, symptoms get worse. You may begin to feel tired and short of breath after getting dressed or walking across the room. Some people have shortness of breath while lying flat.

Fluid buildup from heart failure also causes weight gain, frequent urination, and a cough that is worse at night and when you are lying down. This cough may be a sign of acute pulmonary edema. This is a condition in which too much fluid builds up in your lungs. The condition requires emergency treatment.

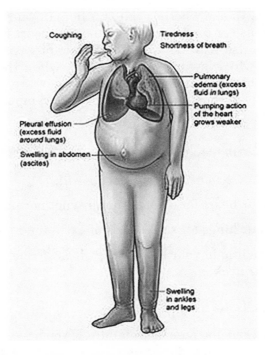

Figure 16.1. *Signs and Symptoms of Heart Failure*

The image shows the major signs and symptoms of heart failure.

Diagnosis of Heart Failure

Your doctor will diagnose heart failure based on your medical and family histories, a physical exam, and test results. The signs and symptoms of heart failure also are common in other conditions. Thus, your doctor will do the following:

- Find out whether you have a disease or condition that can cause heart failure, such as ischemic heart disease, high blood pressure, or diabetes.

- Rule out other causes of your symptoms.

- Find any damage to your heart, and check how well your heart pumps blood.

Early diagnosis and treatment can help people who have heart failure live longer, more active lives.

Medical and Family Histories

Your doctor will ask whether you or others in your family have or have had a disease or condition that can cause heart failure.

Your doctor also will ask about your symptoms. She or he will want to know which symptoms you have, when they occur, how long you have had them, and how severe they are. Your answers will help show whether and how much your symptoms limit your daily routine.

Physical Exam

During the physical exam, your doctor will:

- Listen to your heart for sounds that are not normal.

- Listen to your lungs for the sounds of extra fluid buildup.

- Look for swelling in your ankles, feet, legs, abdomen, and the veins in your neck.

Diagnostic Tests

No single test can diagnose heart failure. If you have signs and symptoms of heart failure, your doctor may recommend one or more tests.

Your doctor also may refer you to a cardiologist. A cardiologist is a doctor who specializes in diagnosing and treating heart diseases and conditions.

Electrocardiogram

An electrocardiogram (EKG) is a simple, painless test that detects and records the heart's electrical activity. The test shows how fast your heart is beating and its rhythm (steady or irregular). An EKG also records the strength and timing of electrical signals as they pass through your heart.

An EKG may show whether the walls in your heart's pumping chambers are thicker than normal. Thicker walls can make it harder for your heart to pump blood. An EKG also can show signs of a previous or current heart attack.

Chest X-Ray

A chest X-ray takes pictures of the structures inside your chest, such as your heart, lungs, and blood vessels. This test can show whether your heart is enlarged, you have fluid in your lungs, or you have lung disease.

Brain Natriuretic Peptide Blood Test

A brain natriuretic peptide blood test checks the level of a hormone in your blood called "brain natriuretic peptide" (BNP). The level of this hormone rises during heart failure.

Echocardiography

An echocardiography (echo) uses sound waves to create a moving picture of your heart. The test shows the size and shape of your heart and how well your heart chambers and valves work.

An echo also can identify areas of poor blood flow to the heart, areas of heart muscle that are not contracting normally, and heart muscle damage caused by lack of blood flow.

An echo might be done before and after a stress test. A stress echo can show how well blood is flowing through your heart. The test also can show how well your heart pumps blood when it beats.

Doppler Ultrasound

A Doppler ultrasound uses sound waves to measure the speed and direction of blood flow. This test often is done with an echo test to give a more complete picture of blood flow to the heart and lungs.

Doctors often use Doppler ultrasound to help diagnose right-side heart failure.

Holter Monitor

A Holter monitor records your heart's electrical activity for a full 24- or 48-hour period, while you go about your normal daily routine.

You wear small patches called "electrodes" on your chest. Wires connect the patches to a small, portable recorder. The recorder can be clipped to a belt, kept in a pocket, or hung around your neck.

Nuclear Heart Scan

A nuclear heart scan shows how well blood is flowing through your heart and how much blood is reaching your heart muscle.

During a nuclear heart scan, a safe, radioactive substance called a "tracer" is injected into your bloodstream through a vein. The tracer travels to your heart and releases energy. Special cameras outside of your body detect the energy and use it to create pictures of your heart.

A nuclear heart scan can show where the heart muscle is healthy and where it is damaged.

A positron emission tomography (PET) scan is a type of nuclear heart scan. It shows the level of chemical activity in areas of your heart. This test can help your doctor see whether enough blood is flowing to these areas. A PET scan can show blood flow problems that other tests might not detect.

Cardiac Catheterization

During cardiac catheterization, a long, thin, flexible tube called a "catheter" is put into a blood vessel in your arm, groin (upper thigh), or neck and threaded to your heart. This allows your doctor to look inside your coronary (heart) arteries.

During this procedure, your doctor can check the pressure and blood flow in your heart chambers, collect blood samples, and use X-rays to look at your coronary arteries.

Coronary Angiography

Coronary angiography usually is done with cardiac catheterization. A dye that can be seen on X-ray is injected into your bloodstream through the tip of the catheter.

The dye allows your doctor to see the flow of blood to your heart muscle. Angiography also shows how well your heart is pumping.

Stress Test

Some heart problems are easier to diagnose when your heart is working hard and beating fast. During stress testing, you exercise to make your heart work hard and beat fast.

You may walk or run on a treadmill or pedal a bicycle. If you cannot exercise, you may be given medicine to raise your heart rate.

Heart tests, such as nuclear heart scanning and an echo, often are done during stress testing.

Cardiac Magnetic Resonance Imaging

Cardiac magnetic resonance imaging (MRI) uses radio waves, magnets, and a computer to create pictures of your heart as it is beating. The test produces both still and moving pictures of your heart and major blood vessels.

A cardiac MRI can show whether parts of your heart are damaged. Doctors also have used MRI in research studies to find early signs of heart failure, even before symptoms appear.

Thyroid Function Tests

Thyroid function tests show how well your thyroid gland is working. These tests include blood tests, imaging tests, and tests to stimulate the thyroid. Having too much or too little thyroid hormone in the blood can lead to heart failure.

Treatment of Heart Failure

Early diagnosis and treatment can help people who have heart failure live longer, more active lives. Treatment for heart failure depends on the type and severity of heart failure.

The goals of treatment for all stages of heart failure include:

- Treating the condition's underlying cause, such as ischemic heart disease, high blood pressure, or diabetes
- Reducing symptoms
- Stopping the heart failure from getting worse
- Increasing your lifespan and improving your quality of life (QOL)

Treatments usually include heart-healthy lifestyle changes, medicines, and ongoing care. If you have severe heart failure, you also may need medical procedures or surgery.

Heart-Healthy Lifestyle Changes

Your doctor may recommend heart-healthy lifestyle changes if you have heart failure. Heart-healthy lifestyle changes include:

- Heart-healthy eating
- Aiming for a healthy weight
- Physical activity
- Quitting smoking

Medicines

Your doctor will prescribe medicines based on the type of heart failure you have, how severe it is, and your response to certain medicines. The following medicines are commonly used to treat heart failure:

- ACE inhibitors lower blood pressure and reduce strain on your heart. They also may reduce the risk of a future heart attack.

- Aldosterone antagonists trigger the body to remove excess sodium through urine. This lowers the volume of blood that the heart must pump.

- Angiotensin receptor blockers relax your blood vessels and lower blood pressure to decrease your heart's workload.

- Beta-blockers slow your heart rate and lower your blood pressure to decrease your heart's workload.

- Digoxin makes the heart beat stronger and pump more blood.

- Diuretics (fluid pills) help reduce fluid buildup in your lungs and swelling in your feet and ankles.

- Isosorbide dinitrate/hydralazine hydrochloride helps relax your blood vessels so your heart does not work as hard to pump blood. Studies have shown that this medicine can reduce the risk of death in Black individuals. More studies are needed to find out whether this medicine will benefit other racial groups.

Take all medicines regularly, as your doctor prescribes. Do not change the amount of your medicine or skip a dose unless your doctor tells you to. You should still follow a heart-healthy lifestyle, even if you take medicines to treat your heart failure.

Ongoing Care

You should watch for signs that heart failure is getting worse. For example, weight gain may mean that fluids are building up in your body. Ask your doctor how often you should check your weight and when to report weight changes.

Getting medical care for other related conditions is important. If you have diabetes or high blood pressure, work with your healthcare team to control these conditions. Have your blood sugar level and blood pressure checked. Talk with your doctor about when you should have tests and how often to take measurements at home.

Try to avoid respiratory infections, such as the flu and pneumonia. Talk with your doctor or nurse about getting flu and pneumonia vaccines.

Many people who have severe heart failure may need treatment in a hospital from time to time. Your doctor may recommend oxygen therapy, which can be given in a hospital or at home.

Medical Procedures and Surgery

As heart failure worsens, lifestyle changes and medicines may no longer control your symptoms. You may need a medical procedure or surgery.

In heart failure, the right and left sides of the heart may no longer contract at the same time. This disrupts the heart's pumping. To correct this problem, your doctor might implant a cardiac resynchronization therapy (CRT) device (a type of pacemaker) near your heart. This device helps both sides of your heart contract at the same time, which can decrease heart failure symptoms.

Some people who have heart failure have very rapid, irregular heartbeats. Without treatment, these heartbeats can cause sudden cardiac arrest (SCA). Your doctor might implant an implantable cardioverter defibrillator (ICD) near your heart to solve this problem. An ICD checks your heart rate and uses electrical pulses to correct irregular heart rhythms.

People who have severe heart failure symptoms at rest, despite other treatments, may need:

- A mechanical heart pump, such as a left ventricular assist device. This device helps pump blood from the heart to the rest of the body. You may use a heart pump until you have surgery or as a long-term treatment.

- Heart transplant. A heart transplant is an operation in which a person's diseased heart is replaced with a healthy heart from a deceased donor. Heart transplants are done as a life-saving measure for end-stage heart failure when medical treatment and less drastic surgery have failed.

Living with Heart Failure

Currently, heart failure has no cure. You will likely have to take medicine and follow a treatment plan for the rest of your life.

Despite treatment, symptoms may get worse over time. You may not be able to do many of the things that you did before you had heart failure. However, if you take all the steps your doctor recommends, you can stay healthier longer.

Follow Your Treatment Plan

Treatment can relieve your symptoms and make daily activities easier. It also can reduce the chance that you will have to go to the hospital. Thus, it is important that you follow your treatment plan.

- Take your medicines as your doctor prescribes. If you have side effects from any of your medicines, tell your doctor. She or he might adjust the dose or type of medicine you take to relieve side effects.

- Make all of the lifestyle changes that your doctor recommends.

- Get advice from your doctor about how active you can and should be. This includes advice on daily activities, work, leisure time, sex, and exercise. Your level of activity will depend on the stage of your heart failure (how severe it is).

- Keep all of your medical appointments, including visits to the doctor and appointments to get tests and lab work. Your doctor needs the results of these tests to adjust your medicine doses and help you avoid harmful side effects.

Take Steps to Prevent Heart Failure from Getting Worse

Certain actions can worsen your heart failure, such as:

- Forgetting to take your medicines

- Not following your diet (for example, eating salty foods)

- Drinking alcohol

These actions can lead to a hospital stay. If you have trouble following your diet, talk with your doctor. She or he can help arrange for a dietitian to work with you. Avoid drinking alcohol.

People who have heart failure often have other serious conditions that require ongoing treatment. If you have other serious conditions, you are likely taking medicines for them as well as for heart failure.

Taking more than one medicine raises the risk of side effects and other problems. Make sure your doctors and your pharmacist have a complete list of all of the medicines and over-the-counter (OTC) products that you are taking.

Tell your doctor right away about any problems with your medicines. Also, talk with your doctor before taking any new medicine prescribed by another doctor or any new OTC medicines or herbal supplements.

Plan Ahead

If you have heart failure, it is important to know:

- When to seek help. Ask your doctor when to make an office visit or get emergency care.

- Phone numbers for your doctor and hospital

- Directions to your doctor's office and hospital and people who can take you there

- All of medicines you are taking

Emotional Issues and Support

Living with heart failure may cause fear, anxiety, depression, and stress. Talk about how you feel with your healthcare team. Talking to a professional counselor also can help. If you are very depressed, your doctor may recommend medicines or other treatments that can improve your QOL.

Joining a patient support group may help you adjust to living with heart failure. You can see how other people who have the same symptoms have coped with them. Talk with your doctor about local support groups or check with an area medical center.

Support from family and friends also can help relieve stress and anxiety. Let your loved ones know how you feel and what they can do to help you.

Chapter 17

Arrhythmias

Chapter Contents

Section 17.1

What Is an Arrhythmia?

This section includes text excerpted from
"Arrhythmia," National Heart, Lung, and Blood
Institute (NHLBI), March 15, 2019.

An arrhythmia is a problem with the rate or rhythm of the heartbeat. During an arrhythmia, the heart can beat too fast, too slowly, or with an irregular rhythm. When a heart beats too fast, the condition is called "tachycardia." When a heart beats too slowly, the condition is called "bradycardia."

Arrhythmia is caused by changes in heart tissue and activity or in the electrical signals that control your heartbeat. These changes can be caused by damage from disease, injury, or genetics. Often there are no symptoms, but some people feel an irregular heartbeat. You may feel faint or dizzy or have difficulty breathing.

The most common test used to diagnose an arrhythmia is an electrocardiogram (EKG or ECG). Your doctor will run other tests as needed. She or he may recommend medicines, the placement of a device that can correct an irregular heartbeat, or surgery to repair nerves that are overstimulating the heart. If arrhythmia is left untreated, the heart may not be able to pump enough blood to the body. This can damage the heart, the brain, or other organs.

Types of Arrhythmias

Arrhythmias differ from normal heartbeats in speed or rhythm. Arrhythmias are also grouped by where they occur—in the upper chambers of the heart, in its lower chambers, or between the chambers. The main types of arrhythmia are bradyarrhythmias; premature, or extra, beats; supraventricular arrhythmias; and ventricular arrhythmias.

Bradyarrhythmia

Bradyarrhythmia is a slow arrhythmia in a heart that beats too slowly—a condition called "bradycardia." For adults, this means slower than 60 beats per minute. Some people, especially people who are young or physically fit, may normally have slow heart rates. For them, bradycardia is not dangerous and does not cause symptoms.

Premature or Extra Heartbeat

A premature heartbeat happens when the signal to beat comes early. It can feel like your heart skipped a beat. The premature, or extra, heartbeat creates a short pause, which is followed by a stronger beat when your heart returns to its regular rhythm. These extra heartbeats are the most common type of arrhythmia. They are called "ectopic heartbeats" and can trigger other arrhythmias.

Supraventricular Arrhythmia

Arrhythmias that start in the heart's upper chambers, called the "atrium," or at the gateway to the lower chambers are called "supraventricular arrhythmias." Supraventricular arrhythmias are known by their fast heart rates, or tachycardia. Tachycardia occurs when the heart, at rest, goes above 100 beats per minute. The fast pace is sometimes paired with an uneven heart rhythm. Sometimes, the upper and lower chambers beat at different rates.

Types of supraventricular arrhythmias include:

- **Atrial fibrillation (AF).** This is one of the most common types of arrhythmia. The heart can race at more than 400 beats per minute.

- **Atrial flutter (AFL).** Atrial flutter can cause the upper chambers to beat 250 to 350 times per minute. The signal that tells the upper chambers to beat may be disrupted when it encounters damaged tissue, such as a scar. The signal may find an alternate path, creating a loop that causes the upper chamber to beat repeatedly. As with atrial fibrillation, some but not all of these signals travel to the lower chambers. As a result, the upper chambers and lower chambers beat at different rates.

- **Paroxysmal supraventricular tachycardia (PSVT).** In PSVT, electrical signals that begin in the upper chambers and travel to the lower chambers cause extra heartbeats. This arrhythmia begins and ends suddenly. It can happen during vigorous physical activity. It is usually not dangerous and tends to occur in young people.

Ventricular Arrhythmia

These arrhythmias start in the heart's lower chambers. They can be very dangerous and usually require medical care right away.

Ventricular tachycardia (VT) is a fast, regular beating of the ventricles that may last for only a few seconds or for much longer. A few beats of VT often do not cause problems. However, episodes that last for more than a few seconds can be dangerous. VT can turn into other more serious arrhythmias, such as ventricular fibrillation, or v-fib.

V-fib occurs if disorganized electrical signals make the ventricles quiver instead of pumping normally. Without the ventricles pumping blood to the body, sudden cardiac arrest (SCA) and death can occur within a few minutes. Torsades de pointes is a type of arrhythmia that causes a unique pattern on an EKG and often leads to v-fib.

What Causes Arrhythmia

Arrhythmia is caused by changes to heart tissue. It can also occur suddenly as a result of exertion or stress, imbalances in the blood, medicines, or problems with electrical signals in the heart. Typically, an arrhythmia is set off by a trigger, and the irregular heartbeat can continue if there is a problem in the heart. Sometimes, the cause of an arrhythmia is unknown.

Changes to the Heart

The following conditions may cause arrhythmia:

- Changes to the heart's anatomy
- Reduced blood flow to the heart or damage to the heart's electrical system
- Restoring blood flow as part of treating a heart attack
- Stiffening of the heart tissue, known as "fibrosis," or "scarring"

Exertion or Strain

Strong emotional stress, anxiety, anger, pain, or a sudden surprise can make the heart work harder, raise blood pressure, and release stress hormones. Sometimes these reactions can lead to arrhythmias. If you have heart disease, physical activity can trigger arrhythmia due to an excess of hormones such as adrenaline. Sometimes vomiting or coughing can trigger arrhythmia.

Imbalances in the Blood

An excess or deficiency of electrolytes, hormones, or fluids can alter your heartbeat.

- An excess of thyroid hormone can cause the heart to beat faster, and thyroid deficiency can slow your heart rate.

- Dehydration can cause the heart to race.

- Low blood sugar, from an eating disorder or higher insulin levels in someone who has diabetes, can lead to slow or extra heartbeats.

- Low levels of potassium, magnesium, or calcium can trigger arrhythmia. These electrolyte disturbances can occur after a heart attack or surgery.

Medicines

Certain medicines can cause arrhythmia. These include medicines to treat high blood pressure (HBP) and other conditions, including arrhythmia, depression, and psychosis. Some people also need to be careful about taking certain antibiotics and over-the-counter (OTC) medicines, such as allergy and cold medicines.

Problems with the Electrical Signals in the Heart

An arrhythmia can occur if the electrical signals that control the heartbeat are delayed or blocked. This can happen when the nerve cells that produce electrical signals do not work properly or when the electrical signals do not travel normally through the heart. Another part of the heart could start to produce electrical signals, disrupting a normal heartbeat.

Disorders of electrical signaling in the heart are called "conduction disorders."

Risk Factors for Arrhythmia

You may have an increased risk of arrhythmia because of your age, environment, family history and genetics, habits in your daily life, certain medical conditions, race or ethnicity, sex, or surgery.

Age

The chances of having arrhythmia grow as we age, in part because of changes in heart tissue and in how the heart works over time. Older people are also more likely to have health conditions, including heart disease, that raise the risk of arrhythmia.

Some types of arrhythmia happen more often in children and young adults, including arrhythmias due to congenital heart defects (CHD) or inherited conduction disorders.

Environment

Some research suggests that exposure to air pollutants, especially particulates and gases, is linked to a short-term risk of arrhythmia.

Family History and Genetics

You may have an increased risk of some types of arrhythmia if your parent or other close relative has had arrhythmia too. Also, some inherited types of heart disease can raise your risk of arrhythmia. With some conduction disorders, gene mutations cause the ion channels that transmit signals through heart cells to work incorrectly or stop working.

Lifestyle Habits

Your risk for arrhythmia may be higher because of certain lifestyle habits, including:

- Drinking alcohol

- Smoking

- Using illegal drugs, such as cocaine or amphetamines

Other Medical Conditions

Arrhythmias are more common in people who have diseases or conditions that weaken the heart, but many conditions can raise the risk for arrhythmia. These include:

- Aneurysms

- Autoimmune disorders, such as rheumatoid arthritis (RA) and lupus

- Diabetes, which increases the risk of high blood pressure and coronary heart disease (CHD)

- Diseases of the heart and blood vessels, including a heart that is larger than normal and heart inflammation

- Eating disorders, such as bulimia and anorexia, which cause electrolyte imbalance and severe malnutrition

- Heart attack

- Heart failure, which weakens the heart and changes the way electrical signals move through the heart

- Heart tissue that is too thick or stiff or that has not formed normally. Arrhythmias can be more common among people who have had surgery to repair a congenital heart defect.

- High blood pressure

- Influenza, or flu

- Kidney disease

- Heart valves. Leaking or narrowed heart valves make the heart work too hard and can lead to heart failure.

- Low blood sugar

- Lung diseases, such as chronic obstructive pulmonary disease (COPD)

- Musculoskeletal disorders (MSD)

- Obesity

- Overactive or underactive thyroid gland, caused by too much or too little thyroid hormone in the body. The most common cause of excess thyroid hormone is Graves' disease.

- Sepsis, a toxic immune response to infection

- Sleep apnea, which can stress the heart by preventing it from getting enough oxygen

Race or Ethnicity

Studies suggest that White Americans may be more likely than African Americans to have some arrhythmias, such as atrial fibrillation (AF); although, African Americans have higher rates of high blood pressure and other arrhythmia risk factors.

Sex

Some studies suggest that men are more likely to have AF than women. However, women taking certain medicines appear to be at a higher risk of a certain type of arrhythmia. Certain times of the menstrual cycle also appear to increase women's risk of some arrhythmia events. If you are a pregnant woman, you may notice that an existing arrhythmia occurs more often. Benign extra beats are also more common during pregnancy. In some cases, the complications that can develop with arrhythmia also differ by sex.

Surgery

You may be at a higher risk of developing atrial flutter in the early days and weeks after surgery involving the heart, lungs, or esophagus.

Screening and Prevention of Arrhythmia

If you or your child is at increased risk of arrhythmia, the doctor may want to do a screening to assess the risk of a life-threatening event. Sometimes, screening is required to participate in competitive sports. If your child carries a genetic risk of arrhythmia, your child's doctor may recommend regular screening to monitor your child's heart or other family members' health. The doctor may also ask about risk factors and may suggest genetic testing if your child, parent, or other family member has a known or suspected arrhythmia or other heart condition. Heart-healthy lifestyle changes and other precautions can help decrease the risk of triggering arrhythmia.

Screening Tests

Your doctor may recommend screening tests based on your risk factors, such as age or family history.

- **An electrocardiogram (EKG or ECG)** is the main test for detecting arrhythmia. An EKG records the heart's electrical activity. Your doctor may do the test while you are at rest or may do a stress test, which records the heart's activity when it is working hard. Your doctor may also give you a portable monitor to wear for a day or several days if no arrhythmia was detected during testing in the clinic. If you have a child who is at risk of arrhythmia because of a genetic condition, the doctor may recommend regular testing for your child and her or his siblings.

- **Genetic testing** can help you understand your risk when a family member has been diagnosed with a genetic condition. Testing is especially important if your newborn or another close relative died suddenly and had a genetic risk. Your doctor may also suggest genetic testing if you have a history of fainting or have survived cardiac arrest or near drowning.

- **Imaging tests,** such as cardiac magnetic resonance imaging (MRI), can help detect scarring or other problems that can increase your risk of arrhythmia.

Prevention Strategies

Prevention strategies that your doctor may recommend, including:

- **Avoiding triggers,** such as caffeine or stimulant medicines, that can cause arrhythmias or make them worse. Your doctor can also help if you are trying to avoid illegal drugs.

- **Getting an implantable or wearable cardioverter defibrillator (ICD)** to prevent SCA from arrhythmia if you have heart disease. Defibrillators can correct arrhythmias by sending an electric shock to the heart.

- **Making heart-healthy lifestyle changes**, such as heart-healthy eating, being physically active, aiming for a healthy weight, quitting smoking, and managing stress

- **Monitoring you after surgery,** if you are having heart surgery. The surgical team may also use medicine and maintain or supplement electrolyte levels during or after the procedure to prevent arrhythmia.

If you are the parents of a child with an inherited condition that increases the risk of arrhythmia, discuss prevention strategies with your pediatrician as part of your child's care.

- If your child is a newborn, follow safe sleep recommendations to help reduce the risk of sudden infant death syndrome (SIDS).

- Your doctor may recommend routine assessments of your child's heart activity to detect patterns or symptoms of arrhythmia that emerge over time.

Signs, Symptoms, and Complications of Arrhythmia

An arrhythmia may not cause any obvious signs or symptoms. You may notice something that occurs only occasionally, or your symptoms may become more frequent over time. Keep track of when and how often arrhythmia occurs, what you feel, and whether these things change over time. They are all important clues your doctor can use. If left untreated, arrhythmia can lead to life-threatening complications, such as stroke, heart failure, or SCA.

Signs and Symptoms

You may be able to feel a slow or irregular heartbeat, or you may notice pauses between heartbeats. If you have palpitations, you may feel as if your heart skipped a beat or may notice it pounding or racing. These are all symptoms of arrhythmia.

More serious signs and symptoms include:

- Anxiety

- Blurred vision

- Chest pain

- Difficulty breathing

- Fainting or nearly fainting

- Foggy thinking

- Fatigue

- Sweating

- Weakness, dizziness, and light-headedness

Complications

Arrhythmias that are unrecognized or left untreated can cause sometimes life-threatening complications affecting the heart and brain.

- **Cognitive impairment and dementia.** Alzheimer disease (AD) and vascular dementia are more common in people who have arrhythmia. This may be due to reduced blood flow to the brain over time.

- **Heart failure.** Repeat arrhythmias can lead to a rapid decline in the ability of the lower chambers to pump blood. Heart failure is especially likely to develop or to grow worse as a result of arrhythmia when you already have heart disease.

- **Stroke**. This can occur in some patients who have AF. With arrhythmia, blood can pool in the atria, causing blood clots to form. If a clot breaks off and travels to the brain, it can cause a stroke.

- **Sudden cardiac arrest**. The heart may suddenly and unexpectedly stop beating as a result of ventricular fibrillation.

- **Sudden infant death syndrome.** SIDS can be attributed to an inherited conduction disorder that causes arrhythmia.

- **Worsening arrhythmia.** Some arrhythmias trigger another type of arrhythmia or get worse over time.

Diagnosis of Arrhythmia

To diagnose arrhythmia, your doctor will ask you about your symptoms, your medical history, and any signs of arrhythmia in your family. Your doctor may also do an EKG and a physical exam as part of your diagnosis. Additional tests may be necessary to rule out another cause or to help your doctor decide on treatment.

Medical History

To diagnose an arrhythmia, your doctor will ask about your eating and physical activity habits, family history, and other risk factors for arrhythmia. Your doctor may ask whether you have any other signs or symptoms. This information can help your doctor determine whether you have complications or other conditions that may be causing you to have arrhythmia.

Physical Exam

During a physical exam, your doctor may take these steps:

- Check for swelling in your legs or feet, which could be a sign of an enlarged heart or heart failure
- Check your pulse to find out how fast your heart is beating.
- Listen to the rate and rhythm of your heartbeat.
- Listen to your heart for a heart murmur.
- Look for signs of other diseases, such as thyroid disease, that could be causing the arrhythmia.

Diagnostic Tests and Procedures

Your doctor may order some of the following tests to diagnose arrhythmia:

- **Blood tests** to check the level of certain substances in the blood, such as potassium and thyroid hormone, that can increase your risk of arrhythmia
- **Cardiac catheterization** to see whether you have complications from heart disease

- **Chest X-ray** to show whether your heart is larger than normal

- **Echocardiography (echo)** to provide information about the size and shape of your heart and how well it is working. Echocardiography may also be used to diagnose fetal arrhythmia in the womb.

- **EKG, or ECG,** to see how fast the heart is beating and whether its rhythm is steady or irregular. This is the most common test used to diagnose arrhythmias.

- **Electrophysiology study (EPS):** to look at the electrical activity of the heart. The study uses a wire to electrically stimulate your heart and trigger an arrhythmia. If your doctor has already detected another condition that raises your risk, an EPS can help her or him assess the possibility that an arrhythmia will develop. An EPS also allows your doctor to see whether a treatment, such as medicine, will stop the problem.

- **Holter or event monitor** to record your heart's electrical activity over long periods of time while you do your normal activities

- **Implantable loop recorder** to detect abnormal heart rhythms. It is placed under the skin and continuously records your heart's electrical activity. The recorder can transmit data to the doctor's office to help with monitoring. An implantable loop recorder helps doctors figure out why a person may be having palpitations or fainting spells, especially if these symptoms do not happen very often.

- **Sleep study** to see whether sleep apnea is causing your arrhythmia

- **Stress test or exercise stress** test to detect arrhythmias that happen while the heart is working hard and beating fast. If you cannot exercise, you may be given medicine to make your heart work hard and beat fast.

- **Tilt table testing** to help find the cause of fainting spells. You lie on a table that moves from a lying-down position to an upright position. The change in position may cause you to faint. Your doctor watches your symptoms, heart rate, EKG reading, and blood pressure throughout the test.

- **Ultrasound** to diagnose a suspected fetal arrhythmia in the womb

Treatment of Arrhythmia

Common arrhythmia treatments include heart-healthy lifestyle changes, medicines, surgically implanted devices that control the heartbeat, and other procedures that treat abnormal electrical signals in the heart.

Healthy Lifestyle Changes

Your doctor may recommend that you adopt the following lifelong heart-healthy lifestyle changes to help lower your risk for conditions, such as high blood pressure and heart disease, which can lead to arrhythmia.

- Aiming for a healthy weight

- Being physically active

- Heart-healthy eating

- Managing stress

- Quitting smoking

Medicines

Your doctor may give you medicine for your arrhythmia. Some medicines are used in combination with each other or together with a procedure or a pacemaker. If the dose is too high, medicines to treat arrhythmia can cause an irregular rhythm. This happens more often in women.

- **Adenosine** to slow a racing heart. Adenosine acts quickly to slow electrical signals. It can cause some chest pain, flushing, and shortness of breath, but any discomfort typically passes soon.

- **Atropine** to treat a slow heart rate. This medicine may cause difficulty swallowing.

- **Beta-blockers** to treat high blood pressure or a fast heart rate or to prevent repeat episodes of arrhythmia. Beta-blockers can cause digestive trouble, sleep problems, and sexual dysfunction and can make some conduction disorders worse.

- **Blood thinners** to reduce the risk of blood clots forming. This helps prevent stroke. With blood-thinning medicines, there is a risk of bleeding.

- **Calcium channel blockers** to slow a rapid heart rate or the speed at which signals travel. Typically, they are used to control arrhythmias of the upper chambers. In some cases, calcium channel blockers can trigger ventricular fibrillation. They can also cause digestive trouble, swollen feet, or low blood pressure.

- **Digitalis, or digoxin**, to treat a fast heart rate. This medicine can cause nausea and may trigger arrhythmias.

- **Potassium channel blockers** to slow the heart rate. They work by lengthening the time it takes for heart cells to recover after firing, so that they do not fire and squeeze as often. Potassium channel blockers can cause low blood pressure or another arrhythmia.

- **Sodium channel blockers** to block transmission of electrical signals, lengthen cell recovery periods, and make cells less excitable. However, these drugs can increase risks of SCA in people who have heart disease.

Procedures

If medicines do not treat your arrhythmia, your doctor may recommend one of these procedures or devices.

- Cardioversion

- Catheter ablation

- Implantable cardioverter defibrillators

- Pacemakers

Other Treatments

Treatment may also include managing any underlying condition, such as an electrolyte imbalance, high blood pressure, heart disease, sleep apnea, or thyroid disease.

Your doctor may use supplements to treat magnesium or electrolyte deficiencies. Electrolytes can also be an alternative to medicines that treat arrhythmia if your doctor is concerned that those medicines might trigger an arrhythmia.

Your doctor may also perform certain techniques to slow your heart rate. The exercises stimulate your body's natural relaxation processes. They do this by affecting the vagus nerve, which helps control the heart rate. Techniques can include:

- Having you cough or gag

- Having you hold your breath and bear down, which is called the "Valsalva maneuver" (VM)

- Having you lie down

- Putting a towel dipped in ice-cold water over your face

Living with Arrhythmias

If you have been diagnosed and treated for arrhythmia, make sure to follow your treatment plan. Your ongoing care may focus on reducing the chance that you will have another episode or a complication. Keep your regular appointments with your doctor. Ask about heart-healthy lifestyle changes that you can make to keep your arrhythmia from happening again or getting worse.

Receive Routine Follow-Up Care

How often you need to see your doctor for follow-up care will depend on your symptoms and treatment.

- **Get regular vaccinations**, including a flu shot every year.

- **Follow your doctor's recommendations** for adopting lifelong lifestyle changes, such as heart-healthy eating, being physically active, quitting smoking, managing stress, and aiming for a healthy weight. Your doctor may also recommend that you reduce or stop drinking alcohol and consuming coffee, tea, soda, chocolate, or other sources of caffeine, to avoid triggering arrhythmia.

- **Keep all of your medical appointments**. Bring a list of all the medicines you take to every doctor and emergency room visit. This will help your doctors know exactly what medicines you are taking, which can help prevent medicine errors.

- **See your doctor for regular checkups** if you are taking blood-thinning medicines. Your doctor may recommend blood thinners to prevent stroke, even if your heart rhythm has returned to normal. You may need routine blood tests to check how the medicines are working or the effect they are having on your organs.

- **Take your medicines as prescribed.** Your doctor may also ask you to check your pulse regularly to monitor the effectiveness of the medicines.

- **Tell your doctor if you have side effects from your medicines,** such as depression, light-headedness, or palpitations. Some of the medicines can cause low blood pressure or a slow heart rate or can make heart failure worse.

- **Tell your doctor if your symptoms are getting worse or if you have new symptoms.** Over time, arrhythmias can become more common, last longer, or get worse. This can sometimes make arrhythmia resistant to medicines. Some arrhythmias can also make it more likely for other types of arrhythmia to develop.

Monitor Your Condition

To monitor your condition, your doctor may recommend the following tests.

- **Blood tests** to check the effects of medicines you are taking

- **Echocardiography (echo)** to check your heart function if you have underlying heart disease

- **EKGs** to monitor changes in heart rhythm

- **Holter or event monitors** to record your heart's electrical activity over several days

- **Smartphone-based monitors** to record heart rhythms and detect when atrial fibrillation occurs. A band that can record a 30-second EKG has been approved by the U.S. Food and Drug Administration (FDA.)

Learn the Warning Signs of Serious Complications and Have a Plan

Arrhythmia can lead to serious complications, such as SCA and severe bleeding in the brain. If you suspect any of the following in yourself or someone else, call 911 immediately:

- **Bleeding in the brain or digestive system.** If you take too high a dose of blood-thinning medicines, it may cause bleeding in the brain or digestive system. Signs and symptoms may include bright red vomit; bright red blood in your stool or black, tarry stools; severe pain in the abdomen or head; sudden, severe changes in your vision or ability to move your arms or legs; or memory loss. A lot of bleeding after a fall or injury or easy bruising or bleeding may mean that your blood is too thin. Excessive bleeding is bleeding that will not stop after you apply pressure to a wound for 10 minutes. Call your doctor right away if you have any of these signs.

- **Heart attack.** Signs of heart attack include mild or severe chest pain or discomfort in the center of the chest or upper abdomen that lasts for more than a few minutes or goes away and comes back. It can feel like pressure, squeezing, fullness, heartburn, or indigestion. There may also be pain down the left arm. Women may also have chest pain and pain down the left arm, but they are more likely to have other symptoms, such as shortness of breath, nausea, vomiting, unusual tiredness, and pain in the back, shoulders, or jaw.

- **Stroke.** If you think someone may be having a stroke, act F.A.S.T. and do the following simple test.

    F—Face: Ask the person to smile. Does one side of the face droop?

    A—Arms: Ask the person to raise both arms. Does one arm drift downward?

    S—Speech: Ask the person to repeat a simple phrase. Is their speech slurred or strange?

    T—Time: If you observe any of these signs, call 911 immediately. Every minute matters.

- **Sudden cardiac arrest.** Usually, the first sign of SCA is fainting. At the same time, no heartbeat can be felt. Some people may have a racing heartbeat or feel dizzy or light-headed just before they faint. Within an hour before cardiac arrest, some people experience chest pain, shortness of breath, nausea, or vomiting. Call 911 right away if someone has signs or symptoms of SCA. Look for a defibrillator nearby and follow the instructions.

Learn about Other Precautions to Help You Stay Safe

If you have arrhythmia, you will need to learn ways to care for your condition at home. You will also need to avoid activities that may trigger your arrhythmia.

- **Ask your doctor whether you can continue your daily activities** without any changes. Your doctor may recommend low or moderate activity; avoiding competitive sports;

175

eliminating activities that might trigger an arrhythmia, such as swimming or diving; or participating in activities with a partner.

- **Carry a medical device ID card** with information about your defibrillator or pacemaker and contact information for the healthcare provider who oversees your care. Medical bracelets with information about your condition can also be helpful in the event of an emergency.

- **Check with your doctor before taking over-the-counter medicines, nutritional supplements, or cold and allergy medicines.** Some of these products can trigger rapid heart rhythms or interact poorly with heart rhythm medicines.

- **Learn how to take your pulse.** Discuss with your doctor what pulse rate is normal for you. Keep a record of changes in your pulse rate, and share this information with your doctor.

- **Lie down** if you feel dizzy or faint or if you feel palpitations. Do not try to walk or drive. Let your doctor know about these symptoms.

- **Talk to your doctor about techniques that you can do at home** if you notice your heart racing. These include breathing out without letting your breath escape or putting a cold, wet towel over your face.

Section 17.2

Atrial Fibrillation

This section includes text excerpted from "Atrial Fibrillation," National Heart, Lung, and Blood Institute (NHLBI), March 15, 2019.

What Is Atrial Fibrillation?

Atrial fibrillation (AF) is one of the most common types of arrhythmias, which are irregular heart rhythms. AF causes the heart to beat much faster than normal, and the upper and lower chambers of the heart do not work together. When this happens, the lower chambers do not fill completely or pump enough blood to the lungs and body. This can make you feel tired or dizzy, or you may notice heart palpitations or chest pain. Blood also pools in the heart, which increases your risk of having a stroke or other complications. AF can also occur without any signs or symptoms. Untreated fibrillation can lead to serious and even life-threatening complications.

Sometimes, atrial fibrillation goes away on its own. For some people, atrial fibrillation is an ongoing heart problem that lasts for years. Over time, it may happen more often and last longer. Treatment restores normal heart rhythms, helps control symptoms, and prevents complications. Your doctor may recommend medicines, medical procedures, and lifestyle changes to treat your AF.

Types of Atrial Fibrillation

Atrial fibrillation is a type of arrhythmia. There are four main types of AF—paroxysmal, persistent, long-term persistent, and permanent atrial fibrillation. The type of AF that you have depends on how often AF occurs and how it responds to treatment.

Paroxysmal Atrial Fibrillation

You may experience a brief event—a paroxysm—of AF. It may pass without symptoms, or you may feel it strongly. It usually stops in less than 24 hours, but it may last up to a week. Paroxysmal atrial fibrillation (PAF) can happen repeatedly.

You may need treatment, or your symptoms may go away on their own. When this kind of AF alternates with a heartbeat that is slower than normal, it is called "tachy-brady syndrome."

Persistent Atrial Fibrillation

Persistent atrial fibrillation is a condition in which the abnormal heart rhythm lasts for more than a week. It may ultimately stop on its own but probably will need treatment.

Long-Term Persistent Atrial Fibrillation

With this condition, the abnormal heart rhythms last for more than a year without going away.

Permanent Atrial Fibrillation

Sometimes atrial fibrillation does not get better, even when you have tried several times to restore a normal heart rhythm with other medicines or other treatments. At this point, your AF is considered permanent.

Causes of Atrial Fibrillation

Changes to the heart's tissue and its electrical signals most often cause AF. To understand AF, it helps to know how the heart works. When the heart's tissue or signaling is damaged, the regular pumping of the heart muscle becomes fast and irregular. Most often, damage to the heart is the result of other conditions, such as high blood pressure and ischemic heart disease. Other factors can also raise your risk of AF.

Changes in Heart Tissue

Usually, the cells of the heart fire and contract together. However, when aging, heart disease, infection, genetics, or other factors change heart tissue, that pattern breaks down. This can happen because of fibrosis, inflammation, a thinning or thickening of the heart walls, lack of blood flow to the heart, or an abnormal buildup of proteins, cells, or minerals in heart tissue.

Changes in Electrical Signaling

Usually, a trigger heartbeat sets off AF. Electrical signals from this trigger may then cause the heart to beat slower or faster than usual because of changes in heart tissue. Sometimes, the signals create an atypical loop, telling the heart to contract over and over. This can create the fast, chaotic beating that defines AF.

Variations in the heart's electrical signaling can be due to differences in heart anatomy, premature or extra heartbeats, normal heart rate adjustments, patches of faster or slower tissue, and repeated stimulation of certain tissue patches.

Risk Factors for Atrial Fibrillation

Age, family history and genetics, lifestyle, heart disease or other medical conditions, race, sex, and a history of surgery can all raise your risk of developing the structural and electrical anomalies that cause AF. Even in a healthy heart, a fast or slow heart rate—from exercising or sleeping, for example—can trigger atrial fibrillation.

Age

The risk of atrial fibrillation increases as you age, especially after the age of 65. AF is rare in children, but it does occur, especially in boys and in children who are obese.

Family History and Genetics

If someone in your family has had AF, you have a higher risk of developing AF too. Scientists have found some genes with mutations that raise the risk of AF. Some of these genes influence fetal organ development or heart cell ion channels. Sometimes, these genetic patterns are also linked to heart disease. Some genetic factors may raise the risk of AF in combination with such factors as age, weight, or sex.

Lifestyle Habits

Some lifestyle habits can raise or lower your risk of AF, including the following:

- **Alcohol.** Drinking large amounts of alcohol, especially binge drinking, raises your risk of AF. Even modest amounts of alcohol can trigger AF in some people.

- **Illegal drugs.** Some street drugs, such as cocaine, can trigger AF or make it worse.

- **Physical activity.** Some competitive athletes and people—men, in particular—participating in endurance sports or exerting themselves at work may have a higher risk of AF. At the same time, moderate physical activity can have a protective effect. Physical fitness appears to be linked to a lower risk of AF.

- **Smoking.** Studies have found that smoking increases the risk of AF. The risk appears to be higher the longer you smoke and decreases if you quit. Exposure to secondhand smoke, even in the womb, can increase a child's risk of developing AF.

- **Stress.** Stressful situations, panic disorders, and other types of emotional stress may be linked to a higher risk of AF.

Other Medical Conditions

Many other medical conditions can increase your risk of AF, especially heart problems. As you age, having more than one condition may increase your risk. Conditions that raise the risk of AF include:

- Chronic kidney disease (CKD)

- Conduction disorders

- Congenital heart defect (CHD)

- Diabetes

- Heart attack

- Heart failure

- Heart inflammation

- Heart tissue that is too thick or stiff

- Heart valve disease

- High blood pressure

- Hyperthyroidism, an overactive thyroid gland

- Ischemic heart disease

- Lung diseases, including chronic obstructive pulmonary disease (COPD)

- Obesity

- Sarcoidosis

- Sleep apnea

- Venous thromboembolism (VTE)

Race or Ethnicity

In the United States, AF is more common among Whites than among African Americans, Hispanic Americans, or Asian Americans. Although people of European ancestry are more likely to develop the condition, African Americans with AF are more likely to have complications, such as stroke, heart failure, or ischemic heart disease.

Surgery

You may be at risk for AF in the early days and weeks after surgery of the heart, lungs, or esophagus. Surgery to correct a congenital heart defect can also raise the risk of AF. This can happen years after a childhood surgery or when you have surgery as an adult to correct a lifelong condition.

Screening and Prevention of Atrial Fibrillation

Typically, doctors screen for AF only when you have symptoms. However, your doctor may check for signs of AF as part of your regular medical care. Screening tests include checking your pulse or recording your heart's electrical activity. Your doctor may recommend healthy lifestyle changes to help you lower your risk of developing AF.

Screening Tests and Results

Screening may be part of your regular care if you are 65 years of age or older or if you have other risk factors.

- Your doctor may check your pulse. Even without symptoms, your heart may have an irregular speed or faulty rhythm that your doctor can detect.
- If you have had a stroke and there is no clear cause, your doctor may recommend screening for AF with a Holter or event monitor.
- Several devices are now available to detect and record your heart's rhythm similar to an electrocardiogram (EKG). These devices may also email the data to your doctor.

Prevention Strategies

To help you lower your risk of AF, your doctor may recommend certain heart-healthy lifestyle changes, including aiming for a healthy weight, being physically active, controlling your blood sugar, limiting alcohol, lowering your blood pressure, managing stress, and quitting smoking.

In addition, some illegal drugs, such as cocaine, can trigger AF or make it worse. Ask your doctor for help avoiding these triggers to prevent arrhythmia.

If you are having heart surgery, your medical team will monitor you. To prevent arrhythmia, your doctor may recommend antiarrhythmic medicine or treatment to maintain or supplement electrolyte levels during or after the procedure.

Signs, Symptoms, and Complications of Atrial Fibrillation

You may or may not notice AF. It often occurs with no signs or symptoms. If you do have symptoms, you may notice something that occurs only occasionally. Or, your symptoms may be frequent or serious. If you have heart disease that is worsening, you may notice more symptoms of AF. If your atrial fibrillation is undetected or left untreated, serious and even life-threatening complications can arise. They include stroke and heart failure.

Signs and Symptoms

The most common symptom of AF is fatigue. Other signs and symptoms include:

- Heart palpitations

- Difficulty breathing, especially when lying down

- Chest pain

- Hypotension, or low blood pressure

- Dizziness or fainting

Keep track of when and how often your symptoms occur, what you feel, and whether these things change over time. They are all important clues for your doctor.

Complications

When it is undetected or untreated, AF can lead to serious complications. This is especially significant for African Americans. Even though White individuals have AF at higher rates, research has found that many of its complications—including stroke, heart disease, and heart failure—are more common among African Americans. Some complications of AF include:

- **Blood clots.** With AF, the heart may not be able to pump the blood out properly, causing it to pool and form an abnormal blood clot in the heart. A piece of the clot—a type of embolus— can break off and travel through the blood to different parts of the body, blocking blood flow to the brain, lungs, intestine, spleen, or kidneys. AF may also increase the risk of venous thromboembolism (VTE), which is a blood clot that forms in a vein.

- **Cognitive impairment and dementia.** Some studies suggest that impaired cognition, Alzheimer disease (AD), and vascular dementia occur more often among people with AF. This may be due to blockages in the blood vessels of the brain or reduced blood flow to the brain.

- **Heart attack.** The risk of a heart attack from AF is highest among women and African Americans and especially in the first year after AF is diagnosed.

- **Heart failure.** AF raises your risk of heart failure because the heart is beating fast and unevenly. The heart's chambers do not fill completely with blood and cannot pump enough blood to the lungs and body. AF may also make your heart failure symptoms worse.

- **Stroke.** If an embolus travels to the brain, it can cause a stroke. For some people, AF has no symptoms, and a stroke is the first sign of the condition. If you have AF, the risk of a stroke is higher if you are a woman.

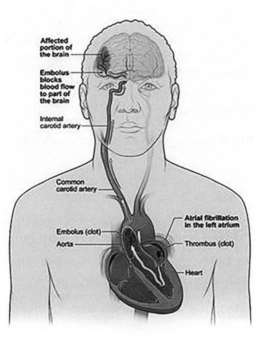

Figure 17.1. *Atrial Fibrillation and Stroke*

The illustration shows how a stroke can occur during atrial fibrillation (AF). A blood clot can form in the left atrium of the heart. If an embolus, or a piece of the clot, breaks off and travels to an artery in the brain, it can block blood flow through the artery. The lack of blood flow to the portion of the brain fed by the artery causes a stroke.

- **Sudden cardiac arrest (SCA).** With AF, there is an increased risk that the heart may suddenly and unexpectedly stop beating if you have another serious heart condition.

Diagnosis of Atrial Fibrillation

A doctor will diagnose AF based on your medical and family history, a physical exam, the results from an electrocardiogram, and possibly other tests and procedures. If you have AF, your doctor will also look for any disease that may be causing it and assess your risk of developing dangerous blood clots. This will help her or him plan the best way to treat you.

Medical History

To help diagnose atrial fibrillation, your doctor will ask about your eating and physical activity habits, family history, and other risk factors for AF and heart disease. Your doctor may ask whether you have any other signs or symptoms. This information can help your doctor determine whether you have complications or other conditions that may be causing you to have AF.

Physical Examination

Your doctor will do a complete examination of your heart and lungs, including:

- Checking for signs of too much thyroid hormone, such as a thyroid gland that is larger than normal
- Checking for swelling in your legs or feet, which could be a sign of heart failure or a heart that is larger than normal
- Checking your pulse to find out how fast your heart is beating
- Listening to the rhythm of your heartbeat
- Listening to your lungs to check for signs of heart failure or infection
- Measuring your blood pressure

Diagnostic Tests

To diagnose atrial fibrillation, your doctor will likely do an EKG first to record your heart's electrical activity. If the diagnosis is unclear from the EKG or your doctor would like more information, your doctor may order additional testing:

- **Blood tests** to check the level of substances in the blood, such as potassium and thyroid hormone.

- **Echocardiography (echo)** to show areas of poor blood flow to the heart, areas of heart muscle that are not contracting normally, and previous injury to the heart muscle caused by poor blood flow. It may also identify harmful blood clots in the heart's chambers.

Other Tests

Your doctor may order other tests to record abnormal heart rhythms that happen under specific conditions or outside of the clinic, confirm whether you have atrial fibrillation or another arrhythmia, and figure out which treatment is best. These tests may include:

- **Chest X-ray** to look for signs of complications from AF, such as fluid buildup in the lungs or a heart that is larger than normal.

- **Electrophysiology study (EPS)** to record your heart's electrical signals if your doctor wants more detail about what is causing a particular EKG reading or to distinguish among possible types of arrhythmias.

- **Holter and event monitors** to record your heart's electrical activity over long periods of time while you do normal, day-to-day activities. These portable EKG monitors can help assess the cause of symptoms, such as palpitations or feeling dizzy, that happen outside the doctor's office. Most portable monitors will send data directly to your doctor.

- **Loop recorder** to record the heart's electrical activity. Some loop recorder models are worn externally, and some require minor surgery to place the device under the skin in the chest area. Implanted devices can record data for months and are used to detect patterns in abnormal heart rhythms that do not happen very often.

- **Sleep study** to see if sleep apnea is causing your symptoms.

- **Stress test** or exercise stress test to look at changes in your heart's activity that occur with increase in heart rate, and recovery after exercise. If you cannot exercise, you may be given medicine to make your heart work hard and beat fast.

- **Transesophageal echocardiography (TEE)** to detect blood clots that may be forming in the heart's upper chambers because of AF. It uses sound waves to take pictures of your heart through the esophagus.

- **Walking test** to measure your heart activity while you walk for six minutes. This can help determine how well your body can control your heart rate under normal circumstances.

Treatment of Atrial Fibrillation

Atrial fibrillation is treated with lifestyle changes, medicines, procedures, and surgery to help prevent blood clots, slow your heartbeat, or restore your heart's normal rhythm.

Your doctor may also treat you for an underlying disorder that is causing or raising the risk of AF, such as sleep apnea or an overactive thyroid gland.

Lifestyle Changes

Your doctor may recommend adopting heart-healthy lifestyle changes, such as the following:

- Heart-healthy eating patterns, such as the DASH eating plan, which reduces salt intake to help lower blood pressure

- Being physically active

- Getting help if you are trying to stop using street drugs

- Limiting or avoiding alcohol or other stimulants that may increase your heart rate

- Managing stress

- Quitting smoking. For free help and support to quit smoking, you can call the National Cancer Institute's (NCI) Smoking Quitline at 877-448-7848.

Medicines

Your doctor may consider treating your AF with medicines to slow your heart rate or to make your heart's rhythm more even:

- **Beta-blockers,** such as metoprolol, carvedilol, and atenolol, to help slow the rate at which the heart's lower chambers pump blood throughout the body. Rate control is important because it allows the ventricles enough time to fill with blood completely. With this approach, the abnormal heart rhythm continues, but you may feel better and have fewer symptoms. Beta-blockers are usually taken by mouth, but they may be delivered through a tube in an emergency situation. If the dose is too high, it can cause the heart to beat too slowly. These medicines can also make chronic obstructive pulmonary disease (COPD) and arrhythmia worse.

- **Blood thinners** to prevent blood clots and lower the risk of stroke. These medicines include warfarin, dabigatran, heparin, and clopidogrel. You may not need to take blood thinners if you are not at risk of a stroke. Blood-thinning medicines carry a risk of bleeding. Other side effects include indigestion and heart attack.

- **Calcium channel blockers** to control the rate at which the heart's lower chambers pump blood throughout the body. They include diltiazem and verapamil.

- **Digitalis, or digoxin,** to control the rate blood is pumped throughout the body. It should be used with caution, as its use can lead to other arrhythmias.

- **Other heart rhythm medicines** to slow a heart that is beating too fast or change an abnormal heart rhythm to a normal, steady rhythm. Rhythm control is an approach recommended for people who continue to have symptoms or otherwise are not getting better with rate-control medicines. Rhythm control also may be used for people who have only recently started having AF or for highly physically active people and athletes. These medicines may be used alone or in combination with electrical cardioversion. Or your doctor may prescribe some of these medicines for you to take on an as-needed basis when you feel symptoms of AF. Some heart rhythm medicines can make arrhythmia worse. Other side effects include effects on the liver, lung, and other organs; low blood pressure; and indigestion.

- Your doctor may recommend treatments for an underlying cause or to reduce AF risk factors. For example, she or he may prescribe medicines to treat an overactive thyroid, lower high blood pressure, or manage high blood cholesterol.

Procedures or Surgery

Your doctor may recommend a procedure or surgery, especially if lifestyle changes and medicine alone did not improve your symptoms. Typically, your doctor will consider a surgical procedure to treat your AF only if you will be having surgery to treat some other heart condition.

- **Catheter ablation** to destroy the tissue that is causing the arrhythmia. Ablation is not always successful and in rare cases, may lead to serious complications, such as stroke. The risk that AF will reoccur is highest in the first few weeks after the procedure. If this happens, your doctor may repeat the procedure. In some cases, your doctor will place a pacemaker at the time of the procedure to make sure your heart beats correctly once the tissue causing problems is destroyed.

- **Electrical cardioversion** to restore your heart rhythm using low-energy shocks to your heart. This may be done in an emergency or if medicines have not worked.

- **Pacemaker** to reduce AF when it is triggered by a slow heartbeat. Typically, a pacemaker is used to treat AF only when it is diagnosed along with another arrhythmia. For example, if you are diagnosed with a slow heart rate or sick sinus syndrome, a pacemaker implanted for that condition can also prevent AF. If you have surgery for a pacemaker, you will need to take blood-thinning medicines.

- **Plugging, closing, or cutting off the left atrial appendage** to prevent clots from forming in the area and causing a stroke. Your doctor may do this at the same time as surgical ablation. It can be difficult to close off the appendage entirely, and leaking can contribute to ongoing clotting risk.

- **Surgical ablation** to destroy heart tissue generating faulty electrical signals. The surgeon usually does surgical ablation at the same time as surgery to repair heart valves, but in some cases, surgical ablation can be done on its own.

Living with Atrial Fibrillation

If you have been diagnosed with AF, it is important that you continue your treatment. Follow-up care can help your doctor check your condition and talk to you about how to prevent repeat events and what to do in an emergency. Sometimes, AF may go back to a normal heart rhythm without treatment.

Receive Routine Follow-Up Care

How often you need to see your doctor for follow-up care will depend on your symptoms and treatment.

- **Keep all your medical appointments.** Bring a list of all the medicines you are taking to every doctor and emergency room visit. This will help your doctor know exactly what medicines you are taking.

- **Take your medicines as prescribed.** If you are taking medicines to treat your AF, your doctor will monitor their effects, including the dose, your body's electrolyte levels, and the medicines' effects on other organs.

- **Tell your doctor if your medicines are causing side effects,** if your symptoms are getting worse, or if you have new symptoms.

- **Ask your doctor about physical activity, weight control, and alcohol use.** Find out what steps you can take to manage your condition. If you use illegal drugs, ask your doctor for help stopping.

- **Check with your doctor before taking over-the-counter (OTC) medicines, nutritional supplements, or cold and allergy medicines.** Some of these products can trigger rapid heart rhythms or interact poorly with other medicines. In addition, the effect of blood thinners can be enhanced by medicines to treat arrhythmia.

- **If you have had an ablation, your doctor will want to see you regularly for three months** to check on the healing process, to check for the reappearance of AF events, and to make adjustments to blood-thinning medicines as needed. You will continue to take blood thinners for several months and maybe much longer. Report any lasting pain, for example at the site, or any other signs of a complication. Your doctor will want to see you at least once a year after the initial follow-up period.

- **If you are taking warfarin, it is important to monitor the dose by measuring how quickly your blood clots.** Your doctor will do blood tests every week at first, then monthly once the level has stabilized. You may be able to do this yourself at home. You will need to avoid certain other medicines and watch what you eat. Some foods, such as leafy green vegetables, may interfere with warfarin.

Monitor Your Condition

Regular visits to the clinic give your doctor a chance to see how well medicines are controlling your AF, monitor your ongoing risks of clotting or bleeding, and see how well you are healing from any procedures. Your doctor may also ask you to wear a heart rhythm monitor and to send data in between visits to see how well your treatment is working and to detect any repeat events.

- **Electrocardiogram.** Regular EKG monitoring can help your doctor detect a repeat AF event or assess your response to changes in dose or medicine, or to ending treatment with medicines. Your doctor may record an EKG during your regular visits or recommend a portable monitor. A band that can record a 30-second EKG has also been approved by the U.S. Food and Drug Administration (FDA).

- **Stress tests** or a six-minute walking test can help your doctor see whether your medicine prevents AF while you are doing typical everyday activities.

- **Blood tests** can check the effect of certain heart rhythm medicines on your thyroid, kidneys, or liver. The blood thinner warfarin also requires regular testing to make sure the dose is correct. In some cases, your doctor may talk to you about devices available for monitoring your blood-thinning medicines at home. Blood thinners can be stopped or adjusted if you are going into surgery.

Prevent Repeat Atrial Fibrillation

To help prevent a repeat episode of AF, your doctor may recommend the following:

- **Medicine that you can take at home** and as needed to correct your heart rhythm. Before giving you this medicine, the doctor will ask you to take a dose and try to trigger an event to see if the medicine prevents it effectively. You can take this medicine if you start feeling symptoms of AF.

- **Treatment for an underlying condition,** such as sleep apnea, high blood pressure, and diabetes

- **Heart-healthy lifestyle changes,** including aiming for a healthy weight. Combining weight loss with physical activity and the management of other risk factors, such as high blood pressure, diabetes, alcohol use, and smoking, can improve symptoms more than weight loss alone.

Learn the Warning Signs of Serious Complications and Have a Plan

Atrial fibrillation can lead to serious complications, such as SCA and stroke. Risks of treatment with blood thinners include severe bleeding in the brain. If you suspect any of the following in you or someone else, call 911 immediately:

- **Bleeding in the brain, digestive system, or urinary tract.** This can happen if you take a dose of blood-thinning medicines that is too high. Signs and symptoms may include bright red vomit; bright red blood in your stool or black, tarry stools; blood in your urine; severe pain in the abdomen or head; sudden, severe changes in your vision or ability to move your arms or legs; or memory loss. A lot of bleeding after a fall or injury, or easy bruising or bleeding, may mean that your blood is too thin. Excessive bleeding is bleeding that will not stop after you apply pressure to a wound for ten minutes. Call your doctor right away if you have any of these signs.

- **Heart attack.** Signs of heart attack include mild or severe chest pain or discomfort in the center of the chest or upper abdomen that lasts for more than a few minutes or goes away and comes back. It can feel like pressure, squeezing, fullness, heartburn, or indigestion. There may also be pain down the left arm. Women may also have chest pain and pain down the left arm, but they are more likely to have less typical symptoms, such as shortness of breath, nausea, vomiting, unusual tiredness, and pain in the back, shoulders, or jaw.

- **Stroke.** If you think someone may be having a stroke, act F.A.S.T. and do the following simple test:

  F—Face: Ask the person to smile. Does one side of the face droop?

A—Arms: Ask the person to raise both arms. Does one arm drift downward?

S—Speech: Ask the person to repeat a simple phrase. Is their speech slurred or strange?

T—Time: If you observe any of these signs, call 911 immediately. Every minute matters.

- **Sudden cardiac arrest.** Usually, the first sign of SCA is fainting. At the same time, no heartbeat can be felt. Some people may have a racing heartbeat or feel dizzy or light-headed just before they faint. Within an hour before cardiac arrest, some people have chest pain, shortness of breath, nausea, or vomiting. Call 911 right away if someone has signs or symptoms of SCA. Look for a defibrillator nearby, and follow the instructions.

Section 17.3

Brugada Syndrome

This section includes text excerpted from "Brugada Syndrome," Genetic and Rare Diseases Information Center (GARD), National Center for Advancing Translational Sciences (NCATS), March 16, 2016.

Brugada syndrome is a heart condition that causes a disruption of the normal rhythm in the heart's lower chambers (ventricular arrhythmia). Signs and symptoms usually develop in adulthood, but the diagnosis may be made at any age. Symptoms and complications often occur during rest or sleep, and may include fainting, seizures, difficulty breathing, or sudden death. Brugada syndrome may be caused by a mutation in any of at least 16 genes (most commonly the *SCN5A* gene) and is inherited in an autosomal dominant manner. An acquired (nongenetic) form has been associated with certain drugs, abnormally high blood levels of calcium or potassium, or very low levels of potassium. In some cases, the cause of Brugada syndrome is unknown. Treatment may include use of an implantable cardioverter defibrillator (ICD).

Symptoms of Brugada Syndrome

While symptoms of Brugada syndrome usually develop in adult-hood, they can develop at any age. Symptoms associated with irregular heartbeat (arrhythmia) can cause fainting, seizures, difficulty breathing, or sudden death. These symptoms and complications usually occur during rest or sleep. Sudden cardiac arrest (SCA) may be the initial symptom of Brugada syndrome in as many as one-third of affected people. The risk of cardiac arrest is much lower in people with no symptoms. After diagnosis, specific tests may provide an estimate of the risk of ventricular arrhythmias and sudden cardiac death in each person.

Inheritance of Brugada Syndrome

The genetic form of Brugada syndrome (not the acquired form) is inherited in an autosomal dominant manner. This means that having one mutated copy of the responsible gene in each cell is enough to cause signs or symptoms. Almost all people with Brugada syndrome have a parent with the condition. In about 1 percent of cases, an affected person has a new mutation in the responsible gene and has no family history of the condition. Each child of an affected person has a 50 percent chance to inherit the mutated gene.

Asymptomatic parents of an affected person should be evaluated with electrocardiography (ECG or EKG), and any family history of sudden death should be discussed. If genetic testing reveals a mutation in the affected person, genetic testing of the parents is recommended. A family history may appear to be negative due to reduced penetrance, death of a parent before symptoms start, or late onset of symptoms in an affected parent.

Prognosis for Brugada Syndrome

The long-term outlook (prognosis) for people with Brugada syndrome varies because the condition is very unpredictable. The condition manifests primarily during adulthood and causes a high risk of ventricular arrhythmias and sudden death. The average age of sudden death is approximately 40 years of age. Affected people with a history of SCA and/or fainting have an increased risk for subsequent episodes compared to people with no symptoms.

Section 17.4

Heart Block

Heart block—also known as "atrioventricular (AV) block"—is a condition where the electrical signals that normally cause the heart muscle to contract are prevented from performing this function, resulting in an abnormally slow heartbeat. Ordinarily, a heartbeat begins with an electrical signal generated by the sinoatrial (SA) node, a group of specialized cells located in the upper right atrium chamber of the heart. This signal travels downward to the atrioventricular (AV) node, an electrical relay station located between the heart's upper and lower chambers. Finally, the current passes through special fibers into the lower chambers or ventricles, causing the heart muscle to contract and pump blood through the body. When the conduction of electrical signals through the heart is delayed or interrupted, partial or total heart block occurs.

Causes and Symptoms of Heart Block

In fact, the risk of acquired heart block increases as people get older and become more susceptible to heart disease. Heart block can be caused by many different types of heart disease, as well as by certain other types of medical conditions. Some of the most common causes of acquired heart block include the following:

- Heart attack
- Coronary artery disease (CAD)
- Heart failure
- Cardiomyopathy (enlarged heart)
- Rheumatic heart disease
- Heart valve abnormalities or structural heart disorders
- Injury during open heart surgery
- Side effects of some medications
- Exposure to toxic substances
- Lyme disease

Even though people with some types of heart block do not experience any symptoms, others may experience fainting, dizziness, fatigue, shortness of breath, or chest pain. These symptoms sometimes indicate other heart problems, so emergency medical attention may be warranted if they appear suddenly.

Diagnosis and Treatment of Heart Block

Heart block is often diagnosed as part of a regular medical examination, when a doctor detects an arrhythmia while listening to the patient's heartbeat or an abnormally slow heart rhythm while taking their pulse. If heart block is suspected, the patient will likely be referred to a cardiologist for further evaluation. The specialist will typically inquire about the patient's symptoms, family history of heart disease, and any medications they may be taking. The doctor may then order an electrocardiogram (EKG) to monitor electrical activity in the patient's heart, as well as perform tests to rule out other types of arrhythmias.

There are several different types of heart block that differ in terms of severity, symptoms, and treatment.

- **First-degree heart block.** This condition is fairly common and rarely causes symptoms or requires treatment. It often occurs in well-trained athletes and healthy teenagers, as well as people who take certain medications. In first-degree heart block, all of the electrical signals reach the ventricles, although their progress is slowed as they pass through the conduction system.

- **Type I second-degree heart block.** This condition sometimes causes dizziness or other symptoms and may require monitoring or treatment. It can occur in people with normal conduction systems during sleep. In this type of heart block, the delay before electrical impulses reach the ventricles grows longer and longer until conduction failure occurs, resulting in a brief pause in the heartbeat.

- **Type II second-degree heart block.** In this condition, some electrical signals fail to reach the ventricles. Although it is less common than Type I, it typically causes more severe symptoms and is considered a more serious condition. A pacemaker is often recommended to regulate the heartbeat in people with Type II heart block.

- **Third-degree or complete heart block.** This condition occurs when no electrical signals successfully reach the ventricles. In the absence of impulses from the right atrium, the lower chambers typically generate ventricular escape beats, which serve as a sort of backup system. Since these beats occur very slowly, people with third-degree heart block usually experience severe symptoms of fatigue, light-headedness, and fainting.

Most cases of first-degree heart block do not require treatment. In addition, some cases of acquired heart block may improve with treatment of the underlying medical condition. For instance, heart block that occurs following a heart attack may resolve itself during recovery, or heart block that is caused by medication may go away if the dosage is lowered or the prescription is changed.

The main form of treatment for third-degree heart block—and some cases of second-degree heart block—is a pacemaker. A pacemaker is a small device that is inserted beneath the skin on the chest or abdomen. It generates electrical impulses to help regulate the heartbeat. Although people with pacemakers can usually pursue normal activities, it is important to avoid things that may prevent the pacemaker from working properly. Examples include devices that produce strong electrical currents or magnetic fields, such as airport screening devices and magnetic resonance imaging (MRI) scanners. Most people with pacemakers wear a medical ID bracelet or carry a card that describes their pacemaker and lists things that may interfere with its operation.

References

1. "Heart Block," Cleveland Clinic, 2016.

2. "Heart Block," Heart Rhythm Society (HRS), 2016.

Section 17.5

Long QT Syndrome

This section includes text excerpted from "Long QT Syndrome," National Heart, Lung, and Blood Institute (NHLBI), June 12, 2017.

What Is Long QT Syndrome?

Long QT syndrome (LQTS) is a disorder of the heart's electrical activity. It can cause sudden, uncontrollable, dangerous arrhythmias in response to exercise or stress. Arrhythmias are problems with the rate or rhythm of the heartbeat.

People who have LQTS also can have arrhythmias for no known reason. However, not everyone who has LQTS has dangerous heart rhythms. When they do occur, though, they can be fatal.

What Does "Long QT" Mean?

The term "long QT" refers to an abnormal pattern seen on an electrocardiogram (EKG). An EKG is a test that detects and records the heart's electrical activity.

With each heartbeat, an electrical signal spreads from the top of your heart to the bottom. As it travels, the signal causes the heart to contract and pump blood. An EKG records electrical signals as they move through your heart.

Data from the EKG are mapped on a graph, so your doctor can study your heart's electrical activity. Each heartbeat is mapped as five distinct electrical waves: P, Q, R, S, and T.

Electrocardiogram

The electrical activity that occurs between the Q and T waves is called the "QT interval." This interval shows electrical activity in the heart's lower chambers, the ventricles.

The timing of the heart's electrical activity is complex, and the body carefully controls it. Normally, the QT interval is about a third of each heartbeat cycle. However, in people who have LQTS, the QT interval lasts longer than normal.

A long QT interval can upset the careful timing of the heartbeat and trigger dangerous heart rhythms.

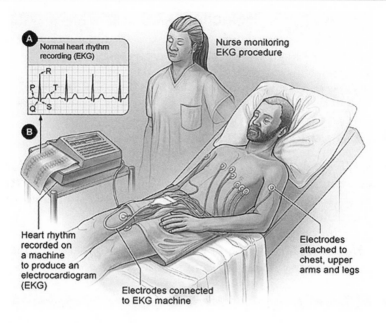

Figure 17.2. *Electrocardiogram*

The image shows the standard setup for an EKG. In figure A, a normal heart rhythm recording shows the electrical pattern of a regular heartbeat. In figure B, a patient lies in a bed with EKG electrodes attached to his chest, upper arms, and legs. A nurse monitors the painless procedure.

Causes of Long QT Syndrome

Long QT syndrome can be inherited or acquired. "Inherited" means you are born with the condition and have it your whole life. Inherited conditions are passed from parents to children through their genes. "Acquired" means you are not born with the condition, but you develop it during your lifetime.

Inherited Long QT Syndrome

Faulty genes cause inherited LQTS. These genes control the production of certain types of ion channels in your heart. Faulty genes may cause the body to make too few ion channels, ion channels that do not work well, or both.

There are seven known types of inherited LQTS (types 1 through 7). The most common types are LQTS 1, 2, and 3.

Some types of LQTS involve faulty or lacking potassium ion or sodium ion channels.

If you have LQTS 1 or LQTS 2, the flow of potassium ions through the ion channels in your heart cells is not normal. This may cause problems when you exercise or when you have strong emotions.

You may develop a rapid, uncontrollable heart rhythm that prevents your heart from pumping blood. This type of heart rhythm can be fatal if it is not quickly brought under control.

If you have LQTS 3, the flow of sodium ions through ion channels in your heart cells is not normal. This can trigger a rapid, uncontrollable heart rhythm that can be fatal. In LQTS 3, problems usually occur when your heart beats slower than normal, such as during sleep.

Acquired Long QT Syndrome

Some medicines and conditions can cause acquired LQTS.

Medication-Induced Long QT Syndrome

More than 50 medicines have been found to cause LQTS. Some common medicines that may cause the disorder include:

- Antihistamines and decongestants
- Diuretics (pills that remove excess water from your body)
- Antibiotics
- Antiarrhythmic medicines
- Antidepressant and antipsychotic medicines
- Cholesterol-lowering medicines and some diabetes medicines

Some people who have medication-induced LQTS also may have an inherited form of the disorder. They may not have symptoms unless they take medicines that lengthen the QT interval or lower potassium levels in the blood. When LQTS does not cause symptoms, it is called "silent LQTS."

Other Causes of Acquired Long QT Syndrome

Severe diarrhea or vomiting that causes a major loss of potassium or sodium ions from the bloodstream may cause LQTS. The disorder lasts until these ion levels return to normal.

The eating disorders anorexia nervosa and bulimia and some thyroid disorders may cause a drop in potassium ion levels in the blood, causing LQTS.

Risk Factors for Long QT Syndrome

Long QT syndrome is a rare disorder. Experts think that about 1 in 7,000 people has LQTS. But no one knows for sure, because LQTS often goes undiagnosed.

Long QT syndrome causes about 3,000 to 4,000 sudden deaths in children and young adults each year in the United States. Unexplained sudden deaths in children are rare. When they do occur, LQTS often is the cause.

Inherited LQTS usually is first detected during childhood or young adulthood. Half of all people who have LQTS have their first abnormal heart rhythm by the time they are 12 years of age, and 90 percent by the time they are 40 years of age. The condition rarely is diagnosed after the age of 40.

In boys who have LQTS, the QT interval (which can be seen on an EKG test) often returns toward normal after puberty. If this happens, the risk of LQTS symptoms and complications decreases.

Long QT syndrome is more common in women than men. Women who have LQTS are more likely to faint or die suddenly from the disorder during menstruation and shortly after giving birth.

Children who are born deaf also are at increased risk for LQTS. This is because the same genetic problem that affects hearing also affects the function of ion channels in the heart.

Major Risk Factors

You are at risk of having LQTS if anyone in your family has ever had it. Unexplained fainting or seizures, drowning or near drowning, and unexplained sudden death are all possible signs of LQTS.

You are also at risk for LQTS if you take medicines that make the QT interval longer. Your doctor can tell you whether your prescription or over-the-counter (OTC) medicines might do this.

You also may develop LQTS if you have excessive vomiting or diarrhea or other conditions that cause low blood levels of potassium or sodium. These conditions include the eating disorders anorexia nervosa and bulimia, as well as some thyroid disorders.

Signs, Symptoms, and Complications of Long QT Syndrome

Major Signs and Symptoms

If you have long QT syndrome, you can have sudden and dangerous arrhythmias (abnormal heart rhythms). Signs and symptoms of

LQTS-related arrhythmias often first occur during childhood and include:

- **Unexplained fainting.** This happens because the heart is not pumping enough blood to the brain. Fainting may occur during physical or emotional stress. Fluttering feelings in the chest may occur before fainting.

- **Unexplained drowning or near drowning.** This may be due to fainting while swimming.

- **Unexplained sudden cardiac arrest (SCA) or death.** SCA is a condition in which the heart suddenly stops beating for no obvious reason. People who have SCA die within minutes unless they receive treatment. In about one out of ten people who have LQTS, SCA or sudden death is the first sign of the disorder.

Other Signs and Symptoms

Often, people who have LQTS 3 develop an abnormal heart rhythm during sleep. This may cause noisy gasping while sleeping.

Silent Long QT Syndrome

Sometimes, long QT syndrome does not cause any signs or symptoms. This is called "silent LQTS." For this reason, doctors often advise family members of people who have LQTS to be tested for the disorder, even if they have no symptoms.

Medical and genetic tests may reveal whether these family members have LQTS and what type of the condition they have.

Diagnosis of Long QT Syndrome

Cardiologists diagnose and treat LQTS. Cardiologists are doctors who specialize in diagnosing and treating heart diseases and conditions. To diagnose LQTS, your cardiologist will consider your electrocardiogram (ECG) results, medical history and the results from a physical exam, and genetic test results.

Electrocardiogram

An electrocardiogram (EKG) is a simple test that detects and records the heart's electrical activity. This test may show a long QT interval and other signs that suggest LQTS. Often, doctors first discover a long QT interval when an EKG is done for another suspected heart problem.

Not all people who have LQTS will always have a long QT interval on an EKG. The QT interval may change from time to time; it may be long sometimes and normal at other times. Thus, your doctor may want you to have several EKG tests over a period of days or weeks. Or, your doctor may have you wear a device called a "Holter monitor."

A Holter monitor records the heart's electrical activity for a full 24- or 48-hour period. It can detect heart problems that occur for only a few minutes out of the day.

You wear small patches called "electrodes" on your chest. Wires connect the patches to a small, portable recorder. You can clip the recorder to a belt, keep it in a pocket, or hang it around your neck.

While you wear the monitor, you do your usual daily activities. You also keep a notebook, noting any symptoms you have and the time they occur. You then return both the recorder and the notebook to your doctor to read the results. Your doctor can see how your heart was beating at the time you had symptoms.

Some people have a long QT interval only while they exercise. For this reason, your doctor may recommend that you have a stress test.

During a stress test, you exercise to make your heart work hard and beat fast. An EKG is done while you exercise. If you cannot exercise, you may be given medicine to increase your heart rate.

Medical History and Physical Exam

Your doctor will ask whether you have had any symptoms of an abnormal heart rhythm. Symptoms may include:

- Unexplained fainting

- A fluttering feeling in your chest, which is the result of your heart beating too fast

- Loud gasping during sleep

- Your doctor may ask what over-the-counter, prescription, or other drugs you take. She or he also may want to know whether anyone in your family has been diagnosed with or has had signs of LQTS.

Your doctor will check you for signs of conditions that may lower blood levels of potassium or sodium. These conditions include the eating disorders; anorexia nervosa and bulimia, excessive vomiting or diarrhea, and certain thyroid disorders.

Genetic Tests

Genetic blood tests can detect some forms of inherited LQTS. If your doctor thinks that you have LQTS, she or he may suggest genetic testing. Genetic blood tests usually are suggested for family members of people who have LQTS as well.

However, genetic tests do not always detect LQTS. So, even if you have the disorder, the tests may not show it.

Also, some people who test positive for LQTS do not have any signs or symptoms of the disorder. These people may have silent LQTS. Less than ten percent of these people will faint or suddenly die from an abnormal heart rhythm.

Even if you have silent LQTS, you may be at increased risk of having an abnormal heart rhythm while taking medicines that affect potassium ion channels or blood levels of potassium.

Types of Inherited Long QT Syndrome

If you have inherited LQTS, it may be helpful to know which type you have. This will help you and your doctor plan your treatment and decide which lifestyle changes you should make.

To find out what type of LQTS you have, your doctor will consider:

- Genetic test results

- The types of situations that trigger an abnormal heart rhythm

- How well you respond to medicine

Treatment of Long QT Syndrome

The goal of treating LQTS is to prevent life-threatening, abnormal heart rhythms and fainting spells.

Treatment is not a cure for the disorder and may not restore a normal QT interval on an electrocardiogram (EKG). However, treatment greatly improves the chances of survival.

Specific Types of Treatment

Your doctor will recommend the best treatment for you based on:

- Whether you have had symptoms, such as fainting or SCA

- What type of LQTS you have

- How likely it is that you will faint or have SCA

203

- What treatment you feel most comfortable with

People who have LQTS without symptoms may be advised to:

- **Make lifestyle changes that reduce the risk of fainting or SCA.** Lifestyle changes may include avoiding certain sports and strenuous exercise, such as swimming, which can cause abnormal heart rhythms.

- **Avoid medicines that may trigger abnormal heart rhythms.** This may include some medicines used to treat allergies, infections, high blood pressure (HBP), high blood cholesterol, depression, and arrhythmias.

- **Take medicines,** such as beta-blockers, which reduce the risk of symptoms by slowing the heart rate.

The type of medicine you take will depend on the type of LQTS you have. For example, doctors usually will prescribe sodium-channel blocker medicines only for people who have LQTS 3.

If your doctor thinks you are at increased risk for LQTS complications, she or he may suggest more aggressive treatments (in addition to medicines and lifestyle changes). These treatments may include:

- **A surgically implanted device,** such as a pacemaker or implantable cardioverter defibrillator (ICD). These devices help control abnormal heart rhythms.

- **Surgery** on the nerves that regulate your heartbeat

People at increased risk are those who have fainted or who have had dangerous heart rhythms from their LQTS.

Lifestyle Changes

If possible, try to avoid things that can trigger abnormal heart rhythms. For example, people who have LQTS should avoid medicines that lengthen the QT interval or lower potassium blood levels.

Many people who have LQTS also benefit from adding more potassium to their diets. Check with your doctor about eating more potassium-rich foods (such as bananas) or taking potassium supplements daily.

Medicines

Beta-blockers are medicines that prevent the heart from beating faster in response to physical or emotional stress. Most people who have LQTS are treated with beta-blockers.

Doctors may suggest that people who have LQTS 3 take sodium channel blockers, such as mexiletine. These medicines make sodium ion channels less active.

Medical Devices

Pacemakers and ICDs are small devices that help control abnormal heart rhythms. Both devices use electrical currents to prompt the heart to beat normally. Surgeons implant pacemakers and ICDs in the chest or belly with a minor procedure.

The use of these devices is similar in children and adults. However, because children are still growing, other issues may arise. For example, as children grow, they may need to have their devices replaced.

Surgery

People who are at a high risk of death from LQTS sometimes are treated with surgery. During surgery, the nerves that prompt the heart to beat faster in response to physical or emotional stress are cut.

This type of surgery keeps the heart beating at a steady pace and lowers the risk of dangerous heart rhythms in response to stress or exercise.

Living with Long QT Syndrome

Long QT syndrome usually is a lifelong condition. The risk of having an abnormal heart rhythm that leads to fainting or SCA may lessen as you age. However, the risk never completely goes away.

You will need to take certain steps for the rest of your life to prevent abnormal heart rhythms. You can:

- Avoid things that trigger abnormal heart rhythms.

- Let others know you might faint or your heart might stop beating, and tell them what steps they can take.

- Have a plan in place for how to handle abnormal heart rhythms.

If an abnormal heart rhythm does occur, you will need to seek treatment right away.

Avoid Triggers

If exercise triggers an abnormal heart rhythm, your doctor may tell you to avoid any strenuous exercise, especially swimming. Ask your doctor what types and amounts of exercise are safe for you.

If you have a pacemaker or implantable cardioverter defibrillator, avoid contact sports that may dislodge these devices. You may want to exercise in public or with a friend who can help you if you faint.

Avoid medicines that can trigger an abnormal heart rhythm. This includes some medicines used to treat allergies, infections, high blood pressure, high blood cholesterol, depression, and arrhythmias. Talk with your doctor before taking any prescription, over-the-counter, or other medicines or drugs.

Seek medical care right away for conditions that lower the sodium or potassium level in your blood. These conditions include anorexia nervosa, bulimia, excessive vomiting or diarrhea, and certain thyroid disorders.

If you have LQTS 2, try to avoid unexpected noises, such as loud or jarring alarm clock buzzers and telephone ringers.

Inform Others

You may want to wear a medical ID necklace or bracelet that states that you have LQTS. This will help alert medical personnel and others about your condition if you have an emergency.

Let your roommates, coworkers, or other people with whom you have regular contact know that you have a condition that might cause you to faint or go into cardiac arrest. Tell them to call 911 right away if you faint.

Consider asking a family member and/or coworker to learn cardio-pulmonary resuscitation (CPR) in case your heart stops beating.

You also may want to keep an automated external defibrillator (AED) with you at home or at work. This device uses electric shocks to restore a normal heart rhythm.

Someone at your home and/or workplace should be trained on how to use the AED, just in case your heart stops beating. If a trained person is not available, an untrained person also can use the AED to help save your life.

If you have LQTS 3 and you sleep alone, you may want to have an intercom in your bedroom that is connected to someone else's bedroom. This will let others detect the noisy gasping that often occurs if you have an abnormal heart rhythm while lying down.

Ongoing Healthcare Needs

You should see your cardiologist (heart specialist) regularly. She or he will adjust your treatment as needed. For example, if you still faint often while using less aggressive treatments, your doctor may suggest other treatment options.

Emotional Issues and Support

Living with LQTS may cause fear, anxiety, depression, and stress. Talk about how you feel with your healthcare team. Talking to a professional counselor also can help. If you are very depressed, your doctor may recommend medicines or other treatments that can improve your quality of life (QOL).

Joining a patient support group may help you adjust to living with LQTS. You can see how other people have coped with the condition. Talk with your doctor about local support groups or check with an area medical center.

Support from family and friends also can help relieve stress and anxiety. Let your loved ones know how you feel and what they can do to help you.

Some people learn they have LQTS because they are tested after a family member dies suddenly from LQTS. Grief counseling may help you cope if this has happened to you. Talk with your doctor about finding a grief counselor.

Section 17.6

Sick Sinus Syndrome

This section includes text excerpted from "Sick Sinus Syndrome," Genetics Home Reference (GHR), National Institutes of Health (NIH), March 19, 2019.

Sick sinus syndrome (SSS), also known as "sinus node dysfunction," is a group of related heart conditions that can affect how the heart beats. "Sick sinus" refers to the sinoatrial (SA) node, which is an area of specialized cells in the heart that functions as a natural pacemaker. The SA node generates electrical impulses that start each heartbeat. These signals travel from the SA node to the rest of the heart, signaling the heart (cardiac) muscle to contract and pump blood. In people with

SSS, the SA node does not function normally. In some cases, it does not produce the right signals to trigger a regular heartbeat. In others, abnormalities disrupt the electrical impulses and prevent them from reaching the rest of the heart.

Sick sinus syndrome tends to cause the heartbeat to be too slow (bradycardia), although occasionally the heartbeat is too fast (tachycardia). In some cases, the heartbeat rapidly switches from being too fast to being too slow, a condition known as "tachycardia-bradycardia syndrome." Symptoms related to abnormal heartbeats can include dizziness, light-headedness, fainting (syncope), a sensation of fluttering or pounding in the chest (palpitations), and confusion or memory problems. During exercise, many affected individuals experience chest pain, difficulty breathing, or excessive tiredness (fatigue). Once symptoms of SSS appear, they usually worsen with time. However, some people with the condition never experience any related health problems.

Sick sinus syndrome occurs most commonly in older adults, although it can be diagnosed in people of any age. The condition increases the risk of several life-threatening problems involving the heart and blood vessels. These include a heart rhythm abnormality called "atrial fibrillation" (AF), heart failure, cardiac arrest, and stroke.

Frequency of Sick Sinus Syndrome

Sick sinus syndrome accounts for 1 in 600 patients with heart disease who are over the age of 65. The incidence of this condition increases with age.

Causes of Sick Sinus Syndrome

Sick sinus syndrome can result from genetic or environmental factors. In many cases, the cause of the condition is unknown.

Genetic changes are an uncommon cause of SSS. Mutations in two genes, *SCN5A* and *HCN4*, have been found to cause the condition in a small number of families. These genes provide instructions for making proteins called "ion channels" that transport positively charged atoms (ions) into cardiac cells, including cells that make up the SA node. The flow of these ions is essential for creating the electrical impulses that start each heartbeat and coordinate contraction of the cardiac muscle. Mutations in these genes reduce the flow of ions, which alters the SA node's ability to create and spread electrical signals. These changes lead to abnormal heartbeats and the other symptoms of SSS.

A particular variation in another gene, *MYH6*, appears to increase the risk of developing SSS. The protein produced from the *MYH6* gene forms part of a larger protein called "myosin," which generates the mechanical force needed for cardiac muscle to contract. Researchers believe that the *MYH6* gene variation changes the structure of myosin, which can affect cardiac muscle contraction and increase the likelihood of developing an abnormal heartbeat.

More commonly, SSS is caused by other factors that alter the structure or function of the SA node. These include a variety of heart conditions; other disorders, such as muscular dystrophy (MD); abnormal inflammation; or a shortage of oxygen (hypoxia). Certain medications, such as drugs given to treat abnormal heart rhythms or high blood pressure, can also disrupt SA node function. One of the most common causes of sick sinus syndrome in children is trauma to the SA node, such as damage that occurs during heart surgery.

In older adults, SSS is often associated with age-related changes in the heart. Over time, the SA node may harden and develop scar-like damage (fibrosis) that prevents it from working properly.

Chapter 18

Heart Valve Disease

What Is Heart Valve Disease?

Heart valve disease occurs if one or more of your heart valves do not work well. The heart has four valves: the tricuspid, pulmonary, mitral, and aortic valves.

These valves have tissue flaps that open and close with each heartbeat. The flaps make sure blood flows in the right direction through your heart's four chambers and to the rest of your body.

Healthy Heart Cross-Section

Birth defects, age-related changes, infections, or other conditions can cause one or more of your heart valves to not open fully or to let blood leak back into the heart chambers. This can make your heart work harder and affect its ability to pump blood.

How the Heart Valves Work

At the start of each heartbeat, blood returning from the body and lungs fills the atria (the heart's two upper chambers). The mitral and tricuspid valves are located at the bottom of these chambers. As the blood builds up in the atria, these valves open to allow blood to flow into the ventricles (the heart's two lower chambers).

This chapter includes text excerpted from "Heart Valve Disease," National Heart, Lung, and Blood Institute (NHLBI), November 18, 2013. Reviewed May 2019.

After a brief delay, as the ventricles begin to contract, the mitral and tricuspid valves shut tightly. This prevents blood from flowing back into the atria.

As the ventricles contract, they pump blood through the pulmonary and aortic valves. The pulmonary valve opens to allow blood to flow from the right ventricle into the pulmonary artery. This artery carries blood to the lungs to get oxygen.

At the same time, the aortic valve opens to allow blood to flow from the left ventricle into the aorta. The aorta carries oxygen-rich blood to the body. As the ventricles relax, the pulmonary and aortic valves shut tightly. This prevents blood from flowing back into the ventricles.

Heart Valve Problems

Heart valves can have three basic kinds of problems: regurgitation, stenosis, and atresia.

Regurgitation, or backflow, occurs if a valve does not close tightly. Blood leaks back into the chambers rather than flowing forward through the heart or into an artery.

In the United States, backflow most often is due to prolapse. Prolapse is when the flaps of the valve flop or bulge back into an upper heart chamber during a heartbeat. Prolapse mainly affects the mitral valve.

Stenosis occurs if the flaps of a valve thicken, stiffen, or fuse together. This prevents the heart valve from fully opening. As a result, not enough blood flows through the valve. Some valves can have both stenosis and backflow problems.

Atresia occurs if a heart valve lacks an opening for blood to pass through.

Some people are born with heart valve disease, while others acquire it later in life. Heart valve disease that develops before birth is called "congenital heart valve disease." Congenital heart valve disease can occur alone or with other congenital heart defects (CHD).

Congenital heart valve disease often involves pulmonary or aortic valves that do not form properly. These valves may not have enough tissue flaps, they may be the wrong size or shape, or they may lack an opening through which blood can flow properly.

Acquired heart valve disease usually involves the aortic or mitral valves. Although the valves are normal at first, problems develop over time.

Both congenital and acquired heart valve disease can cause stenosis or backflow.

Causes of Heart Valve Disease

Heart conditions and other disorders, age-related changes, rheumatic fever, or infections can cause acquired heart valve disease. These factors change the shape or flexibility of once-normal heart valves.

The cause of congenital heart valve disease is not known. It occurs before birth as the heart is forming. Congenital heart valve disease can occur alone or with other types of congenital heart defects.

Heart Conditions and Other Disorders

Certain conditions can stretch and distort the heart valves. These conditions include:

- Advanced high blood pressure (HBP) and heart failure, this can enlarge the heart or the main arteries.

- Atherosclerosis in the aorta. Atherosclerosis is a condition in which a waxy substance called "plaque" builds up inside the arteries. The aorta is the main artery that carries oxygen-rich blood to the body.

- Damage and scar tissue due to a heart attack or injury to the heart

Rheumatic Fever

Untreated strep throat or other infections with strep bacteria that progress to rheumatic fever can cause heart valve disease.

When the body tries to fight the strep infection, one or more heart valves may be damaged or scarred in the process. The aortic and mitral valves most often are affected. Symptoms of heart valve damage often do not appear until many years after recovery from rheumatic fever.

Nowadays, most people who have strep infections are treated with antibiotics before rheumatic fever occurs. If you have strep throat, take all of the antibiotics your doctor prescribes, even if you feel better before the medicine is gone.

Heart valve disease caused by rheumatic fever mainly affects older adults who had strep infections before antibiotics were available. It also affects people from developing countries, where rheumatic fever is more common.

Infections

Common germs that enter the bloodstream and get carried to the heart can sometimes infect the inner surface of the heart, including the heart valves. This rare but serious infection is called "infective endocarditis" (IE).

The germs can enter the bloodstream through needles, syringes, or other medical devices and through breaks in the skin or gums. Often, the body's defenses fight off the germs and no infection occurs. Sometimes these defenses fail, which leads to infective endocarditis.

Infective endocarditis can develop in people who already have abnormal blood flow through a heart valve as the result of congenital or acquired heart valve disease. The abnormal blood flow causes blood clots to form on the surface of the valve. The blood clots make it easier for germs to attach to and infect the valve.

Infective endocarditis can worsen existing heart valve disease.

Other Conditions and Factors Linked to Heart Valve Disease

Many other conditions and factors are linked to heart valve disease. However, the role they play in causing heart valve disease often is not clear.

- **Autoimmune disorders.** Autoimmune disorders, such as lupus, can affect the aortic and mitral valves.

- **Carcinoid syndrome.** Tumors in the digestive tract that spread to the liver or lymph nodes can affect the tricuspid and pulmonary valves.

- **Diet medicines.** The use of fenfluramine and phentermine sometimes has been linked to heart valve problems. These problems typically stabilize or improve after the medicine is stopped.

- **Marfan syndrome.** Congenital disorders, such as Marfan syndrome and other connective tissue disorders, can affect the heart valves.

- **Metabolic disorders.** Relatively uncommon diseases (such as Fabry disease) and other metabolic disorders (such as high blood cholesterol) can affect the heart valves.

- **Radiation therapy.** Radiation therapy to the chest area can cause heart valve disease. This therapy is used to treat cancer. Heart valve disease due to radiation therapy may not cause symptoms until years after the therapy.

Risk Factors

Older age is a risk factor for heart valve disease. As you age, your heart valves thicken and become stiffer. Also, people are living longer now than in the past. As a result, heart valve disease has become an increasing problem.

People who have a history of infective endocarditis, rheumatic fever, heart attack, or heart failure—or previous heart valve disease—also are at a higher risk for heart valve disease. In addition, having risk factors for IE, such as intravenous drug use, increases the risk of heart valve disease.

You are also at a higher risk for heart valve disease if you have risk factors for coronary heart disease. These risk factors include high blood cholesterol, high blood pressure, smoking, insulin resistance, diabetes, being overweight or obese, lack of physical activity, and a family history of early heart disease.

Some people are born with an aortic valve that has two flaps instead of three. Sometimes, an aortic valve may have three flaps, but two flaps are fused together and act as one flap. This is called a "bicuspid aortic valve" or a "bicommissural aortic valve" (BAV). People who have this congenital condition are more likely to develop aortic heart valve disease.

Screening and Prevention

To prevent heart valve disease caused by rheumatic fever, see your doctor if you have signs of a strep infection. These signs include a painful sore throat, fever, and white spots on your tonsils. If you do have a strep infection, be sure to take all medicines prescribed to treat it. Prompt treatment of strep infections can prevent rheumatic fever, which damages the heart valves.

It is possible that exercise, a heart-healthy diet, and medicines that lower cholesterol might prevent aortic stenosis. Researchers continue to study this possibility.

Heart-healthy eating, physical activity, other heart-healthy lifestyle changes, and medicines aimed at preventing a heart attack, high blood pressure, or heart failure also may help prevent heart valve disease.

Signs, Symptoms, and Complications
Major Signs and Symptoms

The main sign of heart valve disease is an unusual heartbeat sound called a "heart murmur." Your doctor can hear a heart murmur with a stethoscope.

However, many people have heart murmurs without having heart valve disease or any other heart problems. Others may have heart murmurs due to heart valve disease, but they have no other signs or symptoms.

Heart valve disease often worsens over time, so signs and symptoms may occur years after a heart murmur is first heard. Many people who have heart valve disease do not have any symptoms until they are middle-aged or older.

Other common signs and symptoms of heart valve disease relate to heart failure, which heart valve disease can cause. These signs and symptoms include:

- Unusual fatigue (tiredness)

- Shortness of breath, especially when you exert yourself or when you are lying down

- Swelling in your ankles, feet, legs, abdomen, and veins in the neck

Other Signs and Symptoms

Heart valve disease can cause chest pain that may happen only when you exert yourself. You also may notice a fluttering, racing, or irregular heartbeat. Some types of heart valve disease, such as aortic or mitral valve stenosis, can cause dizziness or fainting.

Diagnosis

Your primary care doctor may detect a heart murmur or other signs of heart valve disease. However, a cardiologist usually will diagnose the condition. A cardiologist is a doctor who specializes in diagnosing and treating heart problems.

To diagnose heart valve disease, your doctor will ask about your signs and symptoms. She or he also will do a physical exam and look at the results from tests and procedures.

Physical Exam

Your doctor will listen to your heart with a stethoscope. She or he will want to find out whether you have a heart murmur that is likely caused by a heart valve problem.

Your doctor also will listen to your lungs as you breathe to check for fluid buildup. She or he will check for swollen ankles and other signs that your body is retaining water.

Tests and Procedures

Echocardiography (echo) is the main test for diagnosing heart valve disease. But, an electrocardiogram (EKG) or chest X-ray commonly is used to reveal certain signs of the condition. If these signs are present, an echo usually is done to confirm the diagnosis.

Your doctor also may recommend other tests and procedures if you are diagnosed with heart valve disease. For example, you may have cardiac catheterization, stress testing, or cardiac magnetic resonance imaging (MRI). These tests and procedures help your doctor assess how severe your condition is so she or he can plan your treatment.

Electrocardiogram

An electrocardiogram detects and records the heart's electrical activity. An EKG can detect an irregular heartbeat and signs of a previous heart attack. It also can show whether your heart chambers are enlarged.

An EKG usually is done in a doctor's office.

Chest X-Ray

A chest X-Ray can show whether certain sections of your heart are enlarged, whether you have fluid in your lungs, or whether calcium deposits are present in your heart.

A chest X-ray helps your doctor learn which type of valve defect you have, how severe it is, and whether you have any other heart problems.

Echocardiography

An echo uses sound waves to create a moving picture of your heart as it beats. A device called a "transducer" is placed on the surface of your chest.

The transducer sends sound waves through your chest wall to your heart. Echoes from the sound waves are converted into pictures of your heart on a computer screen.

An echo can show:

- The size and shape of your heart valves and chambers

- How well your heart is pumping blood

- Whether a valve is narrow or has backflow

Your doctor may recommend transesophageal echo, or TEE, to get a better image of your heart.

During a transesophageal echo, the transducer is attached to the end of a flexible tube. The tube is guided down your throat and into your esophagus (the passage leading from your mouth to your stomach). From there, your doctor can get detailed pictures of your heart.

You will likely be given medicine to help you relax during this procedure.

Cardiac Catheterization

For a cardiac catheterization, a long, thin, flexible tube called a "catheter" is put into a blood vessel in your arm, groin (upper thigh), or neck and threaded to your heart. Your doctor uses X-ray images to guide the catheter.

Through the catheter, your doctor does diagnostic tests and imaging that shows whether backflow is occurring through a valve and how fully the valve opens. You will be given medicine to help you relax, but you will be awake during the procedure.

Your doctor may recommend cardiac catheterization if your signs and symptoms of heart valve disease are not in line with your echo results.

The procedure also can help your doctor assess whether your symptoms are due to specific valve problems or coronary heart disease.

Stress Test

During stress testing, you exercise to make your heart work hard and beat fast while heart tests and imaging are done. If you cannot exercise, you may be given medicine to raise your heart rate.

A stress test can show whether you have signs and symptoms of heart valve disease when your heart is working hard. It can help your doctor assess the severity of your heart valve disease.

Cardiac Magnetic Resonance Imaging

Cardiac magnetic resonance imaging uses a powerful magnet and radio waves to make detailed images of your heart. A cardiac MRI image can confirm information about valve defects or provide more detailed information. An MRI also may be done before heart valve surgery to help your surgeon plan for the surgery.

Living with Heart Valve Disease

Heart valve disease is a lifelong condition. However, many people have heart valve defects or disease but do not have symptoms. For some people, the condition mostly stays the same throughout their lives and does not cause any problems.

For other people, the condition slowly worsens until symptoms develop. If not treated, advanced heart valve disease can cause heart failure or other life-threatening conditions.

Eventually, you may need to have your faulty heart valve(s) repaired or replaced. After repair or replacement, you will still need certain medicines and regular checkups with your doctor.

Ongoing Care

If you have heart valve disease, see your doctor regularly for check-ups and for echocardiography or other tests. This will allow your doctor to check the progress of your heart valve disease.

Call your doctor if your symptoms worsen or you have new symptoms. Also, discuss with your doctor whether heart-healthy lifestyle changes might benefit you. Ask her or him which types of physical activity are safe for you.

Call your doctor if you have symptoms of infective endocarditis (IE). Symptoms of this heart infection include fever; chills; muscle aches; night sweats; problems breathing; fatigue (tiredness); weakness; red spots on the palms and soles; and swelling of the feet, legs, and belly.

Take all of your medicines as prescribed.

Pregnancy and Heart Valve Disease

Mild or moderate heart valve disease during pregnancy usually can be managed with medicines or bed rest. With proper care, the disease usually will not pose heightened risks to the mother or fetus.

Doctors can treat most heart valve conditions with medicines that are safe to take during pregnancy. Your doctor can advise you about which medicines are safe for you.

Severe heart valve disease can make pregnancy or labor and delivery risky. If you have severe heart valve disease, consider having your heart valves repaired or replaced before getting pregnant. This treatment also can be done during pregnancy, if needed. However, this surgery poses danger to both the mother and fetus.

Chapter 19

Heart Murmur

What Is Heart Murmur?

A heart murmur is an unusual sound heard between heartbeats. Murmurs sometimes sound similar to a whooshing or swishing noise.

Types of Heart Murmur

Murmurs may be harmless, also called "innocent," or "abnormal."

- Harmless murmurs may not cause symptoms and can happen when blood flows more rapidly than normal through the heart, such as during exercise, pregnancy, or rapid growth in children.

- Abnormal murmurs may be a sign of a more serious heart condition, such as a congenital heart defect that is present since birth or heart valve disease. Depending on the heart problem causing the abnormal murmurs, the murmurs may be associated with other symptoms, such as shortness of breath, dizziness or fainting, bluish skin, or a chronic cough.

What the Doctor Does upon Diagnosing Heart Murmur

If a heart murmur is detected, your doctor will listen to the loudness, location, and timing of your murmur to find out whether it is

This chapter includes text excerpted from "Heart Murmur," National Heart, Lung, and Blood Institute (NHLBI), December 12, 2016.

harmless or a sign of a more serious condition. If your doctor thinks you may have a more serious condition, your doctor may refer you to a cardiologist, or a doctor who specializes in the heart.

The cardiologist may have you do other tests, such as an electrocardiogram (EKG) or echocardiogram, to look for heart rhythm or structural problems and see how well your heart is working.

Treatment for Heart Murmur

A heart murmur itself does not require treatment. If it is caused by a more serious heart condition, your doctor may recommend treatment for that heart condition.

Treatment may include:

- Medicines

- Cardiac catheterization or surgery

The outlook and treatment for abnormal heart murmurs depend on the type and severity of the heart condition that is causing the murmur.

Chapter 20

Infectious Diseases
of the Heart

Chapter Contents

Section 20.1

Endocarditis

Endocarditis is an inflammation of the endocardium, the membrane that lines the inner chambers of the heart. It generally occurs when bacteria or, less commonly, fungi travel through the bloodstream and cause an infection in this lining or in a heart valve. If left untreated, endocarditis can be deadly.

What Causes Endocarditis

Endocarditis is not common in healthy hearts. It occurs most often in a diseased heart or one with damaged valves, in which the roughened tissue can provide an ideal spot for bacteria or other microorganisms to settle, multiply, and cause an infection. Endocarditis can, on occasion, also be caused by fungi, such as Candida.

Microorganisms can enter bloodstream through:

- Regular activities, such as eating or drinking

- Poor oral hygiene or gum disease

- Certain dental procedures

- Using infected needles for body piercings, tattoos, or to inject drugs

- The use of a catheter

- Cuts on skin or infections, such as a skin sore

- Other medical conditions, including sexually transmitted diseases (STDs) and intestinal disorders

What Are the Signs and Symptoms of Endocarditis?

Symptoms of endocarditis differ from person to person and usually develop slowly over a period of time. In the initial stages, they can be similar to the symptoms of many other illnesses, such as pneumonia or flu. Some more severe symptoms can occur suddenly and may result from damage or inflammation in the heart.

Some of the symptoms of endocarditis include:

- Pale skin

- Night sweats

- Fever and chills

- Joint and muscle pain

- Decreased appetite

- A full feeling in the upper left part of the stomach

- Nausea

- Weight loss

- Swollen feet, legs, or stomach

- Shortness of breath

- Cough

- New or changed heart murmur

- Enlarged spleen, which may be tender to touch

- Blood in urine

    Endocarditis may also cause changes to the skin, such as:

- Red or purple spots under or on fingers or toes

- Broken blood vessels that appear as red spots, called "petechiae," usually found on the whites of the eyes, inside the mouth, or on the chest

These symptoms depend on what causes the infection and whether there are any other underlying heart problems. A person with previous heart surgery or with a history of endocarditis or other heart issues should contact a doctor immediately if any of these symptoms occur, especially if they last for more than three days or if the person feels unusually tired.

What Are the Risk Factors for Endocarditis?

The following are some of the risk factors for developing endocarditis:

- Past history of endocarditis

- Certain types of heart defects, such as congenital defects

- Scarring of a heart valve caused by certain medical conditions, such as rheumatic fever

- Artificial heart valve or pacemaker

- Human immunodeficiency virus (HIV)

- Use of needles to inject drugs, or for tattoos or body piercings

What Are the Complications Associated with Endocarditis?

Endocarditis can lead to numerous complications, including:

- Scarred or otherwise damaged heart valves

- Abnormal heart rhythm, such as atrial fibrillation (AF)

- Blood clots that may travel to the lungs or other parts of the body

- Jaundice, a yellowing of the skin and whites of the eyes

- Stroke or organ damage, often caused by clumps of bacteria and cell fragments that travel to the brain and other organs

- Abscesses (collection of pus) in other parts of body, including the brain, liver, spleen or kidneys

- Heart failure, especially when endocarditis is left untreated, causing the heart to work harder to pump blood

How Is Endocarditis Diagnosed?

A review of medical history and physical signs and symptoms, such as fever, will help the doctor diagnose endocarditis. A change in heart murmur, identified using a stethoscope, is another possible sign of the condition.

Some of the following tests may also be requested to make the diagnosis:

- A blood test will confirm the presence of bacteria, fungi, or other organisms that could cause endocarditis. It can also reveal if other conditions, such as anemia, are causing the infection.

- An echocardiogram, which creates an image of the heart using ultrasound waves, can be used by the doctor to spot signs of damage or abnormal movements in the heart.

- A transesophageal echocardiogram provides another image of the heart by means of an ultrasound device passed through the throat into the esophagus.

- If the doctor thinks that an irregular heartbeat is caused by endocarditis, an electrocardiogram may be ordered to analyze electrical activity of the heart.

- A chest X-ray will help reveal the condition of the heart and lungs, allowing the doctor to determine whether the infection has caused enlargement of the heart or if it has spread to the lungs. X-ray images also help differentiate between endocarditis and a collapsed lung.

- The doctor may order a magnetic resonance imaging (MRI) or computerized tomography (CT) scan of other parts of the body, such as the brain or chest, to see if infection has spread to those areas.

How Is Endocarditis Treated?

Endocarditis is usually treated with antibiotics, and in some cases, in which the infection has damaged the heart valves or caused complications, surgery may be required.

Antibiotics

Antibiotics are prescribed if endocarditis is caused by a bacterial infection. This treatment would continue until the infection subsides, which may take up to six weeks. In some cases, hospitalization may be required so that high doses of intravenous (IV) antibiotics can be administered until the worst of the symptoms have passed.

Surgery

Surgery to treat endocarditis may be required if the heart valves are damaged because of the infection or if the infection persists. The valve may either be repaired or replaced with an artificial valve that is made of animal tissue or synthetic materials. Surgery is sometimes also required if a fungal infection caused the endocarditis, since this is more difficult to treat than a bacterial infection.

How Can Endocarditis Be Prevented?

To prevent endocarditis:

- It is important to practice good oral hygiene to eliminate some of the germs in the mouth. Brush and floss teeth and gums often, and have regular dental checkups.

- Watch out for symptoms of endocarditis, such as unexplained fatigue and fever, especially if there is a history of endocarditis, heart disease, or heart surgery.

- Avoid procedures that may allow transfer of germs to the bloodstream, such as tattooing, body piercing, or IV drug use.

- Seek immediate medical attention if any skin infection develops or if open sores or cuts do not heal properly.

- If antibiotics have been prescribed by a doctor after certain dental or medical procedures, the medication should be taken exactly as directed. Preventive antibiotics may be required for:

  - Previous endocarditis infection

  - Certain heart surgery procedures

  - Artificial heart valve surgery

  - Certain types of congenital heart defects

  - Procedures that involve the respiratory tract, infected skin, or tissue connecting muscle to bone

References

1. Sullivan, Debra Henline. "Endocarditis," Healthline, January 28, 2016.

2. "Endocarditis," Mayo Clinic, June 14, 2014.

Section 20.2

Myocarditis

"Myocarditis," © 2016 Omnigraphics. Reviewed May 2019.

Myocarditis is a disease characterized by inflammation of the heart muscle, called the "myocardium." It is estimated to affect thousands of Americans each year and is caused by a wide variety of factors, including viral and bacterial infections, environmental toxins, autoimmune diseases, and allergic reactions to certain toxins and medications. Myocarditis often produces no symptoms, and because it is relatively uncommon, the best ways to diagnose and treat the condition are still being studied. It usually affects people who are otherwise healthy, including a significant number of young adults. The best way to prevent myocarditis is by seeking immediate medical attention for infections.

What Causes Myocarditis

Myocarditis is primarily caused by viral infections, the most common among them being those that affect the upper respiratory tract. Other less common causes include contagious infections, such as Lyme disease.

Some of the viral infections that can cause myocarditis include hepatitis C, herpes, human immunodeficiency virus (HIV), and parvovirus. Bacterial infections that can lead to myocarditis include chlamydia (a common sexually transmitted disease (STD)), streptococcus (strep), staphylococcus (staph), mycoplasma (bacteria that cause a lung infection), and treponema (the cause of syphilis). The condition can also be brought on by such factors as allergic reactions to certain medicines and toxins, such as drugs, alcohol, spider or snake bites, wasp stings, lead, radiation, and chemotherapy.

Myocarditis can also be caused by autoimmune diseases (in which the immune system attacks the body), such as lupus or rheumatoid arthritis (RA).

What Are the Signs and Symptoms of Myocarditis?

Some of the symptoms of myocarditis include:

- Shortness of breath during exercise, which may also lead to breathing troubles at night
- Irregular heartbeat and, in some cases, fainting
- Heart palpitations
- Light-headedness
- Sharp or stabbing chest pain or pressure
- Fatigue

- Swelling in joints, the legs, or neck veins

- Indications of infection, such as fever, sore throat, muscle aches, headache, or diarrhea

These symptoms often follow a respiratory infection, and if they do occur, it is important to seek medical attention promptly.

What Are the Complications of Myocarditis?

Not treating myocarditis can cause the heart to work harder to pump blood. This can lead to symptoms of heart failure and in serious cases, it may be fatal. Cardiomyopathy and pericarditis are other possible complications of this infection, both of which are leading causes of heart transplants in the United States. Cardiomyopathy is an increase in size, thickness, or rigidity of the heart muscle. Pericarditis is the inflammation of pericardium, or the sac covering the heart.

How Is Myocarditis Diagnosed?

In many cases, myocarditis has no symptoms and is not diagnosed. However, when there are symptoms, the doctor will conduct a physical exam to check for abnormal heartbeat, fluid in the lungs, or swelling in the legs. Some of the following tests may also be conducted:

- A blood test to analyze blood cell count and check for infection or antibodies

- An electrocardiogram to evaluate the electrical activity of the heart

- A chest X-ray to study the shape and size of the heart

- An echocardiogram to inspect the structure of the heart and to measure blood flow

- Occasionally, a cardiac magnetic resonance imaging (MRI) scan or a heart biopsy may be performed to confirm the diagnosis

How Is Myocarditis Treated?

When a person has myocarditis, treatment will be provided for its underlying cause. This will typically include medication to take the load off the heart, improve heart function, and prevent or control further complications.

In the presence of an abnormal heart rhythm, additional treatment, such as a pacemaker or defibrillator, could be required. Hospitalization may be necessary in case of serious complications, such as a blood clots or a weakened heart. Angiotensin-converting enzyme (ACE) inhibitors, calcium channel blockers, and diuretics are some medicines that may be prescribed to help the heart function better. Steroids and other medications may also be used to treat heart inflammation. Often, reduced physical activity for at least six months, rest, and a low-salt diet are recommended.

The cause of myocarditis, overall health of the person, and complications, if any, determine the outlook. The infected person could either recover completely or develop a chronic condition. There is a small possibility that myocarditis may recur and could, in rare cases, lead to dilated cardiomyopathy, an enlargement and weakening of the ventricles, the heart's pumping chambers.

References

1. "Discover Myocarditis Causes, Symptoms, Diagnosis and Treatment," Myocarditis Foundation, n.d.

2. Beckerman, James, "Myocarditis," WebMD, July 14, 2014.

Section 20.3

Pericarditis

Pericarditis is the swelling and irritation that occurs on the thin sac-like membrane, called the "pericardium," that surrounds the heart. It is characterized by symptoms such as sharp chest pains that occur when inflamed layers of the pericardium brush against each other.

When pericarditis is acute, it usually develops suddenly and may last for a few months. It is considered chronic when the symptoms appear more gradually or persist for a longer period of time. In some cases, excess fluid builds up in the space between the pericardial layers, resulting in pericardial effusion, which can affect heart function.

Most cases of pericarditis are mild, and improvement occurs gradually. For more severe cases, medication and, rarely, surgery will be needed. Risks of long-term complications can be reduced by diagnosing and treating the condition in its early stages.

What Causes Pericarditis

It is often difficult to determine what causes pericarditis. When the cause is unknown, it is called "idiopathic pericarditis." In most cases, it occurs due to one of the following causes:

- Infections that are viral, bacterial, fungal, or parasitic in nature

- Traumatic events that caused injury to the chest

- Health complications, such as kidney failure; tumors; acquired immunodeficiency syndrome (AIDS), tuberculosis; or genetic diseases, such as familial Mediterranean fever (FMF)

- Autoimmune diseases, such as lupus, rheumatoid arthritis (RA), and scleroderma

- Dressler's syndrome, in which pericarditis can occur a few weeks after a major heart attack or heart surgery

- Procedures, such as radiation therapy or those performed through the skin, such as radiofrequency ablation (RFA) or cardiac catheterization

- In rare cases, certain medications that suppress the immune system

What Are the Signs and Symptoms of Pericarditis?

Symptoms of acute pericarditis include:

- A sharp, stabbing chest pain that increases when coughing, swallowing, or breathing deeply

- Pain in the shoulder and neck that spreads from the chest

- Trouble breathing when lying down

- Dry cough

- Fatigue

- Heart palpitations

- Swelling in the feet, legs, ankles, or abdomen (a symptom of constrictive pericarditis)

Chronic pericarditis is characterized by continued inflammation that sometimes results in fluid buildup around the heart (pericardial effusion), and chest pain is the most common symptom.

Also called "recurrent pericarditis," chronic pericarditis often results from autoimmune disorders. The attacks can extend over a long period of time and are of two types. The incessant type occurs within six weeks of discontinuing treatment for acute infection, while the intermittent type occurs after six weeks.

Since most symptoms mimic those of other lung and heart conditions, it is important to consult a doctor as soon as symptoms of pericarditis develop. This enables proper diagnosis and treatment and could possibly help identify other health problems as well. If not treated, pericarditis can lead to fatal conditions, such as cardiac tamponade, which compresses the heart so much that it affects its functioning.

What Are the Complications of Pericarditis?

Constrictive pericarditis is a severe condition in people with long-term inflammation and chronic recurrent episodes. It is characterized by stiff, thickened pericardial layers, which make the pericardium less elastic and restrict the heart from expanding as it normally would when filling up with blood. Eventually, the condition results in symptoms of heart failure, such as swelling of the heart, feet, or legs; labored breathing; water retention; and an abnormal heartbeat. These symptoms should improve when constrictive pericarditis is treated.

Pericardial effusion is a condition that occurs when excess fluid builds up in the space between the two pericardial layers. When fluid accumulates rapidly, it leads to cardiac tamponade—a severe compression of the heart that affects its normal functioning and causes a sudden drop in blood pressure. This is a life-threatening condition that requires immediate removal of the fluid using a catheter.

How Is Pericarditis Diagnosed?

Diagnosis of pericarditis begins with an evaluation of the patient's medical history and symptoms, such as chest pain and difficulty breathing. Other risks of pericarditis, including recent viral illnesses; diseases, such as lupus or kidney failure; and previous heart disease or surgery are also analyzed. This is followed by a physical exam in which the doctor places a stethoscope on the chest to listen for such signs as pericardial rub (noise made when affected pericardial layers rub against each other), excess fluid in the pericardial sac, or indications of fluid in the space around lungs.

Some of the diagnostic procedures that may be required are:

- Blood tests to determine whether viral, bacterial, or other types of infections are present

- Chest X-rays to check for enlargement of the heart or congestion in the lungs

- An electrocardiogram to measure electrical impulses and identify changes in the normal rhythm of the heart

- An echocardiogram to analyze signs of constrictive pericarditis or pericardial effusion

- Cardiac magnetic resonance imaging (MRI) and computerized tomography (CT) scans to reveal abnormal changes in the pericardium and to exclude other causes of acute chest pain

- Cardiac catheterization to study the pressure and flow of blood and confirm diagnosis of constrictive pericarditis

- Other laboratory tests to assess heart function, which may include testing for autoimmune diseases and examining the fluid in the pericardium to evaluate sedimentation rate (ESR) and C-reactive protein levels

How Is Pericarditis Treated?

Treatment for pericarditis depends on what causes it and its severity. Mild cases of pericarditis may not require any treatment.

Medication for acute pericarditis typically includes over-the-counter pain relievers and nonsteroidal anti-inflammatory drugs to reduce pain and inflammation and to prevent the infection from recurring weeks or months later. The small number of patients who develop chronic pericarditis may need to take these medications for a number of years.

Frequent follow-up care to assess changes in liver and kidney function may be required for people taking high doses of nonsteroidal anti-inflammatory drugs (NSAIDs). Antibiotics or antifungal medication may be prescribed depending on what causes the infection. Previously, steroids were prescribed to prevent infection from recurring, but in some cases, these caused dependency on the medication to prevent recurrence.

For most people, pericarditis does not usually require surgery. In the case of cardiac tamponade, a procedure called "pericardiocentesis" will be required to drain excess fluid by means of a needle and catheter. A surgical procedure called "pericardial window" is performed if the fluid cannot be drained using the needle. In severe cases, such as constrictive pericarditis, the doctor might suggest a surgical procedure called "pericardiectomy" to surgically remove a portion of the pericardium that has thickened and affects the normal functioning of the heart.

References

1. "Pericarditis," Cleveland Clinic, n.d.

2. "Pericarditis," Mayo Clinic, April 6, 2014.

Chapter 21

Cardiac Tumors

Cardiac tumors are abnormal growths that occur within the heart, heart valves, or lining of the heart. Primary heart tumors originate in the heart, while secondary or metastatic heart tumors develop elsewhere in the body and spread to the heart. Primary tumors are usually noncancerous (benign), while metastatic tumors are always cancerous (malignant). Although cardiac tumors are rare, the condition can be serious or even fatal.

Types of Cardiac Tumors

Primary cardiac tumors are quite rare, occurring an estimated once in every 2,000 people. Yet, there are many different types—including some that are noncancerous and some that are cancerous—that grow in different parts of the heart. Some of the recognized types of primary cardiac tumors include the following:

- **Myxoma** is the most common type, accounting for about half of all noncancerous primary heart tumors in adults, although it can affect people of any age. It occurs most frequently at the atrial septum, which divides the 2 upper chambers of the heart. Inherited genetic conditions, such as Carney complex, cause around 10 percent of myxomas.

- **Rhabdomyoma** is the most common type of noncancerous primary cardiac tumor in infants and children. These tumors

"Cardiac Tumors," © 2016 Omnigraphics. Reviewed May 2019.

237

usually develop within the heart wall from the heart's muscle cells, and they most often occur in groups.

- **Fibromas** also primarily appear in infants and children. These noncancerous primary tumors typically affect the heart valves and develop from the heart's fibrous tissue cells.

- **Lipomas** are noncancerous tumors that can grow in the lining of the heart chambers, on the heart wall, or on the outer surface of the heart.

- **Papillary fibroelastoma** is a benign primary tumor that grows on the heart valves.

- **Paraganglioma and teratoma** are benign tumors that occur where the major blood vessels attach at the base of the heart.

- **Pericardial cysts** are noncancerous primary growths that affect the pericardium membrane that covers the heart.

- **Sarcomas** are the most common type of cancerous primary heart tumor, ranking second only to myxoma in overall prevalence. They tend to develop in the right or left atrium, where they can block blood flow through the heart or spread to the lungs.

- **Mesothelioma** is a type of cancerous primary heart tumor that can develop in the pericardium and spread to the spine or brain.

- **Primary lymphoma**, or cancer of the white blood cells (WBCs), occasionally develops in the hearts of people who have acquired immune deficiency syndrome (AIDS).

- **Secondary cardiac tumors** are cancerous growths that develop in the lungs, breasts, kidneys, liver, blood, or skin and then spread to the heart. Although they are rare, they are between 30 and 40 times more common than primary heart tumors.

Symptoms of Cardiac Tumors

The symptoms of cardiac tumors vary widely depending on the tumor's location, size, and the extent to which it impedes blood flow through the heart. Some people experience no symptoms at all, and their tumors are only discovered when they undergo an echocardiogram or chest X-ray for another reason. Some patients have minor symptoms such as:

- Light-headedness
- Shortness of breath
- Fatigue
- Joint pain or inflammation
- Unexplained fever
- Small red spots on the skin

Some people with cardiac tumors may experience these symptoms only when they are in a certain physical position—such as standing up or lying down—that causes the tumor to block blood flow.

Around half of people with tumors on a heart valve will develop a heart murmur due to restricted blood flow through the valve. Finally, some patients with cardiac tumors present with symptoms of severe heart malfunction, such as abnormal heart rhythms, extremely low blood pressure (hypotension), or heart failure.

Diagnosis of Cardiac Tumors

Diagnosing primary heart tumors can be difficult because they are relatively rare. In addition, the symptoms vary widely and often resemble those of other health conditions. Doctors are more likely to suspect secondary heart tumors in cancer patients who begin experiencing heart problems.

The diagnosis of a cardiac tumor is typically confirmed through an echocardiogram, which involves using ultrasound to produce an image of the heart. Doctors may seek additional information about the tumor by using a computed tomography (CT) scan, magnetic resonance imaging (MRI), or radionuclide imaging. Since imaging results usually enable doctors to determine whether cardiac tumors are benign or malignant, heart biopsies are seldom performed.

Risks of Cardiac Tumors

Diagnosing primary heart tumors can be difficult because they are relatively rare. In addition, the symptoms vary widely and often resemble those of other health conditions. Doctors are more likely to suspect secondary heart tumors in cancer patients who begin experiencing heart problems.

The diagnosis of a cardiac tumor is typically confirmed through an echocardiogram, which involves using ultrasound to produce an image of the heart. Doctors may seek additional information about the tumor by using a computed tomography (CT) scan, magnetic resonance imaging (MRI), or radionuclide imaging. Since imaging results usually enable doctors to determine whether cardiac tumors are benign or malignant, heart biopsies are seldom performed.

Treatment of Cardiac Tumors

The treatment of primary cardiac tumors depends on their size and type, as well as the patient's symptoms and overall health. Small, noncancerous tumors that do not impede blood flow may not require treatment. Infants born with rhabdomyomas, for instance, usually do not need treatment. About half of these tumors regress on their own, while those that remain in place seldom grow any larger.

The preferred treatment for noncancerous primary heart tumors is surgical removal. Although removal often requires complicated open-heart surgery, it can sometimes be performed robotically or through minimally invasive techniques. The patient typically must spend several days in the hospital, followed by several weeks in recovery. Follow-up treatment includes an annual echocardiogram to ensure that the tumor does not return and that no new growths appear.

In cases where a noncancerous primary heart tumor is large, blocks blood flow, or grows into the surrounding tissue, heart transplantation may be the only surgical option available. However, this procedure is performed only in rare circumstances.

Surgery is not an option for primary cancerous heart tumors because they have usually already spread to other parts of the body. Such tumors are usually fatal, although chemotherapy or radiation therapy may help slow the progression of disease. These treatment options may also be used for metastatic cardiac tumors, depending on the type of cancer and the other organs affected.

References

1. "Cardiac Tumors," Cleveland Clinic, 2016.

2. Howlett, Jonathan G. "Overview of Heart Tumors," Merck and Co., Inc., n.d.

Part Three

Blood Vessel Disorders

Chapter 22

Atherosclerosis

What Is Atherosclerosis?

Atherosclerosis is a disease in which plaque builds up inside your arteries. Arteries are blood vessels that carry oxygen-rich blood to your heart and other parts of your body.

Plaque is made up of fat, cholesterol, calcium, and other substances found in the blood. Over time, plaque hardens and narrows your arteries. This limits the flow of oxygen-rich blood to your organs and to other parts of your body.

Atherosclerosis can lead to serious problems, including heart attack, stroke, or even death.

Atherosclerosis-Related Diseases

Atherosclerosis can affect any artery in the body, including arteries in the heart, brain, arms, legs, pelvis, and kidneys. As a result, different diseases may develop based on which arteries are affected.

Ischemic Heart Disease

Ischemic heart disease occurs when the arteries of the heart cannot deliver enough oxygen-rich blood to the tissues of the heart when needed during periods of stress or physical effort.

This chapter includes text excerpted from "Atherosclerosis," National Heart, Lung, and Blood Institute (NHLBI), February 5, 2019.

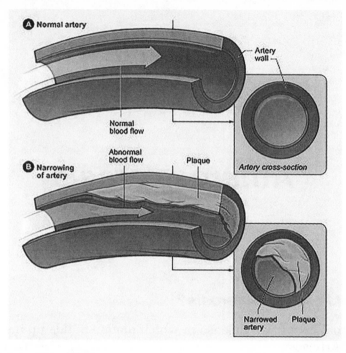

Figure 22.1. *Atherosclerosis*

Figure A shows a normal artery with normal blood flow. The inset image shows a cross-section of a normal artery. Figure B shows an artery with plaque buildup. The inset image shows a cross-section of an artery with plaque buildup.

Coronary heart disease (CHD), also called "coronary artery disease," is a type of ischemic heart disease caused by the buildup of plaque in the coronary arteries that supply oxygen-rich blood to your heart.

This buildup can partially or totally block blood flow in the large arteries of the heart. If blood flow to your heart muscle is reduced or blocked, you may have angina (chest pain or discomfort) or a heart attack.

Coronary microvascular disease (MVD) is another type of ischemic heart disease. It occurs when the heart's tiny arteries do not function normally.

Carotid Artery Disease

Carotid artery disease occurs if plaque builds up in the arteries on each side of your neck (the carotid arteries). These arteries supply oxygen-rich blood to your brain. If blood flow to your brain is reduced or blocked, you may have a stroke.

Peripheral Artery Disease

Peripheral artery disease (PAD) occurs if plaque builds up in the major arteries that supply oxygen-rich blood to your legs, arms, and pelvis.

If blood flow to these parts of your body is reduced or blocked, you may have numbness, pain, and, sometimes, dangerous infections.

Chronic Kidney Disease

Chronic kidney disease (CKD) can occur if plaque builds up in the renal arteries. These arteries supply oxygen-rich blood to your kidneys.

Over time, chronic kidney disease causes a slow loss of kidney function. The main function of the kidneys is to remove waste and extra water from the body.

Causes of Atherosclerosis

The exact cause of atherosclerosis is not known. However, studies show that atherosclerosis is a slow, complex disease that may start in childhood. It develops faster as you age.

Atherosclerosis may start when certain factors damage the inner layers of the arteries. These factors include:

- Smoking

- High amounts of certain fats and cholesterol in the blood

- High blood pressure

- High amounts of sugar in the blood due to insulin resistance or diabetes

Plaque may begin to build up where the arteries are damaged. Over time, plaque hardens and narrows the arteries. Eventually, an area of plaque can rupture.

When this happens, blood cell fragments called "platelets" stick to the site of the injury. They may clump together to form blood clots. Clots narrow the arteries even more, limiting the flow of oxygen-rich blood to your body.

Depending on which arteries are affected, blood clots can worsen angina or cause a heart attack or stroke.

Researchers continue to look for the causes of atherosclerosis. They hope to find answers to questions, such as:

- Why and how do the arteries become damaged?

- How does plaque develop and change over time?

- Why does plaque rupture and lead to blood clots?

Risk Factors for Atherosclerosis

The exact cause of atherosclerosis is not known. However, certain traits, conditions, or habits may raise your risk for the disease. These conditions are known as "risk factors." The more risk factors you have, the more likely it is that you will develop atherosclerosis.

You can control most risk factors and help prevent or delay atherosclerosis. Other risk factors cannot be controlled.

Major Risk Factors

- **Unhealthy blood cholesterol levels.** This includes high low-density lipoprotein (LDL) cholesterol (sometimes called "bad" cholesterol) and low high-density lipoprotein (HDL) cholesterol (sometimes called "good" cholesterol).

- **High blood pressure.** Blood pressure is considered high if it stays at or above 140/90 mmHg over time. If you have diabetes or chronic kidney disease, high blood pressure is defined as 130/80 mmHg or higher. (The mmHg is millimeters of mercury— the units used to measure blood pressure.)

- **Smoking.** Smoking can damage and tighten blood vessels, raise cholesterol levels, and raise blood pressure. Smoking also does not allow enough oxygen to reach the body's tissues.

- **Insulin resistance.** This condition occurs if the body cannot use its insulin properly. Insulin is a hormone that helps move blood sugar into cells, where it is used as an energy source. Insulin resistance may lead to diabetes.

- **Diabetes.** With this disease, the body's blood sugar level is too high because the body does not make enough insulin or does not use its insulin properly.

- **Overweight or obesity.** The terms "overweight" and "obesity" refer to body weight that is greater than what is considered healthy for a certain height.

- **Lack of physical activity.** A lack of physical activity can worsen other risk factors for atherosclerosis, such as unhealthy blood cholesterol levels, high blood pressure, diabetes, and overweight and obesity.

- **Unhealthy diet.** An unhealthy diet can raise your risk for atherosclerosis. Foods that are high in saturated and *trans* fats, cholesterol, sodium (salt), and sugar can worsen other atherosclerosis risk factors.

- **Older age.** As you get older, your risk for atherosclerosis increases. Genetic or lifestyle factors cause plaque to build up in your arteries as you age. By the time you are middle-aged or older, enough plaque has built up to cause signs or symptoms. In men, the risk increases after the age of 45. In women, the risk increases after the age of 55.

- **Family history of early heart disease.** Your risk for atherosclerosis increases if your father or a brother was diagnosed with heart disease before 55 years of age, or if your mother or a sister was diagnosed with heart disease before 65 years of age.

Although age and a family history of early heart disease are risk factors, it does not mean that you will develop atherosclerosis if you have one or both. Controlling other risk factors often can lessen genetic influences and prevent atherosclerosis, even in older adults.

Studies show that an increasing number of children and youth are at risk for atherosclerosis. This is due to a number of causes, including rising childhood obesity rates.

Emerging Risk Factors

Scientists continue to study other possible risk factors for atherosclerosis.

High levels of a protein called "C-reactive protein" (CRP) in the blood may raise the risk for atherosclerosis and heart attack. High levels of CRP are a sign of inflammation in the body.

Inflammation is the body's response to injury or infection. Damage to the arteries' inner walls seems to trigger inflammation and help plaque grow.

People who have low CRP levels may develop atherosclerosis at a slower rate than people who have high CRP levels. Research is under-way to find out whether reducing inflammation and lowering CRP levels also can reduce the risk for atherosclerosis.

High levels of triglycerides in the blood also may raise the risk for atherosclerosis, especially in women. Triglycerides are a type of fat.

Studies are underway to find out whether genetics may play a role in atherosclerosis risk.

Other Factors That Affect Atherosclerosis

Other factors also may raise your risk for atherosclerosis, such as:

- **Sleep apnea.** Sleep apnea is a disorder that causes one or more pauses in breathing or shallow breaths while you sleep. Untreated sleep apnea can raise your risk for high blood pressure, diabetes, and even a heart attack or stroke.

- **Stress.** Research shows that the most commonly reported "trigger" for a heart attack is an emotionally upsetting event, especially one involving anger.

- **Alcohol.** Heavy drinking can damage the heart muscle and worsen other risk factors for atherosclerosis. Men should have no more than two drinks containing alcohol a day. Women should have no more than one drink containing alcohol a day.

Screening and Prevention of Atherosclerosis

Taking action to control your risk factors can help prevent or delay atherosclerosis and its related diseases. Your risk for atherosclerosis increases with the number of risk factors you have.

One step you can take is to adopt a healthy lifestyle, which can include:

Heart-healthy eating. Adopt heart-healthy eating habits, which include eating different fruits and vegetables (including beans and peas), whole grains, lean meats, poultry without skin, seafood, and fat-free or low-fat milk and dairy products. A heart-healthy diet is low in sodium, added sugar, solid fats, and refined grains. Following a heart-healthy diet is an important part of a healthy lifestyle.

Physical activity. Be as physically active as you can. Physical activity can improve your fitness level and your health. Ask your doctor what types and amounts of activity are safe for you.

Quit smoking. If you smoke, quit. Smoking can damage and tighten blood vessels and raise your risk for atherosclerosis. Talk with your doctor about programs and products that can help you quit. Also, try to avoid secondhand smoke.

Weight control. If you are overweight or obese, work with your doctor to create a reasonable weight-loss plan. Controlling your weight helps you control risk factors for atherosclerosis.

Other steps that can prevent or delay atherosclerosis include knowing your family history of atherosclerosis. If you or someone in your family has an atherosclerosis-related disease, be sure to tell your doctor.

If lifestyle changes are not enough, your doctor may prescribe medicines to control your atherosclerosis risk factors. Take all of your medicines as your doctor advises.

Signs, Symptoms, and Complications of Atherosclerosis

Atherosclerosis usually does not cause signs and symptoms until it severely narrows or totally blocks an artery. Many people do not know they have the disease until they have a medical emergency, such as a heart attack or stroke.

Some people may have signs and symptoms of the disease. Signs and symptoms will depend on which arteries are affected.

Coronary Arteries

The coronary arteries supply oxygen-rich blood to your heart. If plaque narrows or blocks these arteries (causing ischemic heart disease), a common symptom is angina. Angina is chest pain or discomfort that occurs when your heart muscle does not get enough oxygen-rich blood.

Angina may feel like pressure or squeezing in your chest. You also may feel it in your shoulders, arms, neck, jaw, or back. Angina pain may even feel like indigestion. The pain tends to get worse with activity and go away with rest. Emotional stress also can trigger the pain.

Other symptoms of ischemic heart disease are shortness of breath and arrhythmias. Arrhythmias are problems with the rate or rhythm of the heartbeat.

Plaque also can form in the heart's smallest arteries. This disease is called "coronary microvascular disease" (MVD). Symptoms of coronary MVD include angina, shortness of breath, sleep problems, fatigue (tiredness), and lack of energy.

Carotid Arteries

The carotid arteries supply oxygen-rich blood to your brain. If plaque narrows or blocks these arteries, you may have symptoms of a stroke. These symptoms may include:

- Sudden weakness

- Paralysis (an inability to move) or numbness of the face, arms, or legs, especially on one side of the body

- Confusion

- Trouble speaking or understanding speech

- Trouble seeing in one or both eyes

- Problems breathing

- Dizziness, trouble walking, loss of balance or coordination, and unexplained falls

- Loss of consciousness

- Sudden and severe headache

Peripheral Arteries

Plaque also can build up in the major arteries that supply oxygen-rich blood to the legs, arms, and pelvis, causing peripheral artery disease.

If these major arteries are narrowed or blocked, you may have numbness, pain, and, sometimes, dangerous infections.

Renal Arteries

The renal arteries supply oxygen-rich blood to your kidneys. If plaque builds up in these arteries, you may develop chronic kidney disease. Over time, chronic kidney disease causes a slow loss of kidney function.

Early kidney disease often has no signs or symptoms. As the disease gets worse, it can cause tiredness, changes in how you urinate (more often or less often), loss of appetite, nausea (feeling sick to the stomach), swelling in the hands or feet, itchiness or numbness, and trouble concentrating.

Diagnosis of Atherosclerosis

Your doctor will diagnose atherosclerosis based on your medical and family histories, a physical exam, and test results.

Specialists Involved

If you have atherosclerosis, a primary care doctor, such as an internist or family practitioner, may handle your care. Your doctor may recommend other healthcare specialists if you need expert care, such as:

- **A cardiologist.** This is a doctor who specializes in diagnosing and treating heart diseases and conditions. You may go to a cardiologist if you have peripheral artery disease or coronary MVD.

- **A vascular specialist.** This is a doctor who specializes in diagnosing and treating blood vessel problems. You may go to a vascular specialist if you have PAD.

- **A neurologist.** This is a doctor who specializes in diagnosing and treating nervous system disorders. You may see a neurologist if you have had a stroke due to carotid artery disease.

- **A nephrologist.** This is a doctor who specializes in diagnosing and treating kidney diseases and conditions. You may go to a nephrologist if you have chronic kidney disease.

Physical Exam

During the physical exam, your doctor may listen to your arteries for an abnormal whooshing sound called a "bruit." Your doctor can hear a bruit when placing a stethoscope over an affected artery. A bruit may indicate poor blood flow due to plaque buildup.

Your doctor also may check to see whether any of your pulses (for example, in the leg or foot) are weak or absent. A weak or absent pulse can be a sign of a blocked artery.

Diagnostic Tests

Your doctor may recommend one or more tests to diagnose atherosclerosis. These tests also can help your doctor learn the extent of your disease and plan the best treatment.

Blood Tests

Blood tests check the levels of certain fats, cholesterol, sugar, and proteins in your blood. Abnormal levels may be a sign that you are at risk for atherosclerosis.

Electrocardiogram

An electrocardiogram (EKG) is a simple, painless test that detects and records the heart's electrical activity. The test shows how fast the heart is beating and its rhythm (steady or irregular). An EKG also records the strength and timing of electrical signals as they pass through the heart.

An EKG can show signs of heart damage caused by congenital heart disease. The test also can show signs of a previous or current heart attack.

Chest X-Ray

A chest X-ray takes pictures of the organs and structures inside your chest, such as your heart, lungs, and blood vessels. A chest X-ray can reveal signs of heart failure.

This test compares the blood pressure in your ankle with the blood pressure in your arm to see how well your blood is flowing. This test can help diagnose PAD.

Echocardiography

An echocardiography (echo) uses sound waves to create a moving picture of your heart. The test provides information about the size and shape of your heart and how well your heart chambers and valves are working.

An echo also can identify areas of poor blood flow to the heart, areas of heart muscle that are not contracting normally, and previous injury to the heart muscle caused by poor blood flow.

Computed Tomography Scan

A computed tomography (CT) scan creates computer-generated pictures of the heart, brain, or other areas of the body. The test can show hardening and narrowing of large arteries.

A cardiac CT scan also can show whether calcium has built up in the walls of the coronary (heart) arteries. This may be an early sign of CHD.

Stress Testing

During stress testing, you exercise to make your heart work hard and beat fast while heart tests are done. If you cannot exercise, you may be given medicine to make your heart work hard and beat fast.

When your heart is working hard, it needs more blood and oxygen. Plaque-narrowed arteries cannot supply enough oxygen-rich blood to meet your heart's needs.

A stress test can show possible signs and symptoms of CHD, such as:

- Abnormal changes in your heart rate or blood pressure

- Shortness of breath or chest pain

- Abnormal changes in your heart rhythm or your heart's electrical activity

As part of some stress tests, pictures are taken of your heart while you exercise and while you rest. These imaging stress tests can show how well blood is flowing in various parts of your heart. They also can show how well your heart pumps blood when it beats.

Angiography

Angiography is a test that uses dye and special X-rays to show the inside of your arteries. This test can show whether plaque is blocking your arteries and how severe the blockage is.

A thin, flexible tube called a "catheter" is put into a blood vessel in your arm, groin (upper thigh), or neck. A dye that can be seen on an X-ray picture is injected through the catheter into the arteries. By looking at the X-ray picture, your doctor can see the flow of blood through your arteries.

Other Tests

Other tests are being studied to see whether they can give a better view of plaque buildup in the arteries. Examples of these tests include magnetic resonance imaging (MRI) and positron emission tomography (PET).

Treatment of Atherosclerosis

Treatments for atherosclerosis may include heart-healthy lifestyle changes, medicines, and medical procedures or surgery. The goals of treatment include:

- Lowering the risk of blood clots forming
- Preventing atherosclerosis-related diseases
- Reducing risk factors in an effort to slow or stop the buildup of plaque
- Relieving symptoms
- Widening or bypassing plaque-clogged arteries

Heart-Healthy Lifestyle Changes

Your doctor may recommend heart-healthy lifestyle changes if you have atherosclerosis. Heart-healthy lifestyle changes include heart-healthy eating, aiming for a healthy weight, managing stress, physical activity and quitting smoking.

Medicines

Sometimes, lifestyle changes alone are not enough to control your cholesterol levels. For example, you also may need statin medications to control or lower your cholesterol. By lowering your blood cholesterol level, you can decrease your chance of having a heart attack or stroke. Doctors usually prescribe statins for people who have:

- Coronary heart disease, peripheral artery disease (PAD), or had a prior stroke
- Diabetes
- High LDL cholesterol levels

Doctors may discuss beginning statin treatment with people who have an elevated risk for developing heart disease or having a stroke. Your doctor also may prescribe other medications to:

- Lower your blood pressure
- Lower your blood sugar levels
- Prevent blood clots, which can lead to heart attack and stroke
- Prevent inflammation

Take all medicines regularly, as your doctor prescribes. Do not change the amount of your medicine or skip a dose unless your doctor tells you to. You should still follow a heart-healthy lifestyle, even if you take medicines to treat your atherosclerosis.

Medical Procedures and Surgery

If you have severe atherosclerosis, your doctor may recommend a medical procedure or surgery.

Percutaneous coronary intervention (PCI), also known as "coronary angioplasty," is a procedure that is used to open blocked or narrowed coronary (heart) arteries. PCI can improve blood flow to the heart and relieve chest pain. Sometimes, a small mesh tube called a "stent" is placed in the artery to keep it open after the procedure.

Coronary artery bypass grafting (CABG) is a type of surgery. In CABG, arteries or veins from other areas in your body are used to bypass, or go around, your narrowed coronary arteries. CABG can improve blood flow to your heart, relieve chest pain, and possibly prevent a heart attack.

Bypass grafting also can be used for leg arteries. For this surgery, a healthy blood vessel is used to bypass a narrowed or blocked artery in one of the legs. The healthy blood vessel redirects blood around the blocked artery, improving blood flow to the leg.

Carotid endarterectomy (CEA) is a type of surgery to remove plaque buildup from the carotid arteries in the neck. This procedure restores blood flow to the brain, which can help prevent a stroke.

Living with Atherosclerosis

Improved treatments have reduced the number of deaths from atherosclerosis-related diseases. These treatments also have improved the quality of life for people who have these diseases.

Adopting a healthy lifestyle may help you prevent or delay atherosclerosis and the problems it can cause. This, along with ongoing medical care, can help you avoid the problems of atherosclerosis and live a long, healthy life.

Researchers continue to look for ways to improve the health of people who have atherosclerosis or may develop it.

Ongoing Care

If you have atherosclerosis, work closely with your doctor and other healthcare providers to avoid serious problems, such as heart attack and stroke.

Follow your treatment plan and take all of your medicines as your doctor prescribes. Your doctor will let you know how often you should schedule office visits or blood tests. Be sure to let your doctor know if you have new or worsening symptoms.

Emotional Issues and Support

Having an atherosclerosis-related disease may cause fear, anxiety, depression, and stress. Talk about how you feel with your doctor. Talking to a professional counselor also can help. If you are very depressed, your doctor may recommend medicines or other treatments that can improve your quality of life (QOL).

Community resources are available to help you learn more about atherosclerosis. Contact your local public-health departments, hospitals, and local chapters of national health organizations to learn more about available resources in your area.

Talk about your lifestyle changes with your family and friends—whoever can provide support or needs to understand why you are changing your habits.

Family and friends may be able to help you make lifestyle changes. For example, they can help you plan healthier meals. Because atherosclerosis tends to run in families, your lifestyle changes may help many of your family members too.

Chapter 23

Carotid Artery Disease

What Is Carotid Artery Disease?

Carotid artery disease is a disease in which a waxy substance called "plaque" builds up inside the carotid arteries. You have two common carotid arteries, one on each side of your neck. They each divide into internal and external carotid arteries.

The internal carotid arteries supply oxygen-rich blood to your brain. The external carotid arteries supply oxygen-rich blood to your face, scalp, and neck.

Carotid Arteries

Carotid artery disease is serious because it can cause a stroke, also called a "brain attack." A stroke occurs if blood flow to your brain is cut off.

If blood flow is cut off for more than a few minutes, the cells in your brain start to die. This impairs the parts of the body that the brain cells control. A stroke can cause lasting brain damage; long-term disability, such as vision or speech problems or paralysis (an inability to move); or death.

This chapter includes text excerpted from "Carotid Artery Disease," National Heart, Lung, and Blood Institute (NHLBI), December 26, 2011. Reviewed May 2019.

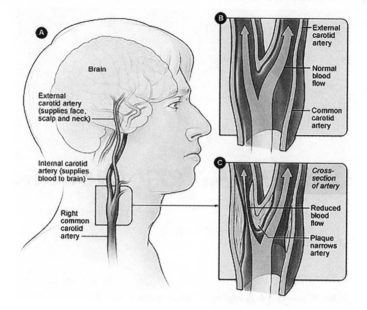

Figure 23.1. *Carotid Arteries*

Figure A shows the location of the right carotid artery in the head and neck. Figure B shows the inside of a normal carotid artery that has normal blood flow. Figure C shows the inside of a carotid artery that has plaque buildup and reduced blood flow.

Causes of Carotid Artery Disease

Carotid artery disease seems to start when damage occurs to the inner layers of the carotid arteries. Major factors that contribute to damage include:

- Smoking

- High levels of certain fats and cholesterol in the blood

- High blood pressure

- High levels of sugar in the blood due to insulin resistance or diabetes

When damage occurs, your body starts a healing process. The healing may cause plaque to build up where the arteries are damaged.

The plaque in an artery can crack or rupture. If this happens, blood cell fragments called "platelets" will stick to the site of the injury and may clump together to form blood clots.

The buildup of plaque or blood clots can severely narrow or block the carotid arteries. This limits the flow of oxygen-rich blood to your brain, which can cause a stroke.

Risk Factors for Carotid Artery Disease

The major risk factors for carotid artery disease, as listed below, also are the major risk factors for coronary heart disease (also called "coronary artery disease") and peripheral artery disease.

- **Diabetes.** With this disease, the body's blood sugar level is too high because the body does not make enough insulin or does not use its insulin properly. People who have diabetes are four times more likely to have carotid artery disease than are people who do not have diabetes.

- **Family history of atherosclerosis.** People who have a family history of atherosclerosis are more likely to develop carotid artery disease.

- **High blood pressure (hypertension).** Blood pressure is considered high if it stays at or above 140/90 mmHg over time. If you have diabetes or chronic kidney disease (CKD), high blood pressure is defined as 130/80 mmHg or higher. (The mmHg is millimeters of mercury—the units used to measure blood pressure.)

- **Lack of physical activity.** Too much sitting (sedentary lifestyle) and a lack of aerobic activity can worsen other risk factors for carotid artery disease, such as unhealthy blood cholesterol levels, high blood pressure, diabetes, and being overweight or obese.

- **Metabolic syndrome.** Metabolic syndrome is the name for a group of risk factors that raise your risk for stroke and other health problems, such as diabetes and heart disease. The five metabolic risk factors are a large waistline (abdominal obesity), a high triglyceride level (a type of fat found in the blood), a low high-density lipoprotein (HDL) cholesterol level, high blood pressure, and high blood sugar. Metabolic syndrome is diagnosed if you have at least three of these metabolic risk factors.

- **Older age.** As you age, your risk for atherosclerosis increases. The process of atherosclerosis begins in youth and typically progresses over many decades before diseases develop.

- **Being overweight or obese.** The terms "overweight" and "obesity" refer to body weight that is greater than what is considered healthy for a certain height.

- **Smoking.** Smoking can damage and tighten blood vessels, lead to unhealthy cholesterol levels, and raise blood pressure. Smoking also can limit how much oxygen reaches the body's tissues.

- **Unhealthy blood cholesterol levels.** This includes high low-density lipoprotein (LDL) ("bad") cholesterol) and low HDL ("good") cholesterol.

- **Unhealthy diet.** An unhealthy diet can raise your risk for carotid artery disease. Foods that are high in saturated and trans fats, cholesterol, sodium, and sugar can worsen other risk factors for carotid artery disease.

Having any of these risk factors does not guarantee that you will develop carotid artery disease. However, if you know that you have one or more risk factors, you can take steps to help prevent or delay the disease.

If you have plaque buildup in your carotid arteries, you also may have plaque buildup in other arteries. People who have carotid artery disease also are at an increased risk for coronary heart disease.

Screening and Prevention of Carotid Artery Disease

Taking action to control your risk factors can help prevent or delay carotid artery disease and stroke. Your risk for carotid artery disease increases with the number of risk factors you have.

One step you can take is to make heart-healthy lifestyle changes, which can include:

- **Heart-healthy eating.** Following heart-healthy eating is an important part of a healthy lifestyle. Dietary Approaches to Stop Hypertension (DASH) is a program that promotes heart-healthy eating.

- **Aiming for a healthy weight.** If you are overweight or obese, work with your doctor to create a reasonable plan for weight loss. Controlling your weight helps you control risk factors for carotid artery disease.

- **Physical activity.** Be as physically active as you can. Physical activity can improve your fitness level and your health. Ask your doctor what types and amounts of activity are safe for you.

- **Quit smoking.** If you smoke, quit. Talk with your doctor about programs and products that can help you quit.

Other steps that can prevent or delay carotid artery disease include knowing your family history of carotid artery disease. If you or someone in your family has carotid artery disease, be sure to tell your doctor.

If lifestyle changes are not enough, your doctor may prescribe medicines to control your carotid artery disease risk factors. Take all of your medicines as your doctor advises.

Signs, Symptoms, and Complications of Carotid Artery Disease

carotid artery disease may not cause signs or symptoms until it severely narrows or blocks a carotid artery. Signs and symptoms may include a bruit, a transient ischemic attack (TIA), or a stroke.

Bruit

During a physical exam, your doctor may listen to your carotid arteries with a stethoscope. She or he may hear a whooshing sound called a "bruit." This sound may suggest a changed or reduced blood flow due to plaque buildup. To find out more, your doctor may recommend tests.

Not all people who have carotid artery disease have bruits.

Transient Ischemic Attack (Mini-Stroke)

For some people, having a TIA, or mini-stroke, is the first sign of carotid artery disease. During a mini-stroke, you may have some or all of the symptoms of a stroke. However, the symptoms usually go away on their own within 24 hours.

Stroke and mini-stroke symptoms may include:

- A sudden, severe headache with no known cause

- Dizziness or loss of balance

- Inability to move one or more of your limbs

- Sudden trouble seeing in one or both eyes

261

- Sudden weakness or numbness in the face or limbs, often on just one side of the body

- Trouble speaking or understanding speech

Even if the symptoms stop quickly, call 911 for emergency help. Do not drive yourself to the hospital. It is important to get checked and to get treatment started as soon as possible.

A mini-stroke is a warning sign that you are at a high risk of having a stroke. You should not ignore these symptoms. Getting medical care can help find possible causes of a mini-stroke and help you manage risk factors. These actions might prevent a future stroke.

Although a mini-stroke may warn of a stroke, it does not predict when a stroke will happen. A stroke may occur days, weeks, or even months after a mini-stroke.

Stroke

The symptoms of a stroke are the same as those of a mini-stroke, but the results are not. A stroke can cause lasting brain damage; long-term disability, such as vision or speech problems or paralysis (an inability to move); or death. Most people who have strokes have not previously had warning mini-strokes.

Getting treatment for a stroke right away is very important. You have the best chance for full recovery if treatment to open a blocked artery is given within four hours of symptom onset. The sooner that treatment occurs, the better your chances of recovery.

Call 911 for emergency help as soon as symptoms occur. Do not drive yourself to the hospital. It is very important to get checked and to get treatment started as soon as possible.

Make those close to you aware of stroke symptoms and the need for urgent action. Learning the signs and symptoms of a stroke will allow you to help yourself or someone close to you lower the risk of brain damage or death due to a stroke.

Diagnosis of Carotid Artery Disease

Your doctor will diagnose carotid artery disease based on your medical history, a physical exam, and test results.

Medical History

Your doctor will find out whether you have any of the major risk factors for carotid artery disease. She or he also will ask whether you have had any signs or symptoms of a mini-stroke or stroke.

Physical Exam

To check your carotid arteries, your doctor will listen to them with a stethoscope. She or he will listen for a bruit. This sound may indicate a changed or reduced blood flow due to plaque buildup. To find out more, your doctor may recommend tests.

Diagnostic Tests

The following tests are common for diagnosing carotid artery disease. If you have symptoms of a mini-stroke or stroke, your doctor may use other tests as well.

Carotid Ultrasound

A carotid ultrasound (also called "sonography") is the most common test for diagnosing carotid artery disease. It is a painless, harmless test that uses sound waves to create pictures of the insides of your carotid arteries. This test can show whether plaque has narrowed your carotid arteries and how narrow they are.

A standard carotid ultrasound shows the structure of your carotid arteries. A Doppler carotid ultrasound shows how blood moves through your carotid arteries.

Carotid Angiography

Carotid angiography is a special type of X-ray. This test may be used if the ultrasound results are unclear or do not give your doctor enough information.

For this test, your doctor will inject a substance (called "contrast dye") into a vein, most often in your leg. The dye travels to your carotid arteries and highlights them on X-ray pictures.

Magnetic Resonance Angiography

A magnetic resonance angiography (MRA) uses a large magnet and radio waves to take pictures of your carotid arteries. Your doctor can see these pictures on a computer screen.

For this test, your doctor may give you contrast dye to highlight your carotid arteries on the pictures.

Computed Tomography Angiography

A computed tomography angiography, or CT angiography, takes X-ray pictures of the body from many angles. A computer combines the pictures into two- and three-dimensional images.

For this test, your doctor may give you contrast dye to highlight your carotid arteries on the pictures.

Treatment Options of Carotid Artery Disease

Treatments for carotid artery disease may include heart-healthy lifestyle changes, medicines, and medical procedures. The goals of treatment are to stop the disease from getting worse and to prevent a stroke. Your treatment will depend on your symptoms, how severe the disease is, and your age and overall health.

Heart-Healthy Lifestyle Changes

Your doctor may recommend heart-healthy lifestyle changes if you have carotid artery disease. Heart-healthy lifestyle changes include:

- Heart-healthy eating
- Aiming for a healthy weight
- Managing stress
- Physical activity
- Quitting smoking

Medicines

If you have a stroke caused by a blood clot, you may be given a clot-dissolving, or clot-busting, medication. This type of medication must be given within four hours of symptom onset. The sooner that treatment occurs, the better your chances of recovery. If you think you are having a stroke, call 911 right away for emergency care.

Medicines to prevent blood clots are the mainstay treatment for people who have carotid artery disease. They prevent platelets from clumping together and forming blood clots in your carotid arteries, which can lead to a stroke. Two common medications are:

- Aspirin
- Clopidogrel

Sometimes, lifestyle changes alone are not enough to control your cholesterol levels. For example, you also may need statin medications to control or lower your cholesterol. By lowering your blood cholesterol level, you can decrease your chance of having a heart attack or stroke. Doctors usually prescribe statins for people who have:

- Diabetes

- Heart disease or have had a stroke

- High LDL cholesterol levels

Doctors may discuss beginning statin treatment with those who have an elevated risk for developing heart disease or having a stroke.

You may need other medications to treat diseases and conditions that damage the carotid arteries. Your doctor also may prescribe medications to:

- Lower your blood pressure

- Lower your blood sugar level

- Prevent blood clots from forming, which can lead to stroke

- Prevent or reduce inflammation

Take all medicines regularly, as your doctor prescribes. Do not change the amount of your medicine or skip a dose unless your doctor tells you to. Your healthcare team will help find a treatment plan that is right for you.

Medical Procedures

You may need a medical procedure if you have symptoms caused by the narrowing of the carotid artery. Doctors use one of two methods to open narrowed or blocked carotid arteries: carotid endarterectomy and carotid artery angioplasty and stenting.

Carotid Endarterectomy

Carotid endarterectomy is mainly for people whose carotid arteries are blocked 50 percent or more.

For the procedure, a surgeon will make an incision in your neck to reach the narrowed or blocked carotid artery. Next, she or he will make a cut in the blocked part of the artery and remove the artery's inner lining that is blocking the blood flow.

Finally, your surgeon will close the artery with stitches and stop any bleeding. She or he will then close the incision in your neck.

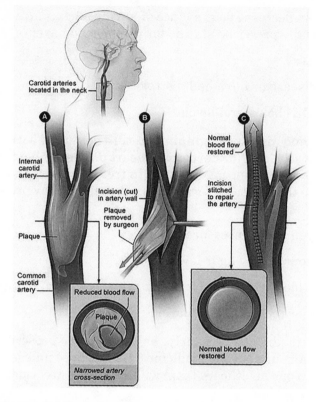

Figure 23.2. *Carotid Endarterectomy*

The illustration shows the process of carotid endarterectomy. Figure A shows a carotid artery with plaque buildup. The inset image shows a cross-section of the narrowed carotid artery. Figure B shows how the carotid artery is cut and how the plaque is removed. Figure C shows the artery stitched up and normal blood flow restored. The inset image shows a cross-section of the artery with plaque removed and normal blood flow restored.

Carotid Artery Angioplasty and Stenting

Doctors use a procedure called "angioplasty" to widen the carotid arteries and restore blood flow to the brain.

A thin tube with a deflated balloon on the end is threaded through a blood vessel in your neck to the narrowed or blocked carotid artery. Once in place, the balloon is inflated to push the plaque outward against the wall of the artery.

A stent (a small mesh tube) is then put in the artery to support the inner artery wall. The stent also helps prevent the artery from becoming narrowed or blocked again.

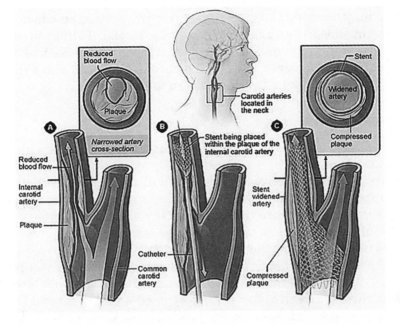

Figure 23.3. *Carotid Artery Stenting*

The illustration shows the process of carotid artery stenting. Figure A shows an internal carotid artery that has plaque buildup and reduced blood flow. The inset image shows a cross-section of the narrowed carotid artery. Figure B shows a stent being placed in the carotid artery to support the inner artery wall and keep the artery open. Figure C shows normal blood flow restored in the stent-widened artery. The inset image shows a cross-section of the stent-widened artery.

Living with Carotid Artery Disease

If you have carotid artery disease, you can take steps to manage the condition, reduce risk factors, and prevent complications. These steps include making heart-healthy lifestyle changes, following your treatment plan, and receiving ongoing care.

Having carotid artery disease raises your risk of having a stroke. Know the warning signs of a stroke—such as weakness and trouble speaking—and what to do if they occur. Call 911 as soon as symptoms start (do not drive yourself to the hospital).

Treatment Plan

Following your treatment plan may help prevent your carotid artery disease from getting worse. It also can lower your risk for stroke and other health problems.

You may need to take medicines to control certain risk factors and to prevent blood clots that could cause a stroke. Taking prescribed medicines and following a healthy lifestyle can help control carotid artery disease. However, they do not cure the disease. You will likely have to stick with your treatment plan for life.

Ongoing Care

If you have carotid artery disease, having ongoing medical care is important.

Most people who have the disease will need to have their blood pressure checked regularly and their blood sugar and blood cholesterol levels tested one or more times a year. If you have diabetes, you will need routine blood sugar tests and other tests.

Testing shows whether these conditions are under control, or whether your doctor needs to adjust your treatment for better results.

If you have had a stroke or have had procedures to restore blood flow in your carotid arteries, you will likely need a yearly carotid Doppler ultrasound test. This test shows how well blood flows through your carotid arteries.

Repeating this test over time will show whether the narrowing in your carotid arteries is getting worse. Results also can show how well treatment procedures have worked.

Follow up with your doctor regularly. The sooner your doctor spots problems, the sooner she or he can prescribe treatment.

Stroke Warning Signs

The signs and symptoms of stroke may include:

• Sudden weakness or numbness in the face or limbs, often on only one side of the body

• The inability to move one or more of your limbs

• Trouble speaking or understanding speech

• Sudden trouble seeing in one or both eyes

• Dizziness or loss of balance

• A sudden, severe headache with no known cause

Learning the signs and symptoms of a stroke will allow you to help yourself or someone close to you lower the risk of damage or death due to a stroke.

Chapter 24

Stroke

What Is a Stroke?

A stroke occurs if the flow of oxygen-rich blood to a portion of the brain is blocked. Without oxygen, brain cells start to die after a few minutes. Sudden bleeding in the brain also can cause a stroke if it damages brain cells.

If brain cells die or are damaged because of a stroke, symptoms occur in the parts of the body that these brain cells control. Examples of stroke symptoms include sudden weakness; paralysis (an inability to move) or numbness of the face, arms, or legs; trouble speaking or understanding speech; and trouble seeing.

A stroke is a serious medical condition that requires emergency care. A stroke can cause lasting brain damage, long-term disability, or even death.

If you think you or someone else is having a stroke, call 911 right away. Do not drive to the hospital or let someone else drive you. Call an ambulance so that medical personnel can begin life-saving treatment on the way to the emergency room. During a stroke, every minute counts.

This chapter includes text excerpted from "Stroke," National Heart, Lung, and Blood Institute (NHLBI), August 14, 2018.

Types of Stroke
Ischemic Stroke

An ischemic stroke occurs if an artery that supplies oxygen-rich blood to the brain becomes blocked. Blood clots often cause the blockages that lead to ischemic strokes.

The two types of ischemic stroke are thrombotic and embolic. In a thrombotic stroke, a blood clot (thrombus) forms in an artery that supplies blood to the brain.

In an embolic stroke, a blood clot or other substance (such as plaque, a fatty material) travels through the bloodstream to an artery in the brain. A blood clot or piece of plaque that travels through the bloodstream is called an "embolus."

With both types of ischemic stroke, the blood clot or plaque blocks the flow of oxygen-rich blood to a portion of the brain.

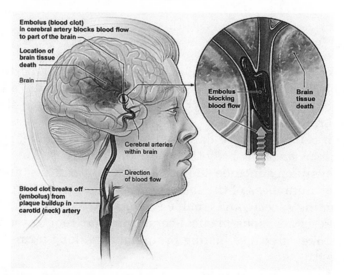

Figure 24.1. *Ischemic Stroke*

The illustration shows how an ischemic stroke can occur in the brain. If a blood clot breaks away from plaque buildup in a carotid (neck) artery, it can travel to and lodge in an artery in the brain. The clot can block blood flow to part of the brain, causing brain tissue death.

Hemorrhagic Stroke

A hemorrhagic stroke occurs if an artery in the brain leaks blood or ruptures (breaks open). The pressure from the leaked blood damages brain cells.

The two types of hemorrhagic stroke are intracerebral and sub-arachnoid. In an intracerebral hemorrhage, a blood vessel inside the brain leaks blood or ruptures.

In a subarachnoid hemorrhage, a blood vessel on the surface of the brain leaks blood or ruptures. When this happens, bleeding occurs between the inner and middle layers of the membranes that cover the brain.

In both types of hemorrhagic stroke, the leaked blood causes swelling of the brain and increased pressure in the skull. The swelling and pressure damages cells and tissues in the brain.

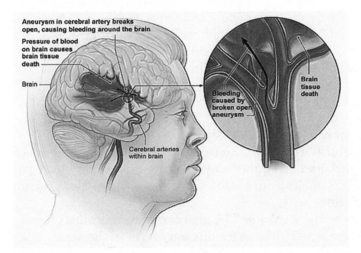

Figure 24.2. *Hemorrhagic Stroke*

Illustration shows how a hemorrhagic stroke can occur in the brain. An aneurysm in a cerebral artery breaks open, which causes bleeding in the brain. The pressure of the blood causes brain tissue death.

Causes of Stroke
Ischemic Stroke and Transient Ischemic Attack

An ischemic stroke or transient ischemic attack (TIA) occurs if an artery that supplies oxygen-rich blood to the brain becomes blocked. Many medical conditions can increase the risk of a ischemic stroke or TIA.

For example, atherosclerosis is a disease in which plaque builds up on the inner walls of the arteries. Plaque hardens and narrows the arteries, which limits the flow of blood to tissues and organs (such as the heart and brain).

Plaque in an artery can crack or rupture. Blood platelets, which are disc-shaped cell fragments, stick to the site of the plaque injury and clump together to form blood clots. These clots can partly or fully block an artery.

Plaque can build up in any artery in the body, including arteries in the heart, brain, and neck. The two main arteries on each side of the neck are called the "carotid arteries." These arteries supply oxygen-rich blood to the brain, face, scalp, and neck.

When plaque builds up in the carotid arteries, the condition is called "carotid artery disease." Carotid artery disease causes many of the ischemic strokes and TIAs that occur in the United States.

An embolic stroke (a type of ischemic stroke) or TIA also can occur if a blood clot or piece of plaque breaks away from the wall of an artery. The clot or plaque can travel through the bloodstream and get stuck in one of the brain's arteries. This stops blood flow through the artery and damages brain cells.

Heart conditions and blood disorders also can cause blood clots that can lead to a stroke or TIA. For example, atrial fibrillation, or AF, is a common cause of embolic stroke.

In atrial fibrillation, the upper chambers of the heart contract in a very fast and irregular way. As a result, some blood pools in the heart. The pooling increases the risk of blood clots forming in the heart chambers.

An ischemic stroke or TIA also can occur because of lesions caused by atherosclerosis. These lesions may form in the small arteries of the brain, and they can block blood flow to the brain.

Hemorrhagic Stroke

Sudden bleeding in the brain can cause a hemorrhagic stroke. The bleeding causes swelling of the brain and increased pressure in the skull. The swelling and pressure damage brain cells and tissues.

Examples of conditions that can cause a hemorrhagic stroke include high blood pressure, aneurysms, and arteriovenous malformations (AVMs).

Blood pressure is the force of blood pushing against the walls of the arteries as the heart pumps blood. If blood pressure rises and stays high over time, it can damage the body in many ways.

Aneurysms are balloon-like bulges in an artery that can stretch and burst. AVMs are tangles of faulty arteries and veins that can rupture within the brain. High blood pressure can increase the risk of hemorrhagic stroke in people who have aneurysms or AVMs.

Risk Factors for Stroke

Certain traits, conditions, and habits can raise your risk of having a stroke or TIA. These traits, conditions, and habits are known as "risk factors."

The more risk factors you have, the more likely you are to have a stroke. You can treat or control some risk factors, such as high blood pressure and smoking. Other risk factors, such as age and gender, you cannot control.

The major risk factors for stroke include:

- **High blood pressure.** High blood pressure is the main risk factor for stroke. Blood pressure is considered high if it stays at or above 140/90 millimeters of mercury (mmHg) over time. If you have diabetes or chronic kidney disease, high blood pressure is defined as 130/80 mmHg or higher.

- **Diabetes.** Diabetes is a disease in which the blood sugar level is high because the body does not make enough insulin or does not use its insulin properly. Insulin is a hormone that helps move blood sugar into cells where it is used for energy.

- **Heart diseases.** Ischemic heart disease, cardiomyopathy, heart failure, and atrial fibrillation can cause blood clots that can lead to a stroke.

- **Smoking.** Smoking can damage blood vessels and raise blood pressure. Smoking also may reduce the amount of oxygen that reaches your body's tissues. Exposure to secondhand smoke also can damage the blood vessels.

- **Age and gender.** Your risk of stroke increases as you get older. At younger ages, men are more likely to have strokes than women. However, women are more likely to die from strokes. Women who take birth control pills also are at slightly higher risk of stroke.

- **Race and ethnicity.** Strokes occur more often in African American, Alaska Native, and American Indian adults than in White, Hispanic, or Asian American adults.

- **Personal or family history of stroke or TIA.** If you have had a stroke, you are at higher risk for another one. Your risk of having a repeat stroke is the highest right after a stroke. A TIA also increases your risk of having a stroke, as does having a family history of stroke.

- **Brain aneurysms or arteriovenous malformations (AVMs).** Aneurysms are balloon-like bulges in an artery that can stretch and burst. AVMs are tangles of faulty arteries and veins that can rupture (break open) within the brain. AVMs may be present at birth, but often are not diagnosed until they rupture.

Other risk factors for stroke, many of which of you can control, include:

- Alcohol and illegal-drug use, including cocaine, amphetamines, and other drugs

- Certain medical conditions, such as sickle cell disease, vasculitis (inflammation of the blood vessels), and bleeding disorders

- Lack of physical activity

- Overweight and Obesity

- Stress and depression

- Unhealthy cholesterol levels

- Unhealthy diet

- Use of nonsteroidal anti-inflammatory drugs (NSAIDs), excluding aspirin, may increase the risk of heart attack or stroke, particularly in patients who have had a heart attack or cardiac bypass surgery. The risk may increase the longer NSAIDs are used. Common NSAIDs include ibuprofen and naproxen.

Following a heart-healthy lifestyle can lower the risk of stroke. Some people also may need to take medicines to lower their risk. Sometimes, strokes can occur in people who do not have any known risk factors.

Screening and Prevention of Stroke

Taking action to control your risk factors can help prevent or delay a stroke. Talk to your doctor about whether you may benefit from aspirin primary prevention or from using aspirin to help prevent your first stroke. The following heart-healthy lifestyle changes can help prevent your first stroke and help prevent you from having another one.

- **Be physically active.** Physical activity can improve your fitness level and health. Talk with your doctor about what types and amounts of activity are safe for you.

- **Do not smoke, or if you smoke or use tobacco, quit.**
  Smoking can damage and tighten blood vessels and raise
  your risk of stroke. Talk with your doctor about programs and
  products that can help you quit. Also, secondhand smoke can
  damage the blood vessels.

- **Aim for a healthy weight.** If you are overweight or obese,
  work with your doctor to create a reasonable weight loss plan.
  Controlling your weight helps you control risk factors for stroke.

- **Make heart-healthy eating choices.** Heart-healthy eating
  can help lower your risk or prevent a stroke.

- **Manage stress.** Use techniques to lower your stress levels.

If you or someone in your family has had a stroke, be sure to tell
your doctor. By knowing your family history of stroke, you may be able
to lower your risk factors and prevent or delay a stroke. If you have
had a TIA, do not ignore it. TIAs are warnings, and it is important
for your doctor to find the cause of the TIA, so you can take steps to
prevent a stroke.

Signs, Symptoms, and Complications of Stroke

The signs and symptoms of a stroke often develop quickly. However,
they can develop over hours or even days.

The type of symptoms depends on the type of stroke and the area
of the brain that is affected. How long symptoms last and how severe
they are, vary among different people.

Signs and symptoms of a stroke may include:

- Sudden weakness

- Paralysis or numbness of the face, arms, or legs, especially on
  one side of the body

- Confusion

- Trouble speaking or understanding speech

- Trouble seeing in one or both eyes

- Problems breathing

- Dizziness, trouble walking, loss of balance or coordination, and
  unexplained falls

- Loss of consciousness

- Sudden and severe headache

A transient ischemic attack has the same signs and symptoms as a stroke. However, TIA symptoms usually last less than 1 to 2 hours (although they may last up to 24 hours). A TIA may occur only once in a person's lifetime or more often.

At first, it may not be possible to tell whether someone is having a TIA or stroke. All stroke-like symptoms require medical care.

If you think you or someone else is having a TIA or stroke, call 911 right away. Do not drive to the hospital or let someone else drive you. Call an ambulance so that medical personnel can begin life-saving treatment on the way to the emergency room. During a stroke, every minute counts.

Stroke Complications

After you have had a stroke, you may develop other complications, such as:

- **Blood clots and muscle weakness.** Being immobile (unable to move around) for a long time can raise your risk of developing blood clots in the deep veins of the legs. Being immobile also can lead to muscle weakness and decreased muscle flexibility.

- **Problems swallowing and pneumonia.** If a stroke affects the muscles used for swallowing, you may have a hard time eating or drinking. You also may be at risk of inhaling food or drink into your lungs. If this happens, you may develop pneumonia.

Loss of bladder control. Some strokes affect the muscles used to urinate. You may need a urinary catheter (a tube placed into the bladder) until you can urinate on your own. Use of these catheters can lead to urinary tract infections (UTIs). Loss of bowel control or constipation also may occur after a stroke.

Diagnosis of Stroke

Your doctor will diagnose a stroke based on your signs and symptoms, your medical history, a physical exam, and test results.

Your doctor will want to find out the type of stroke you have had, its cause, the part of the brain that is affected, and whether you have bleeding in the brain.

If your doctor thinks you have had a TIA, she or he will look for its cause to help prevent a future stroke.

Medical History and Physical Exam

Your doctor will ask you or a family member about your risk factors for stroke. Examples of risk factors include high blood pressure, smoking, heart disease, and a personal or family history of stroke. Your doctor also will ask about your signs and symptoms and when they began.

During the physical exam, your doctor will check your mental alertness and your coordination and balance. She or he will check for numbness or weakness in your face, arms, and legs; confusion; and trouble speaking and seeing clearly.

Your doctor will look for signs of carotid artery disease, a common cause of ischemic stroke. She or he will listen to your carotid arteries with a stethoscope. A whooshing sound called a "bruit" may suggest changed or reduced blood flow due to plaque buildup in the carotid arteries.

Diagnostic Tests and Procedures

Your doctor may recommend one or more of the following tests to diagnose a stroke or TIA.

Brain Computed Tomography

A brain computed tomography scan, or brain CT scan, is a painless test that uses X-rays to take clear, detailed pictures of your brain. This test often is done right after a stroke is suspected.

A brain CT scan can show bleeding in the brain or damage to the brain cells from a stroke. The test also can show other brain conditions that may be causing your symptoms.

Magnetic Resonance Imaging

Magnetic resonance imaging (MRI) uses magnets and radio waves to create pictures of the organs and structures in your body. This test can detect changes in brain tissue and damage to brain cells from a stroke.

An MRI may be used instead of, or in addition to, a CT scan to diagnose a stroke.

Computed Tomography Arteriogram and Magnetic Resonance Arteriogram

A computerized tomography arteriogram (CTA) and magnetic resonance arteriogram (MRA) can show the large blood vessels in the brain. These tests may give your doctor more information about the site of a blood clot and the flow of blood through your brain.

Carotid Ultrasound

A carotid ultrasound is a painless and harmless test that uses sound waves to create pictures of the insides of your carotid arteries. These arteries supply oxygen-rich blood to your brain.

A carotid ultrasound shows whether plaque has narrowed or blocked your carotid arteries.

Your carotid ultrasound test may include a Doppler ultrasound. A Doppler ultrasound is a special test that shows the speed and direction of blood moving through your blood vessels.

Carotid Angiography

A carotid angiography is a test that uses dye and special X-rays to show the insides of your carotid arteries.

For this test, a catheter is put into an artery, usually in the groin (upper thigh). The tube is then moved up into one of your carotid arteries.

Your doctor will inject a substance (called "contrast dye") into the carotid artery. The dye helps make the artery visible on X-ray pictures.

Heart Tests
Electrocardiogram

An electrocardiogram (EKG) is a simple, painless test that records the heart's electrical activity. The test shows how fast the heart is beating and its rhythm (steady or irregular). An EKG also records the strength and timing of electrical signals as they pass through each part of the heart.

An EKG can help detect heart problems that may have led to a stroke. For example, the test can help diagnose atrial fibrillation or a previous heart attack.

Echocardiography

An echocardiography, or echo, is a painless test that uses sound waves to create pictures of your heart.

The test gives information about the size and shape of your heart and how well your heart's chambers and valves are working.

An echo can detect possible blood clots inside the heart and problems with the aorta. The aorta is the main artery that carries oxygen-rich blood from your heart to all parts of your body.

Blood Tests

Your doctor also may use blood tests to help diagnose a stroke.

A blood glucose test measures the amount of glucose (sugar) in your blood. Low blood glucose levels may cause symptoms similar to those of a stroke.

A platelet count measures the number of platelets in your blood. Blood platelets are cell fragments that help your blood clot. Abnormal platelet levels may be a sign of a bleeding disorder (not enough clotting) or a thrombotic disorder (too much clotting).

Your doctor also may recommend blood tests to measure how long it takes for your blood to clot. Two tests that may be used are called "prothrombin time" (PT) and "partial thromboplastin time" (PTT) tests. These tests show whether your blood is clotting normally.

Treatment of Stroke

Treatment for a stroke depends on whether it is ischemic or hemorrhagic. Treatment for a TIA depends on its cause, how much time has passed since symptoms began, and whether you have other medical conditions.

Strokes and TIAs are medical emergencies. If you have stroke symptoms, call 911 right away. Do not drive to the hospital or let someone else drive you. Call an ambulance so that medical personnel can begin lifesaving treatment on the way to the emergency room. During a stroke, every minute counts.

Once you receive immediate treatment, your doctor will try to treat your stroke risk factors and prevent complications by recommending heart-healthy lifestyle changes.

Treating an Ischemic Stroke or Transient Ischemic Attack

An ischemic stroke or TIA occurs if an artery that supplies oxygen-rich blood to the brain becomes blocked. Often, blood clots cause the blockages that lead to ischemic strokes and TIAs. Treatment for an ischemic stroke or TIA may include medicines and medical procedures.

Medicines

If you have a stroke caused by a blood clot, you may be given a clot-dissolving, or clot-busting, medication called "tissue plasminogen activator" (tPA). A doctor will inject the tPA into a vein in your arm. This type of medication must be given within four hours of symptom onset. Ideally, it should be given as soon as possible. The sooner that treatment begins, the better your chances of recovery. Thus, it is important to know the signs and symptoms of a stroke and to call 911 right away for emergency care.

If you cannot have tPA for medical reasons, your doctor may give you antiplatelet medicine that helps stop platelets from clumping together to form blood clots or anticoagulant medicine (blood thinner) that keeps existing blood clots from getting larger. Two common medicines are aspirin and clopidogrel.

Medical Procedures

If you have carotid artery disease, your doctor may recommend a carotid endarterectomy or carotid artery angioplasty. Both procedures open blocked carotid arteries.

Researchers are testing other treatments for ischemic stroke, such as intra-arterial thrombolysis and mechanical clot removal in cerebral ischemia (MERCI).

In intra-arterial thrombolysis, a catheter is put into your groin (upper thigh) and threaded to the tiny arteries of the brain. Your doctor can deliver medicine through this catheter to break up a blood clot in the brain.

MERCI is a device that can remove blood clots from an artery. During the procedure, a catheter is threaded through a carotid artery to the affected artery in the brain. The device is then used to pull the blood clot out through the catheter.

Treating a Hemorrhagic Stroke

A hemorrhagic stroke occurs if an artery in the brain leaks blood or ruptures. The first steps in treating a hemorrhagic stroke are to find the cause of bleeding in the brain and then control it. Unlike ischemic strokes, hemorrhagic strokes are not treated with antiplatelet medicines and blood thinners because these medicines can make bleeding worse.

If you are taking antiplatelet medicines or blood thinners and have a hemorrhagic stroke, you will be taken off the medicine. If high blood pressure is the cause of bleeding in the brain, your doctor may prescribe medicines to lower your blood pressure. This can help prevent further bleeding.

Surgery also may be needed to treat a hemorrhagic stroke. The types of surgery used include aneurysm clipping, coil embolization, and arteriovenous malformation (AVM) repair.

Aneurysm Clipping and Coil Embolization

If an aneurysm (a balloon-like bulge in an artery) is the cause of a stroke, your doctor may recommend aneurysm clipping or coil embolization.

Aneurysm clipping is done to block off the aneurysm from the blood vessels in the brain. This surgery helps prevent further leaking of blood from the aneurysm. It also can help prevent the aneurysm from bursting again. During the procedure, a surgeon will make an incision (cut) in the brain and place a tiny clamp at the base of the aneurysm. You will be given medicine to make you sleep during the surgery. After the surgery, you will need to stay in the hospital's intensive care unit for a few days.

Coil embolization is a less complex procedure for treating an aneurysm. The surgeon will insert a catheter into an artery in the groin. She or he will thread the tube to the site of the aneurysm. Then, a tiny coil will be pushed through the tube and into the aneurysm. The coil will cause a blood clot to form, which will block blood flow through the aneurysm and prevent it from bursting again. Coil embolization is done in a hospital. You will be given medicine to make you sleep during the surgery.

Arteriovenous Malformation Repair

If an arteriovenous malformation repair (AVM) is the cause of a stroke, your doctor may recommend an AVM repair. An AVM is a tangle of faulty arteries and veins that can rupture within the brain. An AVM repair helps prevent further bleeding in the brain.

Doctors use several methods to repair AVMs. These methods include:

- Injecting a substance into the blood vessels of the AVM to block blood flow

- Surgery to remove the AVM

- Using radiation to shrink the blood vessels of the AVM

Treating Stroke Risk Factors

After initial treatment for a stroke or TIA, your doctor will treat your risk factors. She or he may recommend heart-healthy lifestyle changes to help control your risk factors.

Heart-healthy lifestyle changes may include:

- Heart-healthy eating

- Aiming for a healthy weight

- Managing stress

- Physical activity

- Quitting smoking

If heart-healthy lifestyle changes are not enough, you may need medicine to control your risk factors.

Life after a Stroke

The time it takes to recover from a stroke varies—it can take weeks, months, or even years. Some people recover fully, while others have long-term or lifelong disabilities.

Ongoing care, rehabilitation, and emotional support can help you recover and may even help prevent another stroke.

If you have had a stroke, you are at risk of having another one. Know the warning signs and what to do if a stroke or TIA occurs. Call 911 as soon as symptoms start.

Do not drive to the hospital or let someone else drive you. By calling an ambulance, medical personnel can begin lifesaving treatment on the way to the emergency room. During a stroke, every minute counts.

Chapter 25

Aortic Aneurysm

An aortic aneurysm is a balloon-like bulge in the aorta, the large artery that carries blood from the heart through the chest and torso.

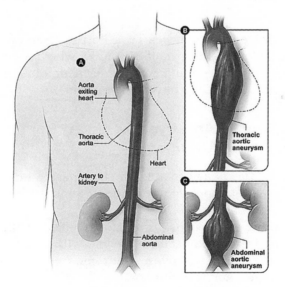

Figure 25.1. *Aortic Aneurysms* (Source: "Aortic Aneurysm," National Heart, Lung, and Blood Institute (NHLBI).)

This chapter includes text excerpted from "Aortic Aneurysm Fact Sheet," Centers for Disease Control and Prevention (CDC), June 16, 2016.

On the right, Figure A shows a normal aorta. Figure B shows a thoracic aortic aneurysm located behind the heart. Figure C shows an abdominal aortic aneurysm located below the arteries that supply blood to the kidneys.

Aortic aneurysms work in two ways:

- The force of blood pumping can split the layers of the artery wall, allowing blood to leak in between them. This process is called "dissection."

- The aneurysm can burst completely, causing bleeding inside the body. This is called a "rupture."

Dissections and ruptures are the cause of most deaths from aortic aneurysms.

In the United States:

- Aortic aneurysms were the primary cause of 9,863 deaths in 2014 and a contributing cause in more than 17,215 deaths in the United States in 2009.

- About two-thirds of people who have an aortic dissection are male.

- The U.S. Preventive Services Task Force (USPSTF) recommends that men between the ages of 65 and 75 who have ever smoked should get an ultrasound screening for abdominal aortic aneurysms, even if they have no symptoms.

Types of Aortic Aneurysm
Thoracic Aortic Aneurysms

A thoracic aortic aneurysm occurs in the chest. Men and women are equally likely to get thoracic aortic aneurysms, which become more common with increasing age.

Thoracic aortic aneurysms are usually caused by high blood pressure or sudden injury. Sometimes, people with inherited connective tissue disorders, such as Marfan syndrome and Ehlers-Danlos syndrome, get thoracic aortic aneurysms.

Signs and symptoms of thoracic aortic aneurysm can include:

- A sharp, sudden pain in the chest or upper back

- Shortness of breath

- Trouble breathing or swallowing

Abdominal Aortic Aneurysms

An abdominal aortic aneurysm occurs below the chest. Abdominal aortic aneurysms happen more often than thoracic aortic aneurysms.

Abdominal aortic aneurysms are more common in men and among people 65 years of age and older. Abdominal aortic aneurysms are less common among Black individuals when compared with White individuals.

Abdominal aortic aneurysms are usually caused by atherosclerosis (hardened arteries), but an infection or injury can also cause them.

Abdominal aortic aneurysms often do not have any symptoms. If an individual does have symptoms, they can include:

- Throbbing or deep pain in the back or side

- Pain in the buttocks, groin, or legs

Other Types of Aneurysms

Aneurysms can occur in other parts of your body. A ruptured aneurysm in the brain can cause a stroke. Peripheral aneurysms—those found in arteries other than the aorta—can occur in the neck, in the groin, or behind the knees. These aneurysms are less likely to rupture or dissect than aortic aneurysms, but they can form blood clots. These clots can break away and block blood flow through the artery.

Risk Factors for Aortic Aneurysm

Diseases that damage your heart and blood vessels also increase your risk for aortic aneurysm. These diseases include:

- High blood pressure

- High cholesterol

- Atherosclerosis

- Smoking

Some inherited connective tissue disorders, such as Marfan syndrome and Ehlers-Danlos syndrome, can also increase your risk for aortic aneurysm. Your family may also have a history of aortic aneurysms that can increase your risk.

Unhealthy behaviors can also increase your risk for aortic aneurysm, especially for people who have one of the diseases listed above. Tobacco use is the most important behavior related to aortic aneurysm.

People who have a history of smoking are three to five times more likely to develop an abdominal aortic aneurysm.

Treating Aortic Aneurysm

The two main treatments for aortic aneurysms are medicines and surgery. Medicines can lower blood pressure and reduce risk for an aortic aneurysm. Surgery can repair or replace the injured section of the aorta.

Chapter 26

Disorders of
the Peripheral Arteries

Chapter Contents

Section 26.1

Fibromuscular Dysplasia

"Fibromuscular Dysplasia,"
© 2016 Omnigraphics. Reviewed May 2019.

Fibromuscular dysplasia (FMD) is a rare medical condition in which abnormal cell growth occurs in the walls of medium and large arteries, causing the arteries to become narrowed (stenosis) or enlarged (aneurysm). There are two main types of fibromuscular dysplasia: multifocal and focal. Patients are classified as having one or the other based on the appearance of the affected arteries in imaging studies, such as angiography. Multifocal FMD is the most common type, affecting around 90 percent of patients. The pattern of alternating areas of narrowing and widening in the affected arteries has been described as a "string of beads." Focal FMD is less common, affecting around 10 percent of patients. The affected arteries have distinct lesions or areas of narrowing.

Fibromuscular dysplasia most commonly affects the renal arteries that supply blood to the kidneys and the carotid arteries in the neck that supply blood to the brain. It occurs more rarely in the mesenteric arteries that supply blood to the intestines, the coronary arteries that supply blood to the heart, and peripheral arteries in the arms and legs. FMD can limit blood flow to vital organs and cause a variety of health complications. Although there is no cure, effective treatments are available.

Causes and Risk Factors for Fibromuscular Dysplasia

Researchers have not identified a definitive cause of FMD. But, they have uncovered several risk factors that appear to increase the likelihood that a person will develop the condition, such as:

- **Hormones.** Since 90 percent of people who develop FMD are women, many researchers believe that hormones may be a factor.

- **Age.** Most people are diagnosed with FMD between the ages of 40 and 60, although it also affects children and older people.

- **Genetics.** Around 10 percent of people with FMD have a relative with the condition, leading researchers to believe that there may be a genetic component. In addition, some people who develop FMD have genetic abnormalities in their blood vessels.

- **Abnormal arteries.** Researchers also suspect that FMD may be caused by abnormally formed arteries, which may result from inadequate oxygen supply to the blood vessel walls, pressure due to the position of the arteries, or trauma to the arteries.

- **Smoking.** Smoking affects the arteries and increases the risk of developing FMD.

Symptoms of Fibromuscular Dysplasia

Many people with fibromuscular dysplasia do not experience symptoms. FMD mainly produces symptoms when stenosis of the arteries restricts blood flow or aneurysms in the arteries tear or rupture. The nature of the symptoms depends on the specific arteries that are affected.

If fibromuscular dysplasia affects the renal arteries, the symptoms may include high blood pressure or poor kidney function. If FMD affects the carotid arteries, the symptoms are likely to include headaches, dizziness, blurred vision, a swooshing sound in the ears, facial weakness or numbness, or neck pain. FMD in the mesenteric arteries may cause pain in the abdomen, especially after eating, or unexplained weight loss. People with FMD in the peripheral arteries may experience numbness, coldness, weakness, or discomfort in the arms or legs during exercise. When FMD affects the coronary arteries, symptoms may include chest pain, shortness of breath, or occasionally a heart attack.

Diagnosis of Fibromuscular Dysplasia

Some people are diagnosed with FMD during routine medical exams when the doctor hears an unusual swooshing noise (bruit) through the stethoscope, indicating a problem with blood flow. Other patients are diagnosed with FMD after undergoing an imaging scan for a different medical problem. Several noninvasive tests can help doctors determine whether arteries are affected by FMD, including Doppler ultrasound, magnetic resonance imaging (MRI), and computed tomography angiography (CTA).

A catheter-based angiography is another test that is commonly used to diagnose FMD. In this procedure, a thin tube is inserted into the artery and dye is injected to allow the doctor to examine it. Once a patient is diagnosed with FMD in a particular artery, the doctor will typically scan the rest of the body to see if it is present in other locations. Most patients with FMD also undergo additional tests to check for an aneurysm in the brain or heart that might pose dangerous health complications.

Complications of Fibromuscular Dysplasia

Fibromuscular dysplasia can cause a variety of health complications, some of which can be life-threatening. One of the most common complications is high blood pressure due to the narrowing of the arteries. High blood pressure is a risk factor for heart disease and stroke. FMD can also cause arterial dissection, or tears in the walls of the arteries that allow blood to leak into the artery wall. When this process occurs in the heart, it is known as "spontaneous coronary artery dissection" (SCAD), and it can cause a heart attack. Aneurysms are another complication of FMD that can have serious health consequences. If an aneurysm ruptures in the brain, it can cause a stroke.

Treatment of Fibromuscular Dysplasia

There are several different options available to treat fibromuscular dysplasia, including medications; procedures, such as angioplasty; and surgery. The most appropriate treatment depends on the location of the affected artery, the severity of the condition, and the patient's overall health.

People with FMD who do not have symptoms may only need to take medication to prevent blood clots, such as daily aspirin, or to control high blood pressure. Common blood-pressure medications include angiotensin-converting enzyme (ACE) inhibitors, angiotensin receptor blockers (ARBs), diuretics, calcium channel blockers, and beta-blockers.

The medical procedure most often used to open arteries that become narrowed or blocked due to FMD is percutaneous transluminal angioplasty (PTA). A catheter with a tiny balloon on the end is inserted into the affected artery and inflated to open up the narrowed section. In the angioplasty procedures commonly performed on patients with blocked coronary arteries, a metal mesh tube called a "stent" is often inserted to keep the artery open. Stents are only used under certain circumstances in patients with FMD, however, such as to prevent an aneurysm from rupturing.

In cases where the artery is blocked or severely damaged, surgery may be required to repair the artery and restore blood flow. Surgical revascularization involves removing the blocked section of the artery or creating a bypass around the blockage. The most commonly performed type of revascularization surgery is an aortorenal bypass, which uses a vein from the leg to replace the renal artery that leads to the kidney.

References

1. "Fibromuscular Dysplasia," Mayo Clinic, 2016.

2. "Fibromuscular Dysplasia (FMD)," Cleveland Clinic, 2016.

Section 26.2

Peripheral Arterial Disease of the Legs

This section includes text excerpted from "Peripheral Artery Disease," National Heart, Lung, and Blood Institute (NHLBI), January 23, 2019.

What Is Peripheral Artery Disease?

Peripheral artery disease (PAD) is a disease in which plaque builds up in the arteries that carry blood to your head, organs, and limbs. Plaque is made up of fat, cholesterol, calcium, fibrous tissue, and other substances in the blood.

When plaque builds up in the body's arteries, the condition is called "atherosclerosis." Over time, plaque can harden and narrow the arteries. This limits the flow of oxygen-rich blood to your organs and other parts of your body.

Peripheral artery disease usually affects the arteries in the legs, but it also can affect the arteries that carry blood from your heart to your head, arms, kidneys, and stomach. This section focuses on PAD that affects blood flow to the legs.

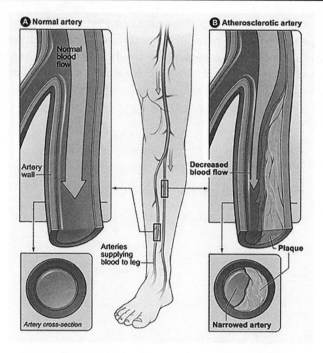

Figure 26.1. *Normal Artery and Artery with Plaque Buildup*

The illustration shows how PAD can affect arteries in the legs. Figure A shows a normal artery with normal blood flow. The inset image shows a cross-section of the normal artery. Figure B shows an artery with plaque buildup that is partially blocking blood flow. The inset image shows a cross-section of the narrowed artery.

Causes of Peripheral Artery Disease

The most common cause of PAD is atherosclerosis. Atherosclerosis is a disease in which plaque builds up in your arteries. The exact cause of atherosclerosis is not known.

The disease may start if certain factors damage the inner layers of the arteries. These factors include:

- Smoking
- High amounts of certain fats and cholesterol in the blood
- High blood pressure
- High amounts of sugar in the blood due to insulin resistance or diabetes

When damage occurs, your body starts a healing process. The healing may cause plaque to build up where the arteries are damaged.

Eventually, a section of plaque can rupture (break open), causing a blood clot to form at the site. The buildup of plaque or blood clots can severely narrow or block the arteries and limit the flow of oxygen-rich blood to your body.

Risk Factors for Peripheral Artery Disease

Peripheral artery disease affects millions of people in the United States. The disease is more common in Blacks than any other racial or ethnic group. The major risk factors for PAD are smoking, older age, and having certain diseases or conditions.

Smoking

Smoking is the main risk factor for PAD, and your risk increases if you smoke or have a history of smoking. Quitting smoking slows the progress of PAD. People who smoke and people who have diabetes are at the highest risk for PAD complications, such as gangrene (tissue death) in the leg from decreased blood flow.

Older Age

Older age also is a risk factor for PAD. Plaque builds up in your arteries as you age. Older age combined with other risk factors, such as smoking or diabetes, also puts you at higher risk for PAD.

Diseases and Conditions

Many diseases and conditions can raise your risk of PAD, including:

- Diabetes
- High blood pressure
- High blood cholesterol
- Ischemic heart disease
- Stroke
- Metabolic syndrome

Screening and Prevention of Peripheral Artery Disease

Taking action to control your risk factors can help prevent or delay PAD and its complications. Know your family history of health problems related to PAD. If you or someone in your family has the disease, be sure to tell your doctor. Controlling risk factors includes the following:

- Be physically active.

- Be screened for PAD. A simple office test, called an "ankle-brachial index" or "ABI," can help determine whether you have PAD.

- Follow heart-healthy eating.

- If you smoke, quit. Talk with your doctor about programs and products that can help you quit smoking.

- If you are overweight or obese, work with your doctor to create a reasonable weight-loss plan.

The lifestyle changes described above can reduce your risk of developing PAD These changes also can help prevent and control conditions that can be associated with PAD, such as ischemic heart disease, diabetes, high blood pressure, high blood cholesterol, and stroke.

Signs, Symptoms, and Complications of Peripheral Artery Disease

Many people who have PAD do not have any signs or symptoms. Even if you do not have signs or symptoms, ask your doctor whether you should get checked for PAD if you are:

- 70 years of age or older

- 50 years of age or older and have a history of smoking or diabetes

- Younger than 50 years of age and have diabetes and one or more risk factors for atherosclerosis

Intermittent Claudication

People who have PAD may have symptoms when walking or climbing stairs, which may include pain, numbness, aching, or heaviness in the leg muscles. Symptoms also may include cramping in the affected leg(s) and in the buttocks, thighs, calves, and feet. Symptoms may ease after resting. These symptoms are called "intermittent claudication."

During physical activity, your muscles need increased blood flow. If your blood vessels are narrowed or blocked, your muscles will not get enough blood, which will lead to symptoms. When resting, the muscles need less blood flow, so the symptoms will go away.

Other Signs and Symptoms

Other signs and symptoms of PAD include:

• Weak or absent pulses in the legs or feet

• Sores or wounds on the toes, feet, or legs that heal slowly, poorly, or not at all

• A pale or bluish color to the skin

• A lower temperature in one leg when compared to the other leg

• Poor nail growth on the toes and decreased hair growth on the legs

• Erectile dysfunction (ED), especially among men who have diabetes

Diagnosis of Peripheral Artery Disease

Peripheral artery disease is diagnosed based on your medical and family histories, a physical exam, and test results.

Peripheral artery disease often is diagnosed after symptoms are reported. A correct diagnosis is important because people who have PAD are at a higher risk for ischemic heart disease, heart attack, stroke, and transient ischemic attack (TIA), also called as "mini-stroke." If you have PAD, your doctor also may want to check for signs of these diseases and conditions.

Specialists Involved

Primary care doctors, such as internists and family doctors, may treat people who have mild PAD For more advanced PAD, a vascular specialist may be involved. This is a doctor who specializes in treating blood vessel diseases and conditions.

A cardiologist also may be involved in treating people who have PAD. Cardiologists treat heart problems, such as heart disease and heart attack, which often affect people who have PAD.

Medical and Family Histories

Your doctor may ask:

- Whether you have any risk factors for PAD. For example, she or he may ask whether you smoke or have diabetes.

- About your symptoms, including any symptoms that occur when walking, exercising, sitting, standing, or climbing

- About your diet

- About any medicines you take, including prescription and over-the-counter medicines

- Whether anyone in your family has a history of heart or blood vessel diseases

Physical Exam

During the physical exam, your doctor will look for signs of PAD. She or he may check the blood flow in your legs or feet to see whether you have weak or absent pulses.

Your doctor also may check the pulses in your leg arteries for an abnormal whooshing sound called a "bruit." She or he can hear this sound with a stethoscope. A bruit may be a warning sign of a narrowed or blocked artery.

Your doctor may compare blood pressure between your limbs to see whether the pressure is lower in the affected limb. She or he also may check for poor wound healing or any changes in your hair, skin, or nails that may be signs of PAD.

Diagnostic Tests
Ankle-Brachial Index

An ankle-brachial index (ABI) often is used to diagnose PAD. The ABI compares blood pressure in your ankle to blood pressure in your arm. This test shows how well blood is flowing in your limbs.

An ankle-brachial index can show whether PAD is affecting your limbs, but it will not show which blood vessels are narrowed or blocked.

A normal ABI result is 1.0 or greater (with a range of 0.90 to 1.30). The test takes about 10 to 15 minutes to measure both arms and both ankles. This test may be done yearly to see whether PAD is getting worse.

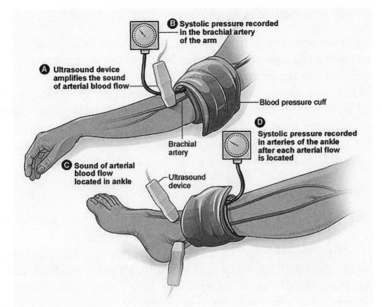

Figure 26.2. *Ankle-Brachial Index*

The illustration shows the ankle-brachial index test. The test compares blood pressure in the ankle to blood pressure in the arm. As the blood pressure cuff deflates, the blood pressure in the arteries is recorded.

Doppler Ultrasound

A Doppler ultrasound looks at blood flow in the major arteries and veins in the limbs. During this test, a handheld device is placed on your body and passed back and forth over the affected area. A computer converts sound waves into a picture of blood flow in the arteries and veins.

The results of this test can show whether a blood vessel is blocked. The results also can help show the severity of PAD.

Treadmill Test

A treadmill test can show the severity of symptoms and the level of exercise that brings them on. You will walk on a treadmill for this test. This shows whether you have any problems during normal walking.

You may have an ABI test before and after the treadmill test. This will help compare blood flow in your arms and legs before and after exercise.

Magnetic Resonance Angiogram

A magnetic resonance angiogram (MRA) uses magnetic and radio wave energy to take pictures of your blood vessels. This test is a type of magnetic resonance imaging (MRI).

An MRA can show the location and severity of a blocked blood vessel. If you have a pacemaker, manufactured joint, stent, surgical clips, mechanical heart valve, or other metallic devices in your body, you might not be able to have an MRA. Ask your doctor whether an MRA is an option for you.

Arteriogram

An arteriogram provides a "road map" of the arteries. Doctors use this test to find the exact location of a blocked artery.

For this test, dye is injected through a needle or catheter (tube) into one of your arteries. This may make you feel mildly flushed. After the dye is injected, an X-ray is taken. The X-ray can show the location, type, and extent of the blockage in the artery.

Some doctors use a newer method of arteriogram that uses tiny ultrasound cameras. These cameras take pictures of the insides of the blood vessels. This method is called "intravascular ultrasound."

Blood Tests

Your doctor may recommend blood tests to check for PAD risk factors. For example, blood tests can help diagnose conditions, such as diabetes and high blood cholesterol.

Treatment of Peripheral Artery Disease

Treatments for peripheral artery disease include heart-healthy lifestyle changes, medicines, and surgery or procedures.

The overall goals of treating PAD include reducing risk of heart attack and stroke, reducing symptoms of claudication, improving mobility and overall quality of life, and preventing complications. Treatment is based on your signs and symptoms, risk factors, and the results of physical exams and tests.

Treatment may slow or stop the progression of the disease and reduce the risk of complications. Without treatment, PAD may progress, resulting in serious tissue damage in the form of sores or gangrene (tissue death) due to inadequate blood flow. In extreme cases of PAD, also referred to as "critical limb ischemia" (CLI), removal (amputation) of part of the leg or foot may be necessary.

Heart-Healthy Lifestyle Changes

Treatment often includes making lifelong heart-healthy lifestyle changes such as:

- Physical activity
- Quitting smoking
- Heart-healthy eating

Surgery or Procedures
Bypass Grafting

Your doctor may recommend bypass grafting surgery if blood flow in your limb is blocked or nearly blocked. For this surgery, your doctor uses a blood vessel from another part of your body or a synthetic tube to make a graft.

This graft bypasses (that is, goes around) the blocked part of the artery. The bypass allows blood to flow around the blockage. This surgery does not cure PAD, but it may increase blood flow to the affected limb.

Angioplasty and Stent Placement

Your doctor may recommend angioplasty to restore blood flow through a narrowed or blocked artery.

During this procedure, a catheter with a balloon at the tip is inserted into a blocked artery. The balloon is then inflated, which pushes plaque outward against the artery wall. This widens the artery and restores blood flow.

A stent (a small mesh tube) may be placed in the artery during angioplasty. A stent helps keep the artery open after angioplasty is done. Some stents are coated with medicine to help prevent blockages in the artery.

Atherectomy

An atherectomy is a procedure that removes plaque buildup from an artery. During the procedure, a catheter is used to insert a small cutting device into the blocked artery. The device is used to shave or cut off plaque.

The bits of plaque are removed from the body through the catheter or washed away in the bloodstream (if they are small enough).

Doctors also can perform atherectomy using a special laser that dissolves the blockage.

Other Types of Treatment

Researchers are studying cell and gene therapies to treat PAD. However, these treatments are not yet available outside of clinical trials.

Living with Peripheral Artery Disease

If you have peripheral artery disease, you are more likely to also have ischemic heart disease, heart attack, stroke, and transient ischemic attack. However, you can take steps to treat and control PAD and lower your risk for these other conditions.

Living with Peripheral Artery Disease Symptoms

If you have PAD, you may feel pain in your calf or thigh muscles after walking. Try to take a break and allow the pain to ease before walking again. Over time, this may increase the distance that you can walk without pain.

Talk with your doctor about taking part in a supervised exercise program. This type of program has been shown to reduce PAD symptoms.

Check your feet and toes regularly for sores or possible infections. Wear comfortable shoes that fit well. Maintain good foot hygiene, and have professional medical treatment for corns, bunions, or calluses.

Ongoing Healthcare Needs and Lifestyle Changes

See your doctor for checkups as she or he advises. If you have PAD without symptoms, you still should see your doctor regularly. Take all medicines as your doctor prescribes.

Heart-healthy lifestyle changes can help prevent or delay PAD and other related problems, such as ischemic heart disease, heart attack, stroke, and transient ischemic attack. Heart-healthy lifestyle changes include physical activity, quitting smoking, and heart-healthy eating.

Section 26.3

Raynaud Phenomenon

This section includes text excerpted from "Raynaud's Phenomenon,"
National Institute of Arthritis and Musculoskeletal and Skin
Diseases (NIAMS), October 30, 2016.

Raynaud phenomenon is a condition that affects your blood vessels.
It causes some areas of your body, especially your hands and feet, to
feel numb and cold in response to cold temperatures or stress. Raynaud
phenomenon is also called "Raynaud disease" or "Raynaud syndrome."

Who Gets Raynaud Phenomenon

Anyone can get Raynaud phenomenon, but some people are more
at risk for developing the disease. Risk factors include:

- **Your sex:** Women are more likely to develop Raynaud
  phenomenon.

- **Where you live:** People who live in cold places are more likely
  to develop Raynaud phenomenon.

- **Certain health conditions:** Certain health conditions increase
  the risk of Raynaud phenomenon.

It is especially common in people who have connective tissue diseases, which affect how blood flows to the organs and other body tissues. Connective tissue diseases include:

- **Lupus,** which causes the immune system to attack healthy
  tissues in the body

- **Scleroderma,** which causes the skin and other tissues in the
  body to harden

- **Sjögren's syndrome,** which causes dryness in the mouth and
  eyes

Other health conditions can also increase your risk of developing
Raynaud phenomenon. These include:

- **Carpal tunnel syndrome,** which affects nerves in the wrists

- **Blood vessel disease,** which causes the blood vessels in the
  legs, arms, and belly to narrow

301

Medicines: Taking certain medicines increases your risk of developing Raynaud phenomenon. These include:

- Medicines used to treat high blood pressure, migraines, or cancer

- Over-the-counter (OTC) cold medicines

- Narcotics

Your job: People with certain jobs may be more likely to develop Raynaud phenomenon. These include:

- People who are around certain chemicals

- People who use tools that vibrate, such as a jackhammer.

Genetics: Some research suggests that Raynaud phenomenon runs in certain families, but more research is needed.

Types of Raynaud Phenomenon

There are two types of Raynaud phenomenon.

- Primary Raynaud phenomenon occurs for an unknown reason. It is the more common form of Raynaud phenomenon.

- Secondary Raynaud phenomenon is caused by another health condition, such as lupus or scleroderma. Secondary Raynaud phenomenon is less common but more serious than the primary form of the disease.

Symptoms of Raynaud Phenomenon

During an attack, your body limits blood flow to the hands and feet. This makes your fingers and toes feel cold and numb. It may also cause your fingers and toes to turn white or blue. Once blood flow to the fingers and toes returns, they may turn red, tingle, and begin to hurt.

The symptoms of the primary form of Raynaud phenomenon usually begins between the ages of 15 and 25. The symptoms of the secondary form of Raynaud phenomenon usually start after the ages of 35 and 40.

For many people, especially those with a primary form of Raynaud phenomenon, the symptoms are mild and not very troublesome. Others have more severe symptoms.

Causes of Raynaud Phenomenon

Doctors do not know exactly what causes Raynaud phenomenon to develop, but they do know some causes of attacks.

Usually, when a person is exposed to cold, the body tries to slow the loss of heat and maintain its temperature. To do so, blood vessels in the surface of the skin move blood from veins near the skin's surface to veins deeper in the body. In people with Raynaud phenomenon, blood vessels in the hands and feet appear to overreact to cold temperatures or stress. They narrow and limit blood supply.

Diagnosis of Raynaud Phenomenon

There is no single test to diagnose Raynaud phenomenon. Doctors usually diagnose Raynaud phenomenon after taking a complete medical history, an exam, and tests. Tests may include:

- Blood tests

- Looking at fingernail tissue with a microscope

If you are diagnosed with Raynaud phenomenon, your doctor will likely perform more tests to determine what form of the disease you have.

- **Nailfold capillaroscopy:** During this test, your doctor will put a drop of oil on your nail folds, the skin at the base of the fingernail. Your doctor will then examine your nail folds under a microscope to look for problems in the tiny blood vessels called "capillaries." If your capillaries are enlarged or malformed, you may have a connective tissue disease.

- **Antinuclear antibody (ANA) test:** In this blood test, the doctor determines whether your body is producing special proteins called "antibodies." These abnormal antibodies are often found in people who have connective tissue diseases or autoimmune disorders.

- **Erythrocyte sedimentation rate (ESR or sed rate):** This blood test measures how quickly your red blood cells fall to the bottom of a test tube of unclotted blood. Red blood cells that fall rapidly may suggest you have inflammation in your body. This is a sign that you may have an inflammatory disease.

Treatment of Raynaud Phenomenon

There are several treatments for Raynaud phenomenon. The goal of treatment is to:

- Reduce how many attacks you have
- Make attacks less severe
- Prevent tissue damage
- Prevent loss of finger and toe tissue

Treatment for Primary Raynaud Phenomenon

People with the primary form of Raynaud phenomenon are rarely treated with medication. Most people with the primary form of Raynaud phenomenon can prevent or manage the disease without medicine. Strategies that you can incorporate into your life include:

- Keep your hands and feet warm and dry.
- Warm your hands and feet with warm water.
- Avoid air conditioning.
- Wear gloves to touch frozen or cold foods.
- Wear many layers of loose clothing and a hat when it is cold.
- Use chemical warmers, such as small heating pouches that can be placed in pockets, mittens, boots, or shoes.
- Talk to your doctor before exercising outside in cold weather.
- Do not smoke.
- Avoid medicines that make symptoms worse.
- Control stress.
- Exercise regularly.

Treatment for Secondary Form of Raynaud Phenomenon

People with the secondary form of Raynaud phenomenon are more likely than those with the primary form to be treated with medicines. If you have the secondary form of Raynaud phenomenon, your doctor may prescribe medicines because severe attacks that cause ulcers or tissue damage are more likely. Medicines used to treat Raynaud phenomenon include:

- Blood pressure medicines

- Medicines that relax blood vessels

Pregnant woman should not take these medicines.

Surgery

If you have a severe case of Raynaud phenomenon, you may need surgery to restore blood flow to parts of the body affected by the disease.

Living with Raynaud Phenomenon

There are steps you can take to decrease the number of Raynaud attacks you have and the severity of these attacks.

- **Keep warm.** Set your thermostat to a higher temperature. You lose a lot of body heat through your head—wear a hat. Keep your feet warm and dry. In cold weather, wear several layers of loose clothing, socks, hats, and gloves or mittens. Keep pocket warmers in your pockets if you are will be outside for a long time. Use insulated drinking glasses when drinking something cold. Put on gloves before handling frozen or refrigerated foods.

- **Avoid rapidly shifting temperatures and damp climates.** Rapidly moving from 90 degrees outside to a 70-degree air-conditioned room can bring on an attack. So can damp rainy weather.

- **Avoid air conditioning.** In warm weather, air conditioning also can bring on attacks.

- **Do not smoke.** The nicotine in cigarettes causes the skin temperature to drop, which may lead to an attack.

- **Avoid medicines that bring on attacks.** Certain medicines cause the blood vessel to narrow, which can bring on an attack. These include beta-blockers, cold preparations, caffeine, narcotics, some migraine headache medications, and some chemotherapy drugs. Talk to your doctor before starting any new medicines. Do not stop any medicines you are taking without talking to your doctor first.

- **Control stress.** Because stress can bring on an attack, learning how to manage or control stress is important. Talk to your doctor about stress reduction techniques.

- **Exercise regularly.** Exercise can improve your overall well-being. In addition, it can increase your energy level, help control your weight, keep your heart healthy, and improve sleep. Talk to your doctor before starting an exercise program.

Section 26.4

Thromboangiitis Obliterans (Buerger Disease)

This section includes text excerpted from "Buerger disease," Genetic and Rare Diseases Information Center (GARD), National Center for Advancing Translational Sciences (NCATS), March 21, 2018.

What Is Buerger Disease?

Buerger disease is a disease in which small and medium-sized blood vessels in the arms and/or legs become inflamed and blocked (vasculitis). This reduces blood flow to affected areas of the body, eventually resulting in damage to the tissues. Symptoms of Buerger disease may include coldness, numbness, tingling or burning, and pain. Symptoms may first be felt in the fingertips or toes, and then move further up the arms or legs. Additional symptoms that may develop include changes in the texture and color of the skin, Raynaud phenomenon, painful muscle cramps, swelling (edema), skin ulcers, and gangrene. Rare complications that have been reported include transient ischemic attacks (TIA) or stroke, and heart attack.

Buerger disease almost always occurs in people who use tobacco, but it is not known exactly how tobacco plays a role in the development of the disease. Some people may have a genetic predisposition to Buerger disease. It is also possible that Buerger disease is an autoimmune disease, as the immune system seems to play a large role in its development. More research is needed to identify the exact underlying causes.

Quitting all forms of tobacco is an essential part of stopping the progression of the disease. There are no definitive treatments, but certain therapies may improve symptoms in some people. Therapies that have been reported with varying success include medications to improve blood flow and reduce the risk of clots, pain medicines, compression of the arms and legs, spinal cord stimulation, and surgery to control pain and increase blood flow. Amputation may be necessary if gangrene or a serious infection develops.

How Common Is Buerger Disease?

Buerger disease has become less common over the past 10 years, given the decrease in smoking prevalence and more strict diagnostic criteria. In 1947, it was estimated to occur in 104 out of 100,000 people. It now is estimated to occur in 12 to 20 out of 100,000 people.

What Causes Buerger Disease

Buerger disease has a strong relationship with cigarette smoking. This association may be due to direct poisoning of cells from some component of tobacco or by hypersensitivity to the same components. Many people with Buerger disease will show hypersensitivities to injection of tobacco extracts into their skin. There may be a genetic component to susceptibility to Buerger disease as well. It is possible that these genetic influences account for the higher prevalence of Buerger disease in people of Israeli, Indian subcontinent, and Japanese descent. Certain human leukocyte antigen (HLA) haplotypes have also been found in association with Buerger disease.

Are There Products Other than Cigarette Tobacco Associated with Buerger Disease?

Data is lacking regarding the association of Buerger disease with drugs or products other than cigarette smoking; however, there have been case reports describing Buerger disease in patients who used other products alone or in combination with tobacco. You can search for these case reports through a service called "PubMed," a searchable database of medical literature. Some articles are available as a complete document, while information on other studies is available as a summary abstract. To obtain the full article, contact a medical/university library (or your local library for interlibrary loan), or order it online. Using "Buerger disease AND" followed by the name of the drug or product of interest as your search term should locate articles. To narrow your search, click on the "Limits" tab under the search box and specify your criteria for locating more relevant articles.

How Is Buerger Disease Treated?

Currently, there is not a cure for Buerger disease; however, there are treatments that can help control it. The most essential part of treatment is to avoid all tobacco and nicotine products. Even one cigarette a day can worsen the disease. A doctor can help a person with Buerger disease learn about safe medications and programs to combat smoking/nicotine addiction. Continued smoking is associated with an overall amputation rate of 40 to 50 percent.

The following treatments may also be helpful, but do not replace smoking/nicotine cessation:

- Medications to dilate blood vessels and improve blood flow (e.g., intravenous Iloprost)
- Medications to dissolve blood clots
- Treatment with calcium channel blockers
- Walking exercises
- Intermittent compression of the arms and legs to increase blood flow to your extremities
- Surgical sympathectomy (a controversial surgery to cut the nerves to the affected area to control pain and increase blood flow)
- Therapeutic angiogenesis (medications to stimulate the growth of new blood vessels)
- Spinal cord stimulation
- Amputation, if infection or gangrene occurs

What Diet Is Recommended for People with Buerger Disease?

There are no specific diet recommendations for people with Buerger disease.

Chapter 27

Peripheral Venous Disorders

Chapter Contents

Section 27.1

Deep Vein Thrombosis and Pulmonary Embolism

This section includes text excerpted from "What Is Venous Thromboembolism?" Centers for Disease Control and Prevention (CDC), January 29, 2019.

Deep vein thrombosis and pulmonary embolism (DVT/PE) are often underdiagnosed and serious, but preventable medical conditions.

Deep vein thrombosis is a medical condition that occurs when a blood clot forms in a deep vein. These clots usually develop in the lower leg, thigh, or pelvis, but they can also occur in the arm.

It is important to know about DVT because it can happen to anybody and can cause serious illness, disability, and in some cases, death. The good news is that DVT is preventable and treatable if discovered early.

Complications of Deep Vein Thrombosis

The most serious complication of DVT happens when a part of the clot breaks off and travels through the bloodstream to the lungs, causing a blockage called a "pulmonary embolism" (PE). If the clot is small, and with appropriate treatment, people can recover from PE. However, there could be some damage to the lungs. If the clot is large, it can stop blood from reaching the lungs and is fatal.

In addition, nearly one-third of people who have a DVT will have long-term complications caused by the damage the clot does to the valves in the vein called "postthrombotic syndrome" (PTS). People with PTS have symptoms, such as swelling; pain; discoloration; and in severe cases, scaling or ulcers in the affected part of the body. In some cases, the symptoms can be so severe that a person becomes disabled.

For some people, DVT and PE can become a chronic illness; about 30 percent of people who have had a DVT or PE are at risk for another episode.

Risk Factors for Deep Vein Thrombosis

Almost anyone can have a DVT. However, certain factors can increase the chance of having this condition. The chance increases even more for someone who has more than one of these factors at the same time.

The following is a list of factors that increase the risk of developing DVT:

- Injury to a vein, often caused by:
  - Fractures
  - Severe muscle injury
  - Major surgery (particularly involving the abdomen, pelvis, hip, or legs)
- Slow blood flow, often caused by:
  - Confinement to bed (e.g., due to a medical condition or after surgery)
  - Limited movement (e.g., a cast on a leg to help heal an injured bone)
  - Sitting for a long time, especially with crossed legs
  - Paralysis
- Increased estrogen, often caused by:
  - Birth control pills
  - Hormone replacement therapy (HRT), sometimes used after menopause
  - Pregnancy, for up to three months after giving birth
- Certain chronic medical illnesses, such as:
  - Heart disease
  - Lung disease
  - Cancer and its treatments
  - Inflammatory bowel disease (Crohn disease or ulcerative colitis)
- Other factors that increase the risk of DVT include:
  - Previous DVT or PE
  - Family history of DVT or PE
  - Age (risk increases as age increases)

- Obesity

- A catheter located in a central vein

- Inherited clotting disorders

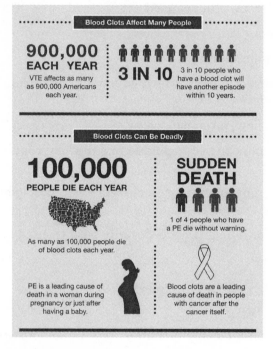

Figure 27.1. *Stats on Blood Clots*

Preventing Deep Vein Thrombosis

The following tips can help prevent DVT:

- Move around as soon as possible after having been confined to bed, such as after surgery, illness, or injury.

- If you are at risk for DVT, talk to your doctor about:

    - Graduated compression stockings (sometimes called "medical compression stockings")

    - Medication (anticoagulants) to prevent DVT

- When sitting for long periods of time, such as when traveling for more than four hours:

    - Get up and walk around every two to three hours.

- Exercise your legs while you are sitting by:
  - Raising and lowering your heels while keeping your toes on the floor
  - Raising and lowering your toes while keeping your heels on the floor
  - Tightening and releasing your leg muscles
  - Wear loose-fitting clothes.
- You can reduce your risk of DVT by maintaining a healthy weight, avoiding a sedentary lifestyle, and following your doctor's recommendations based on your individual risk factors.

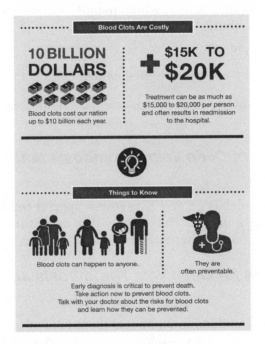

Figure 27.2. *Blood Clots and Economic Burden*

Symptoms of Deep Vein Thrombosis and Pulmonary Embolism

About half of the people with DVT have no symptoms at all. The following are the most common symptoms of DVT that occur in the affected part of the body:

- Swelling

313

- Pain

- Tenderness

- Redness of the skin

If you have any of these symptoms, you should see your doctor as soon as possible.

You can have a PE without any symptoms of a DVT.

Signs and symptoms of PE can include:

- Difficulty breathing

- Faster than normal or irregular heart beat

- Chest pain or discomfort, which usually worsens with a deep breath or coughing

- Coughing up blood

- Very low blood pressure, light-headedness,, or fainting

If you have any of these symptoms, you should seek medical help immediately.

Diagnosis of Deep Vein Thrombosis and Pulmonary Embolism

The diagnosis of DVT or PE requires special tests that can only be performed by a doctor. That is why it is important for you to seek medical care if you experience any of the symptoms of DVT or PE.

Treatments for Deep Vein Thrombosis and Pulmonary Embolism

Medication is used to prevent and treat DVT. Compression stockings are sometimes recommended to prevent DVT and to relieve pain and swelling. These might need to be worn for two years or more after having DVT. In severe cases, the clot might need to be removed surgically.

Immediate medical attention is necessary to treat PE. In cases of severe, life-threatening PE, there are medicines called "thrombolytics" that can dissolve the clot. Other medicines, called "anticoagulants," may be prescribed to prevent more clots from forming. Some people may need to be on medication long-term to prevent future blood clots.

Section 27.2

Varicose Veins and Spider Veins

This section includes text excerpted from "Varicose Veins and Spider Veins," Office on Women's Health (OWH), U.S. Department of Health and Human Services (HHS), March 1, 2019.

What Are Varicose Veins?

Varicose veins are twisted veins that can be blue, red, or skin-colored. The larger veins may appear ropelike and make the skin bulge out.

Varicose veins are often on the thighs; the backs and fronts of the calves; or the inside of the legs, near the ankles and feet. During pregnancy, varicose veins can be around the inner thigh, lower pelvic area, and buttocks.

What Are Spider Veins?

Spider veins, or thread veins, are smaller than varicose veins. They are usually red. They may look similar to tree branches or spider webs. Spider veins can usually be seen under the skin, but they do not make the skin bulge out in the way that varicose veins do.

Spider veins are usually found on the legs or the face.

Who Gets Varicose Veins and Spider Veins

Varicose veins affect almost twice as many women as men and are more common in older women. Spider veins may affect more than half of women.

What Are the Symptoms of Varicose Veins and Spider Veins?

Some women do not have any symptoms with varicose veins and spider veins. If you do have symptoms, your legs may feel extremely tired, heavy, or achy. Your symptoms may get worse after sitting or standing for long periods of time. Your symptoms may get better after resting and putting your legs up.

Other symptoms that may be more common with varicose veins include:

• Throbbing or cramping

- Swelling

- Itching

Changing hormone levels may affect your symptoms. Because of this, you may notice more symptoms during certain times in your menstrual cycle, during pregnancy, or during menopause.

What Causes Varicose Veins and Spider Veins

Problems in the valves in your veins can prevent blood from flowing normally and cause varicose veins or spider veins.

Your heart pumps blood filled with oxygen and nutrients through your arteries to your whole body. Veins then carry the blood from different parts of your body back to your heart. Normally, your veins have valves that act as one-way flaps. But, if the valves do not close correctly, blood can leak back into the lower part of the vein rather than going toward the heart. Over time, more blood gets stuck in the vein, building pressure that weakens the walls of the vein. This causes the vein to grow larger.

Are Some Women More at Risk of Varicose Veins and Spider Veins?

Yes. Varicose veins and spider veins are caused by damaged valves in the veins that prevent blood from flowing normally. Many things can damage your valves, but your risk of varicose veins and spider veins may be higher if you:

- **Have a family or personal history of varicose veins or spider veins.** In one small study, more than half of women with varicose veins had a parent with varicose veins too.

- **Sit or stand for long periods.** Sitting or standing for a long time, especially for more than four hours at a time, may make your veins work harder against gravity to pump blood to your heart.

- Are **overweight or obese.** Being overweight or obese can put extra pressure on your veins. Women who are obese are more likely to have varicose veins than women at a healthy weight.

- **Are pregnant.** During pregnancy, the amount of blood pumping through your body increases to support the fetus. The extra blood causes your veins to swell. Your growing uterus (womb) also puts pressure on your veins. Varicose veins may go away a few months after childbirth, or they may remain and continue to cause symptoms. More varicose veins and spider veins may appear with each additional pregnancy.

- **Are older.** As you get older, the valves in your veins may weaken and not work as well. Your calf muscles also weaken as you age. Your calf muscles normally help squeeze veins and send blood back toward the heart as you walk.

- **Use hormonal birth control or menopausal hormone therapy.** The hormone estrogen may weaken vein valves and lead to varicose veins. Using hormonal birth control— including the pill, a patch, a shot, a vaginal ring, or an intrauterine device (IUD), with estrogen and progesterone, or taking menopausal hormone therapy—may raise your risk of varicose or spider veins.

- **Have a condition that damaged the valves.** Blood clots in the legs or scarring of the veins can damage the valves.

Why Do Varicose Veins and Spider Veins Usually Appear in the Legs?

Varicose veins and spider veins appear most often in the legs. This is because the veins in your legs carry blood to your heart against gravity and for the longest distance of anywhere in the body.

Should You Call Your Doctor or Nurse If You Have Varicose Veins or Spider Veins?

Maybe. If you think you have varicose veins or spider veins and they cause you pain or discomfort, talk to your doctor or nurse. Varicose veins and spider veins usually do not cause symptoms. But, you may want to remove or close varicose veins or spider veins if you have symptoms or if you do not like the way they look.

Talk to your doctor or nurse if varicose veins or spider veins cause you pain or if:

- The vein has become swollen, red, or very tender or warm to the touch, which can be a sign of a blood clot.

- You have sores or a rash on your leg or near your ankle.

- The skin on your ankle or calf changes color.

317

- One of the varicose veins begins to bleed.

- Your symptoms keep you from doing daily activities.

Will You Get Varicose Veins during Pregnancy?

Maybe. During pregnancy, you have more blood pumping through your body to support the fetus. The extra blood can cause your veins to get larger. Your growing uterus (womb) also puts pressure on the veins. Varicose veins may appear around the vagina and buttocks.

For some women, varicose veins shrink or disappear after childbirth. For others, varicose veins stay after childbirth, and symptoms continue to get worse. Women may also get more varicose veins or spider veins with each additional pregnancy.

How Are Varicose Veins and Spider Veins Diagnosed?

Your doctor or nurse will look at your legs while you are standing or sitting down. She or he may ask you about your symptoms, including pain. Sometimes, the doctor or nurse may do other tests to rule out other health problems.

Your doctor or nurse may also do one of the following:

- **Ultrasound.** This test uses sound waves to create pictures of the inside of your body. Your doctor or nurse can check the blood flow in your veins to look for weakened or leaky valves and blood clots.

- **Venogram.** Your doctor or nurse may do this test to get a closer look at blood flow through your veins. A venogram is a type of X-ray that uses a dye (called a "contrast") to help your doctor or nurse see the veins in your legs. A venogram is a type of angiogram, a test often used in heart disease. This test is used only if your doctor or nurse thinks you may have a large blood clot.

How Are Varicose Veins and Spider Veins Treated?

If your symptoms are mild, your doctor or nurse may suggest steps to take at home. Your doctor or nurse may also suggest compression stockings to wear daily and remove at night to make blood flow better in your legs. These steps may help you manage symptoms of existing varicose veins and spider veins. They can also help prevent new varicose veins and spider veins from forming.

If compression stockings do not work or if you have pain or other symptoms that bother you, your doctor or nurse may talk to you about nonsurgical procedures to treat varicose veins and spider veins.

If you have very large or severe varicose veins, you may need surgery.

Is Treatment for Varicose Veins and Spider Veins Permanent?

Maybe. Some treatments for varicose veins seal off or remove the vein permanently. But, over time, new varicose veins or spider veins can develop. You cannot control some risk factors for varicose veins and spider veins, such as your age and family history. If you get new varicose veins or spider veins, you may need to have a surgery or medical procedure again to remove them or block them off.

Wearing gradient compression support stockings may help prevent new varicose veins or spider veins from developing.

What Can You Do at Home to Help Varicose Veins and Spider Veins?

If your varicose veins or spider veins bother you, you can take steps at home or work to make blood flow in your legs better.

- **Get regular physical activity.** Muscles in the legs help your veins push blood back to the heart, against the force of gravity. If you have varicose veins or spider veins in your legs, any exercise that works the muscles in your legs will help prevent new varicose veins or spider veins from forming.

- **Lose weight,** if you are overweight or obese. Extra weight makes it more difficult for your veins to move blood back up to your heart, against the force of gravity. Losing weight may help prevent new varicose veins or spider veins from forming.

- **Do not sit or stand for a long time.** If you have to sit or stand at work or home for a long time, take a break every 30 minutes to stand up and walk around. This makes the muscles in your legs move the blood back up to your heart more than when you are sitting or standing still without moving around.

- **Wear compression stockings.** Compression stockings help increase blood flow from your legs.

- **Put your feet up.** Rest your feet on a stool as much as possible when sitting to help the blood in your legs flow back to your heart.

How Do Compression Stockings Help Treat Varicose Veins and Spider Veins?

Compression stockings put pressure on your veins, which increases blood flow from your legs. There are three kinds of compression stockings:

- **Support pantyhose,** which give the least amount of pressure. These are sold in most stores.

- **Over-the-counter (OTC) gradient compression hose,** which give a little more pressure around the foot, ankle, and lower leg, where pressure is needed most to move the blood back toward your heart. These are sold in medical supply stores and some drugstores.

- **Prescription-strength gradient compression hose,** which offers the greatest amount of pressure to the feet, ankles, and lower legs. You may need a prescription from your doctor to buy them, especially if your insurance plan covers it. You will also need to be fitted by someone who has been trained to do this. This hose is sold in medical supply stores and some drugstores.

Some stronger compression stockings can hurt people with certain medical conditions, such as certain types of heart disease or heart failure. Ask your doctor or nurse if it is safe for you to use prescription-strength compression stockings or what strength would be safe for you.

What Else Can You Do to Treat Varicose Veins and Spider Veins without Having Surgery?

Your doctor or nurse may give you medicine to treat the symptoms of varicose veins, including swelling, pain, and itching.

Other nonsurgical treatments for varicose veins and spider veins include:

- **Sclerotherapy.** Sclerotherapy is the most common treatment for smaller varicose veins and spider veins. The doctor injects a chemical into the vein. The chemical causes the vein walls to swell, stick together, and seal shut. This stops the flow of blood, and the vein turns into scar tissue. Your doctor or nurse may suggest that you wear gradient compression stockings after sclerotherapy to help with healing. In a few weeks, the vein should fade. You may need multiple treatments for it to work. There is also a chance that varicose veins or spider veins may come back.

- **Closure system.** This system works only for veins just beneath the skin's surface. Deeper veins are not treatable with this option. The system closes the vein permanently using a type of adhesive (sticky material) injected into the vein. After the treatment, healthy veins around the closed vein take over the normal flow of blood.

- **Percutaneous (skin surface) laser treatments.** Laser treatments can treat spider veins and varicose veins that are smaller than three millimeters in diameter (about a tenth of an inch). This procedure sends very strong bursts of light through the skin and onto the vein. This makes the vein slowly fade and disappear. You may need several treatments to close spider veins in the legs. There is a chance that varicose veins or spider veins may come back.

- **Endovenous thermal therapy (laser and radiofrequency ablation).** This procedure treats the larger bulging surface veins of the legs. During the procedure, the doctor inserts a small tube into the vein. The doctor places a small probe through the tube. A device at the tip of the probe heats up the inside of the vein and closes it off. The device uses radio waves or laser energy to seal the vein permanently. Healthy veins around the sealed vein take over the normal flow of blood.

What Types of Surgery Do Treat Varicose Veins?

Your doctor or nurse may recommend surgery for very large or severe varicose veins. Types of surgery for varicose veins include:

- **Ambulatory phlebectomy.** This surgery removes varicose veins that are just beneath the skin's surface. The doctor makes tiny cuts in the skin and uses hooks to pull the vein out of the leg. The doctor usually removes the vein in one treatment, and this procedure leaves only tiny scars. Many people can return to normal activity the day after treatment. Healthy veins will then take over the normal flow of blood.

- **Surgical ligation and stripping.** This surgery is for larger varicose veins. With this treatment, problem veins are tied shut and completely removed from the leg through small cuts in the skin. Recovery can take up to a month. Healthy veins take over the normal flow of blood.

Does Insurance Cover Varicose Veins and Spider Veins Treatment?

Maybe. Your insurance plan may cover certain treatments for varicose veins and spider veins, such as compression stockings, medicine, or a procedure if you have symptoms, such as pain or swelling. Insurance may also cover surgery if wearing compression stockings has not helped.

- If you have insurance, check with your insurance provider to find out what is included in your plan.

- If you have Medicare, find out about Medicare coverage for varicose veins.

- If you have Medicaid, the benefits covered are different in each state, but certain benefits must be covered. Check with your state's Medicaid program to find out what is covered.

- If you need health insurance, check to see if you are eligible.

What Can Happen If Varicose Veins and Spider Veins Are Not Treated?

Most varicose veins and spider veins do not cause any health problems. Larger varicose veins may cause aching, throbbing, and discomfort, especially after you have been sitting or standing for long periods of time.

Sometimes, varicose veins can lead to more serious health problems, including:

- **Sores or skin ulcers** caused by long-term collection of blood in the veins. These sores or ulcers are painful and difficult to heal. You may need special care to treat these sores or ulcers.

- **Bleeding from damage to the vein.** The skin over varicose veins can become thin and easily hurt. Any injury to the vein can cause bleeding.

- **Superficial thrombophlebitis,** or blood clots that form in veins just below the skin. These types of blood clots can cause skin redness; a firm, tender, warm vein; and pain and swelling.

Deep vein thrombosis, or blood clots in veins that are deeper under the skin. You may not have any signs or symptoms of DVT, or the blood clot may cause pain, swelling, warmth, and a "pulling" feeling in the calf. Sitting still for a long time, such as when you are traveling for more than eight hours, may increase your risk of a blood clot. The blood clot can then break off and travel to the lungs. It can cause a blockage in the lungs, called a "pulmonary embolism," that makes it difficult to breathe, speeds up your heartbeat, and causes chest pain. It can also lead to death. You can help prevent blood clots during long airplane flights, for example, by wearing compression stockings, staying hydrated, and moving around regularly.

How Can You Prevent Varicose Veins and Spider Veins?

You may not be able to prevent varicose veins and spider veins, especially if they usually happen in your family or when you are pregnant. There are other parts of your life that you cannot control, such as getting older, that can also contribute to varicose veins and spider veins.

There are steps you can take at home, such as exercising and losing extra weight, that can make you healthier and may prevent new varicose veins or spider veins from forming. These steps may also help your legs feel better by relieving pain and discomfort.

Chapter 28

Hereditary Hemorrhagic Telangiectasia

Hereditary hemorrhagic telangiectasia (HHT) is a disorder in which some blood vessels do not develop properly. A person with HHT may form blood vessels without the capillaries (tiny blood vessels that pass blood from arteries to veins) that are usually present between arteries and veins.

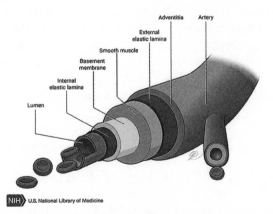

Figure 28.1. *Artery* (Source: "Hereditary Hemorrhagic Telangiectasia," Genetics Home Reference (GHR), National Institutes of Health (NIH).)

This chapter includes text excerpted from "Facts about Hereditary Hemorrhagic Telangiectasia (HHT)," Centers for Disease Control and Prevention (CDC), February 8, 2019.

The space between an artery and a vein is often fragile and can burst and bleed much more easily than other blood vessels. Men, women, and children from all racial and ethnic groups can be affected by HHT and experience the problems associated with this disorder, some of which are serious and potentially life-threatening. Fortunately, if HHT is discovered early, effective treatments are available. However, there is no cure for HHT.

Signs of Hereditary Hemorrhagic Telangiectasia

Nosebleeds are the most common sign of HHT, resulting from small abnormal blood vessels within the inside layer of the nose. Abnormal blood vessels in the skin can appear on the hands, fingertips, face, lips, lining of the mouth, and nose as delicate red or purplish spots that lighten briefly when touched. Bleeding within the stomach or intestines is another possible indicator of HHT that occurs because of abnormal blood vessels lining the digestive tract. Additional signs of HHT include abnormal artery-vein connections within the brain, lungs, and liver, which often do not display any warning signs before rupturing.

Causes of Hereditary Hemorrhagic Telangiectasia

Hereditary hemorrhagic telangiectasia is a genetic disorder. Each person with HHT has one gene that is altered, which causes HHT, as well as one normal gene. It takes only one mutant gene to cause HHT. When someone with HHT has children, each child has a 50 percent chance to receive the mutant gene from her or his parent, and therefore, to have HHT as well. Each child also has a 50 percent chance to receive the normal gene and not be affected with HHT. At least 5 different genes can cause HHT, 3 of which are known.

Diagnosis of Hereditary Hemorrhagic Telangiectasia

Hereditary hemorrhagic telangiectasia can be diagnosed by performing genetic testing. Genetic testing can detect a gene mutation in about ¾ of families with signs of HHT, which, if found, can establish the diagnosis of HHT in individuals and families who are unsure about whether they have HHT. HHT can also be diagnosed by using clinical criteria (presence of signs and a history of signs in a parent, sibling, or child).

Complications and Treatment of Hereditary Hemorrhagic Telangiectasia

The complications of HHT can vary widely, even among people affected by HHT in the same family. Complications and treatment of HHT depend on the parts of the body that are affected by this disorder. Treatment may include controlling bleeding and anemia and preventing complications from abnormal artery-vein connections in the lungs and brain.

Chapter 29

Vasculitis

What Is Vasculitis?

Vasculitis is a condition that involves inflammation in the blood vessels. The condition occurs if your immune system attacks your blood vessels by mistake. This may happen as the result of an infection, a medicine, or another disease or condition.

"Inflammation" refers to the body's response to injury, including injury to the blood vessels. Inflammation may involve pain, redness, warmth, swelling, and loss of function in the affected tissues.

In vasculitis, inflammation can lead to serious problems. Complications depend on which blood vessels, organs, or other body systems are affected.

Types of Vasculitis

There are many types of vasculitis. Each type involves inflamed blood vessels. However, most types differ in whom they affect and the organs that are involved.

The types of vasculitis often are grouped based on the size of the blood vessels they affect.

This chapter includes text excerpted from "Vasculitis," National Heart, Lung, and Blood Institute (NHLBI), April 8, 2011. Reviewed May 2019.

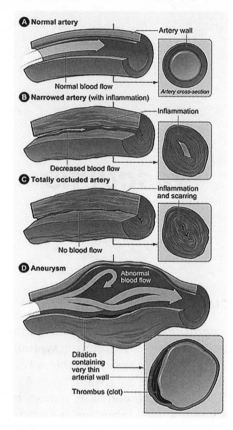

Figure 29.1. *Vasculitis*

Figure A shows a normal artery with normal blood flow. The inset image shows a cross-section of the normal artery. Figure B shows an inflamed, narrowed artery with decreased blood flow. The inset image shows a cross-section of the inflamed artery. Figure C shows an inflamed, blocked (occluded) artery and scarring on the artery wall. The inset image shows a cross-section of the blocked artery. Figure D shows an artery with an aneurysm. The inset image shows a cross-section of the artery with an aneurysm.

Mostly Large Vessel Vasculitis

These types of vasculitis usually, but not always, affect the body's larger blood vessels.

Behçet Disease

Behçet disease can cause recurrent, painful ulcers (sores) in the mouth, ulcers on the genitals, acne-like skin lesions, and eye inflammation called "uveitis."

The disease occurs most often in people between the ages of 20 and 40. Men are more likely to get it, but it also can affect women. Behçet disease is more common in people of Mediterranean, Middle Eastern, and Far Eastern descent, although it rarely affects Black individuals.

Researchers believe that a gene called the *"HLA-B51"* gene may play a role in Behçet disease. However, not everyone who has the gene gets the disease.

Cogan Syndrome

Cogan syndrome can occur in people who have a systemic vasculitis that affects the large blood vessels, especially the aorta and aortic valve. The aorta is the main artery that carries oxygen-rich blood from the heart to the body.

A systemic vasculitis is a type of vasculitis that affects you in a general or overall way.

Cogan syndrome can lead to eye inflammation called "interstitial keratitis." The syndrome also can cause hearing changes, including sudden deafness.

Giant Cell Arteritis

Giant cell arteritis (GCA) usually affects the temporal artery, an artery on the side of your head. This condition also is called "temporal arteritis." Symptoms of this condition can include headaches, scalp tenderness, jaw pain, blurred vision, double vision, and acute (sudden) vision loss.

Giant cell arteritis is the most common form of vasculitis in adults older than 50 years of age. It is more likely to occur in people of Scandinavian origin, but it can affect people of any race.

Polymyalgia Rheumatica

Polymyalgia rheumatica (PMR) commonly affects the large joints in the body, such as the shoulders and hips. PMR typically causes stiffness and pain in the muscles of the neck, shoulders, lower back, hips, and thighs.

Polymyalgia rheumatica usually occurs by itself, but 10 to 20 percent of people who have PMR also develop giant cell arteritis. Also, about half of the people who have giant cell arteritis may develop PMR.

Takayasu Arteritis

Takayasu arteritis (TA) affects medium- and large-sized arteries, particularly the aorta and its branches. The condition sometimes is called "aortic arch syndrome."

Though rare, TA mainly affects teenage girls and young women. The condition is most common in Asians, but it can affect people of all races.

Takayasu arteritis is a systemic disease.

Symptoms of TA may include tiredness and a sense of feeling unwell, fever, night sweats, sore joints, loss of appetite, and weight loss. These symptoms usually occur before other signs develop that point to arteritis.

Mostly Medium Vessel Vasculitis

These types of vasculitis usually, but not always, affect the body's medium-sized blood vessels.

Buerger Disease

Buerger disease, also known as "thromboangiitis obliterans," typically affects blood flow to the hands and feet. In this disease, the blood vessels in the hands and feet tighten or become blocked. As a result, less blood flows to the affected tissues, which can lead to pain and tissue damage.

Rarely, Buerger disease also can affect blood vessels in the brain, abdomen, and heart. The disease usually affects men between the ages of 20 and 40 of Asian or Eastern European descent. The disease is strongly linked to cigarette smoking.

Symptoms of Buerger disease include pain in the calves or feet when walking or pain in the forearms and hands with activity. Other symptoms include blood clots in the surface veins of the limbs and Raynaud phenomenon.

In severe cases, ulcers may develop on the fingers and toes, leading to gangrene. The term "gangrene" refers to the death or decay of body tissues.

Surgical bypass of the blood vessels may help restore blood flow to some areas. Medicines generally do not work well to treat Buerger disease. The best treatment is to stop using tobacco of any kind.

Central Nervous System Vasculitis

Central nervous system (CNS) vasculitis usually occurs as a result of a systemic vasculitis.

Very rarely, vasculitis affects only the brain and/or spinal cord. When it does, the condition is called "isolated vasculitis of the central nervous system" or "primary angiitis of the central nervous system."

Symptoms of CNS vasculitis include headaches, problems thinking clearly; changes in mental function; or stroke-like symptoms, such as muscle weakness and paralysis (an inability to move).

Kawasaki Disease

Kawasaki disease (KS) is a rare childhood disease in which the walls of the blood vessels throughout the body become inflamed. The disease can affect any blood vessel in the body, including arteries, veins, and capillaries.

Kawasaki disease also is known as "mucocutaneous lymph node syndrome." This is because the disease is associated with redness of the mucous membranes in the eyes and mouth, redness of the skin, and enlarged lymph nodes. (Mucous membranes are tissues that line some organs and body cavities.)

Sometimes, the disease affects the coronary arteries, which carry oxygen-rich blood to the heart. As a result, a small number of children who have Kawasaki disease may have serious heart problems.

Polyarteritis Nodosa

Polyarteritis nodosa can affect many parts of the body. This disorder often affects the kidneys, the digestive tract, the nerves, and the skin.

Symptoms often include fever, a general feeling of being unwell, weight loss, and muscle and joint aches, including pain in the calf muscles that develops over weeks or months.

Other signs and symptoms include anemia (a low red blood cell count), a lace- or web-like rash, bumps under the skin, and stomach pain after eating.

Researchers believe that this type of vasculitis is very rare, although the symptoms can be similar to those of other types of vasculitis. Some cases of polyarteritis nodosa seem to be linked to hepatitis B or C infections.

Mostly Small Vessel Vasculitis

These types of vasculitis usually, but not always, affect the body's small blood vessels.

Eosinophilic Granulomatosis with Polyangiitis

Eosinophilic granulomatosis with polyangiitis (EGPA) is a very rare disorder that causes blood vessel inflammation. The disorder is also known as "Churg-Strauss syndrome" or "allergic angiitis" and "granulomatosis."

Eosinophilic granulomatosis with polyangiitis can affect many organs, including the lungs, skin, kidneys, nervous system, and heart. Symptoms can vary widely. They may include asthma, higher than normal levels of white blood cells (WBC) in the blood and tissues, and abnormal lumps known as "granulomas."

Cryoglobulinemia Vasculitis

Cryoglobulinemic vasculitis occurs when abnormal immune proteins (cryoglobulins) thicken the blood and impair blood flow. This causes pain and damage to the skin, joints, peripheral nerves, kidneys, and liver.

Cryoglobulins are abnormal immune proteins in the blood that clump together and thicken the blood plasma. Cryoglobulins can be detected in the laboratory by exposing a sample of blood to cold temperature (below normal body temperature). In cold temperatures, the immune proteins form clumps; but when the blood is rewarmed, the clumps dissolve.

The cause of cryoglobulinemic vasculitis is not always known. In some cases, it is associated with other conditions, such as lymphoma, multiple myeloma, connective tissue diseases, and infection (particularly hepatitis C infection).

IgA Vasculitis

In immunoglobulin A (IgA) vasculitis (also known as "Henoch-Schonlein purpura"), abnormal IgA deposits develop in small blood vessels in the skin, joints, intestines, and kidneys. IgA is a type of antibody (a protein) that normally helps defend the body against infections.

Symptoms of IgA vasculitis include a bruise-like, reddish-purple rash, most often seen on the buttocks, legs, and feet (but can be anywhere on the body); abdominal pain; swollen and painful joints; and blood in the urine. People with IgA vasculitis do not necessarily have all of the symptoms, but nearly all will have the characteristic rash.

IgA vasculitis is most often seen in children between 2 and 11 years of age, but it can affect people of all ages. More than 75 percent of the cases of IgA vasculitis follow an upper respiratory tract infection, a throat infection, or a gastrointestinal (GI) infection.

Most people with IgA vasculitis are well within one to two months and do not have any lasting problems. In rare cases, symptoms can last longer or come back. All IgA vasculitis patients should have a full evaluation by a medical professional.

Hypersensitivity Vasculitis

Hypersensitivity vasculitis affects the skin. This condition also is known as "allergic vasculitis," "cutaneous vasculitis," or "leukocyto-clastic vasculitis."

A common symptom is red spots on the skin, usually on the lower legs. For people who are bedridden, the rash appears on the lower back.

An allergic reaction to a medicine or infection often causes this type of vasculitis. Stopping the medicine or treating the infection usually clears up the vasculitis. However, some people may need to take anti-inflammatory medicines, such as corticosteroids, for a short time. These medicines help reduce inflammation.

Microscopic Polyangiitis

Microscopic polyangiitis affects small blood vessels, particularly those in the kidneys and lungs. The disease mainly occurs in middle-aged people; it affects men slightly more often than women.

The symptoms often are not specific, and they can begin gradually with fever, weight loss, and muscle aches. Sometimes, the symptoms come on suddenly and progress quickly, leading to kidney failure.

If the lungs are affected, coughing up blood may be the first symptom. Sometimes, microscopic polyangiitis occurs with a vasculitis that affects the intestinal tract, the skin, and the nervous system.

The signs and symptoms of microscopic polyangiitis are similar to those of Wegener's granulomatosis (another type of vasculitis). However, microscopic polyangiitis usually does not affect the nose and sinuses or cause abnormal tissue formations in the lungs and kidneys.

The results of certain blood tests can suggest inflammation. These results include a higher-than-normal erythrocyte sedimentation rate (ESR); lower-than-normal hemoglobin and hematocrit levels (which suggest anemia); and higher-than-normal white blood cell (WBC) and platelet counts.

Also, more than half of the people who have microscopic polyangiitis have certain antibodies (proteins) in their blood. These antibodies are called "antineutrophil cytoplasmic autoantibodies" (ANCA). ANCA also occur in people who have Wegener's granulomatosis.

Testing for ANCA cannot be used to diagnose either of these two types of vasculitis. However, testing can help evaluate people who have vasculitis-like symptoms.

Causes of Vasculitis

Vasculitis occurs if your immune system attacks your blood vessels by mistake. What causes this to happen is not fully known.

A recent or chronic (ongoing) infection may prompt the attack. Your body also may attack its own blood vessels in reaction to a medicine.

Sometimes, an autoimmune disorder triggers vasculitis. Autoimmune disorders occur if the immune system makes antibodies (proteins) that attack and damage the body's own tissues or cells. Examples of these disorders include lupus, rheumatoid arthritis (RA), and scleroderma. You can have these disorders for years before developing vasculitis.

Vasculitis also may be linked to certain blood cancers, such as leukemia and lymphoma.

Risk Factors for Vasculitis

Vasculitis can affect people of all ages and races and both sexes. Some types of vasculitis seem to occur more often in people who:

- Have certain medical conditions, such as chronic hepatitis B or C infection

- Have certain autoimmune diseases, such as lupus, rheumatoid arthritis, and scleroderma

- Smoke

Screening and Prevention of Vasculitis

You cannot prevent vasculitis. However, treatment can help prevent or delay the complications of vasculitis.

People who have severe vasculitis are treated with prescription medicines. Rarely, surgery may be done. People who have mild vasculitis may find relief with over-the-counter (OTC) pain medicines, such as acetaminophen, aspirin, ibuprofen, or naproxen.

Signs, Symptoms, and Complications of Vasculitis

The signs and symptoms of vasculitis vary. They depend on the type of vasculitis you have, the organs involved, and the severity of the condition. Some people may have few signs and symptoms. Other people may become very sick.

Sometimes, the signs and symptoms develop slowly, over months. Other times, the signs and symptoms develop quickly, over days or weeks.

Systemic Signs and Symptoms

Systemic signs and symptoms are those that affect you in a general or overall way. Common systemic signs and symptoms of vasculitis are:

- Fever

- Loss of appetite

- Weight loss

- Fatigue (tiredness)

- General aches and pains

Organ- or Body System-Specific Signs and Symptoms

Vasculitis can affect specific organs and body systems, causing a range of signs and symptoms.

Skin. If vasculitis affects your skin, you may notice skin changes. For example, you may have purple or red spots or bumps, clusters of small dots, splotches, bruises, or hives. Your skin also may itch.

Joints. If vasculitis affects your joints, you may ache or develop arthritis in one or more joints.

Lungs. If vasculitis affects your lungs, you may feel short of breath. You may even cough up blood. The results from a chest X-ray may show signs that suggest pneumonia, even though that may not be what you have.

Gastrointestinal tract. If vasculitis affects your GI tract, you may get ulcers (sores) in your mouth or have stomach pain.

In severe cases, blood flow to the intestines can be blocked. This can cause the wall of the intestines to weaken and possibly rupture (burst). A rupture can lead to serious problems or even death.

337

Sinuses, nose, throat, and ears, If vasculitis affects your sinuses, nose, throat, and ears, you may have sinus or chronic (ongoing) middle ear infections. Other symptoms include ulcers in the nose and, in some cases, hearing loss.

Eyes. If vasculitis affects your eyes, you may develop red, itchy, burning eyes. Your eyes also may become sensitive to light, and your vision may blur. Rarely, certain types of vasculitis may cause blindness.

Brain. If vasculitis affects your brain, symptoms may include headaches; problems thinking clearly; changes in mental function; or stroke-like symptoms, such as muscle weakness and paralysis (an inability to move).

Nerves. If vasculitis affects your nerves, you may have numbness, tingling, and weakness in various parts of your body. You also may have a loss of feeling or strength in your hands and feet and shooting pains in your arms and legs.

Diagnosis of Vasculitis

Your doctor will diagnose vasculitis based on your signs and symptoms, your medical history, a physical exam, and test results.

Specialists Involved

Depending on the type of vasculitis you have and the organs affected, your doctor may refer you to various specialists, including:

- A rheumatologist (joint and muscle specialist)

- An infectious disease specialist

- A dermatologist (skin specialist)

- A pulmonologist (lung specialist)

- A nephrologist (kidney specialist)

- A neurologist (nervous system specialist)

- A cardiologist (heart specialist)

- An ophthalmologist (eye specialist)

- A urologist (urinary tract and urogenital system specialist)

Diagnostic Tests and Procedures

Many tests are used to diagnose vasculitis.

Blood Tests

Blood tests can show whether you have abnormal levels of certain blood cells and antibodies (proteins) in your blood. These tests may look at:

- **Hemoglobin and hematocrit.** A low hemoglobin or hematocrit level suggests anemia, a complication of vasculitis. Vasculitis can interfere with the body's ability to make enough red blood cells (RBCs). Vasculitis also can be linked to increased destruction of red blood cells.

- **Antineutrophil cytoplasmic antibodies.** These antibodies are present in people who have certain types of vasculitis.

- **Erythrocyte sedimentation rate (ESR).** A high ESR may be a sign of inflammation in the body.

- The amount of **C-reactive protein (CRP)** in your blood. A high CRP level suggests inflammation.

Biopsy

A biopsy often is the best way for your doctor to make a firm diagnosis of vasculitis. During a biopsy, your doctor will take a small sample of your body tissue to study under a microscope. She or he will take the tissue sample from a blood vessel or an organ.

A pathologist will study the sample for signs of inflammation or tissue damage. A pathologist is a doctor who specializes in identifying diseases by studying cells and tissues under a microscope.

Blood Pressure

People who have vasculitis should have their blood pressure checked routinely. Vasculitis that damages the kidneys can cause high blood pressure.

Urinalysis

For this test, you will provide a urine sample for analysis. This test detects abnormal levels of protein or blood cells in the urine. Abnormal levels of these substances can be a sign of vasculitis affecting the kidneys.

Electrocardiogram

An electrocardiogram (EKG) is a simple, painless test that records the heart's electrical activity. You might have this test to show whether vasculitis is affecting your heart.

Echocardiography

An echocardiography (echo) is a painless test that uses sound waves to create a moving picture of your heart. The test gives information about the size and shape of your heart and how well your heart chambers and valves are working.

Chest X-Ray

A chest X-ray is a painless test that creates pictures of the structures inside your chest, such as your heart, lungs, and blood vessels. Abnormal chest X-ray results may show whether vasculitis is affecting your lungs or your large arteries (such as the aorta or the pulmonary arteries).

Lung Function Tests

Lung function tests measure how much air you can breathe in and out, how fast you can breathe air out, and how well your lungs deliver oxygen to your blood.

Lung function tests can help your doctor find out whether airflow into and out of your lungs is restricted or blocked.

Abdominal Ultrasound

An abdominal ultrasound uses sound waves to create a picture of the organs and structures in your abdomen. The picture may show whether vasculitis is affecting your abdominal organs.

Computed Tomography Scan

A computed tomography (CT) scan is a type of X-ray that creates more detailed pictures of your internal organs than a standard X-ray. The results from this test can show whether you have a type of vasculitis that affects your abdominal organs or blood vessels.

Magnetic Resonance Imaging

A magnetic resonance imaging (MRI) test uses radio waves, magnets, and a computer to create detailed pictures of your internal organs.

Other Advanced Imaging Techniques

Several new imaging techniques are now being used to help diagnose vasculitis. Duplex ultrasonography combines an image of the structure of the blood vessel with a color image of the blood flow through that vein or artery. 18F-fluorodeoxyglucose positron emission tomography (FDG-PET) identifies areas that show higher glucose metabolism, leading to problems in the blood vessels.

Angiography

Angiography is a test that uses dye and special X-rays to show blood flowing through your blood vessels.

The dye is injected into your bloodstream. Special X-ray pictures are taken while the dye flows through your blood vessels. The dye helps highlight the vessels on the X-ray pictures.

Doctors use angiography to help find out whether blood vessels are narrowed, swollen, deformed, or blocked.

Treatment of Vasculitis

Treatment for vasculitis will depend on the type of vasculitis you have, which organs are affected, and the severity of the condition.

People who have severe vasculitis are treated with prescription medicines. Rarely, surgery may be done. People who have mild vasculitis may find relief with over-the-counter pain medicines, such as acetaminophen, aspirin, ibuprofen, or naproxen.

The main goal of treating vasculitis is to reduce inflammation in the affected blood vessels. This usually is done by reducing or stopping the immune response that caused the inflammation.

Types of Treatment

Common prescription medicines used to treat vasculitis include corticosteroids and cytotoxic medicines.

Corticosteroids help reduce inflammation in your blood vessels. Examples of corticosteroids are prednisone, prednisolone, and methylprednisolone.

Doctors may prescribe cytotoxic medicines if vasculitis is severe or if corticosteroids do not work well. Cytotoxic medicines kill the cells that are causing the inflammation. Examples of these medicines are azathioprine, methotrexate, and cyclophosphamide.

341

Your doctor may prescribe both corticosteroids and cytotoxic medicines.

Other treatments may be used for certain types of vasculitis. For example, the standard treatment for Kawasaki disease is high-dose aspirin and immune globulin. Immune globulin is a medicine that is injected into a vein.

Certain types of vasculitis may require surgery to remove aneurysms that have formed as a result of the condition. An aneurysm is an abnormal bulge in the wall of a blood vessel.

Living with Vasculitis

The outcome of vasculitis is hard to predict. It will depend on the type of vasculitis you have, which organs are affected, and the severity of the condition.

If vasculitis is diagnosed early and responds well to treatment, it may go away or go into remission. "Remission" means the condition is not active, but it can come back, or "flare," at any time.

Flares can be hard to predict. You may have a flare when you stop treatment or change your treatment. Some types of vasculitis seem to flare more often than others. Also, some people have flares more often than others.

Sometimes, vasculitis is chronic (ongoing) and never goes into remission. Long-term treatment with medicines often can control chronic vasculitis, but no cure has been found. Rarely, vasculitis does not respond well to treatment. This can lead to disability or even death.

Ongoing Care

The medicines used to treat vasculitis can have side effects. For example, long-term use of corticosteroids may lead to weight gain, diabetes, weakness, a decrease in muscle size, and osteoporosis (a bone-thinning condition). Long-term use of these medicines also may increase your risk of infection.

Your doctor may adjust the type or dose of medicine you take to lessen or prevent the side effects. If your vasculitis goes into remission, your doctor may carefully withdraw your medicines. However, she or he will still need to carefully watch you for flares.

While you are being treated for vasculitis, you will need to see your doctor regularly. Talk with your doctor about any new symptoms and other changes in your health, including side effects of your medicines.

Emotional Issues and Support

Living with a chronic condition may cause fear, anxiety, depression, and stress. Talk about how you feel with your healthcare team. Talking to a professional counselor also can help. If you are very depressed, your doctor may recommend medicines or other treatments that can improve your quality of life (QOL).

Joining a patient support group may help you adjust to living with vasculitis. You can see how other people who have the same symptoms have coped with them. Talk with your doctor about local support groups or check with an area medical center.

Support from family and friends also can help relieve stress and anxiety. Let your loved ones know how you feel and what they can do to help you.

Part Four

Cardiovascular Disorders in Specific Populations

Chapter 30

Cardiovascular Disease in Children

Chapter Contents

Section 30.1

Basic Facts about Congenital Heart Defects

This section includes text excerpted from "Congenital Heart Defects," National Heart, Lung, and Blood Institute (NHLBI), May 2, 2018.

Congenital heart defects, or diseases, are problems with the heart's structure that are present at birth. They may change the normal flow of blood through the heart. Congenital heart defects are the most common type of birth defect.

Congenital heart defects affect nearly 1 percent of—or about 40,000—births per year in the United States. The prevalence of some congenital heart defects, especially mild types, is increasing, while the prevalence of other types has remained stable. Researchers estimated that about 1 million U.S. children and about 1.4 million U.S. adults were living with congenital heart defects. Overall, there are slightly more adults living with congenital heart defects than children.*

* Excerpted from "Data and Statistics on Congenital Heart Defects," Centers for Disease Control and Prevention (CDC), November 2, 2018.

There are many types of congenital heart defects. The most common defects involve the inside walls of the heart, the valves of the heart, or the large blood vessels that carry blood to and from the heart. Some defects require no treatment, but some require treatment soon after birth. Because diagnosis and treatment of congenital heart defects have improved, more babies are surviving, and now many adults are living with congenital heart defects.

Types of Congenital Heart Defects

There are many types of congenital heart defects. They range from simple to complex and critical. Simple defects, such as atrial septal defect (ASD) and ventricular septal defects (VSD), may have no symptoms and may not require surgery. Complex or critical defects, such as hypoplastic left heart syndrome (HLHS) may have severe, life-threatening symptoms. Babies born with a critical congenital heart defect typically have low levels of oxygen soon after birth and need surgery within the first year of life.

Atrial Septal Defect

An atrial septal defect is a hole in the wall between the atria, which are the two upper chambers of the heart. The hole causes blood to flow from the left atrium and mix with the right atrium, instead of going to the rest of the body. Atrial septal defect is considered a simple congenital heart defect because the hole may close on its own as the heart grows during childhood, and repair may not be necessary.

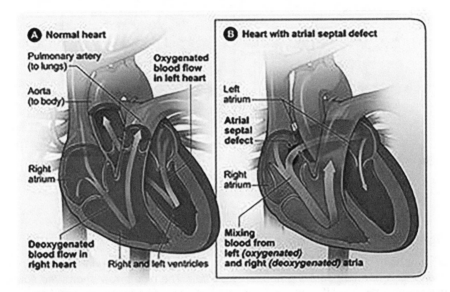

Figure 30.1. *Atrial Septal Defect*

Cross-section of a normal heart and a heart with an atrial septal defect. Figure A shows the structure and blood flow inside a normal heart. The blue arrow shows the flow of oxygen-poor blood as it is pumped from the body into the right atrium and then to the right ventricle. From there, it pumps through the pulmonary artery to the lungs, where it picks up oxygen. The oxygen-rich blood, shown by the red arrows, flows from the lungs through the pulmonary veins into the left atrium. Figure B shows a heart with an atrial septal defect. The hole allows oxygen-rich blood from the left atrium to mix with the oxygen-poor blood from the right atrium. The mixed blood is shown with a purple arrow.

Pulmonary Stenosis

Pulmonary stenosis is a narrowing of the valve through which blood leaves the heart on its way to the lungs. Many children with pulmonary stenosis do not need treatment.

Patent Ductus Arteriosus

This common type of simple congenital heart defect occurs when a connection between the heart's two major arteries does not close properly after birth. This leaves an opening through which blood can flow when it should not. Small openings may close on their own.

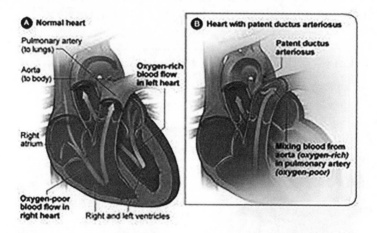

Figure 30.2. *Patent Ductus Arteriosus*

Normal heart and heart with patent ductus arteriosus (PDA). Figure A shows the interior of a normal heart and normal blood flow. The blue arrow shows the flow of oxygen-poor blood as it is pumped from the body into the right atrium and then to the right ventricle. From there, it pumps through the pulmonary artery to the lungs, where it picks up oxygen. The oxygen-rich blood, shown with a red arrow, flows from the lungs through the pulmonary veins into the left atrium. Figure B shows a heart with patent ductus arteriosus. The defect connects the aorta with the pulmonary artery, a connection that should have closed to form the ligamentum arteriosum (see Figure A) at birth. The hole allows oxygen-rich blood from the left atrium to mix with the oxygen-poor blood from the right atrium. The mixed blood is shown with a purple arrow

Ventricular Septal Defect

A ventricular septal defect is a hole in the wall between the ventricles, which are the two lower chambers of the heart. Blood may flow from the left ventricle and mix with blood in the right ventricle, instead of going to the rest of the body. If the hole is large, this may make the heart and lungs work harder and may cause fluid to build up in the lungs.

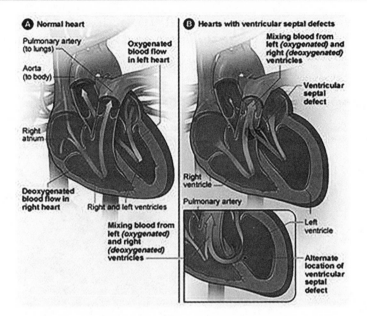

Figure 30.3. *Ventricular Septal Defect*

Cross-section of a normal heart and a heart with a ventricular septal defect. Figure A shows the structure and blood flow inside a normal heart. The blue arrow shows the flow of oxygen-poor blood as it is pumped from the body into the right atrium and then to the right ventricle. From there, it pumps through the pulmonary artery to the lungs, where it picks up oxygen. The oxygen-rich blood, shown with a red arrow, flows from the lungs through the pulmonary veins into the left atrium. Figure B shows two common locations for a ventricular septal defect. The defect, or hole, allows oxygen-rich blood from the left ventricle to mix with oxygen-poor blood in the right ventricle before the blood flows into the pulmonary artery. The mixed blood is shown with a purple arrow

Tetralogy of Fallot

This is the most common complex congenital heart defect. Tetralogy of Fallot is a combination of four defects:

- Pulmonary stenosis

- A large ventricular septal defect

- An overriding aorta. With this defect, the aorta is located between the left and right ventricles, directly over the ventricular septal defect. As a result, oxygen-poor blood from the right ventricle can flow directly into the aorta instead of into the pulmonary artery.

351

- Right ventricular hypertrophy (RVH). In this case, the muscle of the right ventricle is thicker than usual because it has to work harder than normal.

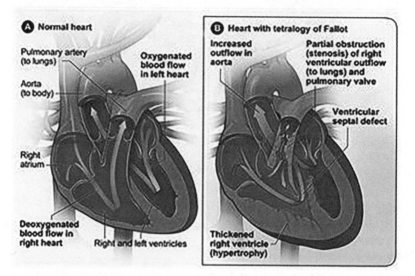

Figure 30.4. *Tetralogy of Fallot*

Cross-Section of a Normal Heart and a Heart with Tetralogy of Fallot. Figure A shows the structure and blood flow inside a normal heart. The blue arrow shows the flow of oxygen-poor blood as it is pumped from the body into the right atrium and then to the right ventricle. From there, it pumps through the pulmonary artery to the lungs, where it picks up oxygen. The oxygen-rich blood, shown with a red arrow, flows from the lungs through the pulmonary veins into the left atrium. Figure B shows a heart with the four defects of tetralogy of Fallot, which includes pulmonary stenosis, ventricular septal defect, an overriding aorta, shown in the figure as increased output in the aorta; and a thickened right ventricular hypertrophy. These defects can cause the heart to work harder or allow oxygen-rich blood to mix with oxygen-poor blood. The mixed blood is shown with a purple arrow

Other Critical Congenital Heart Defects

Common congenital heart defects include:

- Coarctation of the aorta
- Double outlet right ventricle (DORV)
- D-transposition of the great arteries (D-TGA)
- Ebstein anomaly

- Hypoplastic left heart syndrome

- Interrupted aortic arch (IAA)

- Pulmonary atresia with intact ventricular septum (PAIVS)

- Single ventricle

- Total anomalous pulmonary venous return (TAPVR)

- Tricuspid atresia

- Truncus arteriosus (TA)

Causes of Congenital Defects

Congenital heart defects happen because the heart does not develop normally while the fetus is growing in the womb. Doctors often do not know why congenital heart defects occur. Researchers do know that genetics can sometimes play a role though.

Genetics

It is common for congenital heart defects to occur because of changes in the child's deoxyribonucleic acid (DNA). The changes in the DNA may or may not have come from the parents.

Rarely, congenital heart defects are caused by particular genes that are inherited from the parents. This means that a parent who has a congenital heart defect may have an increased risk of having a child with the defect.

Risk Factors for Congenital Heart Defects

Congenital heart defects are the most common type of birth defect, occurring in about one percent of live births in the United States. If your child has a congenital heart defect, you may think you did something wrong during your pregnancy to cause the problem.

However, doctors often do not know why congenital heart defects occur. Although, researchers do know that the risk of having a baby with a congenital heart defect is influenced by family history and genetics; the mother's health; sex; and exposure to environmental factors during pregnancy, such as smoke or certain medicines. Other medical conditions can also raise your risk for having a baby with a congenital heart defect.

Family History and Genetics

Congenital heart disease (CHD) is not usually passed along to your children, but there is some risk. The risk is increased if your baby's other parent or one of your other children has a congenital heart defect.

Environmental Factors

Exposure to certain substances during pregnancy may increase your risk of having a baby with a congenital heart defect.

- Smoking during pregnancy or exposure to secondhand smoke

- Taking some medicines—such as angiotensin-converting enzyme (ACE) inhibitors for high blood pressure and retinoic acids for acne treatment—in the first trimester

Other Medical Conditions

Some medical conditions increase the risk of having a baby with a congenital heart defect, such as:

- **Diabetes.** Your risk is higher if you have diabetes before pregnancy, or if you are diagnosed with diabetes while you are in your first trimester. However, a diagnosis of gestational diabetes, which occurs later in the pregnancy, is not a major risk factor.

- **Phenylketonuria.** This rare, inherited disorder affects how your body processes a protein called "phenylalanine," which is found in many foods. Getting phenylketonuria under control before getting pregnant can reduce your risk of having a baby with a congenital heart defect.

- **Rubella.** Infection with the rubella virus, also known as "German measles," during pregnancy increases your risk.

Sex

Congenital heart defects can occur in either sex. Congenital heart defects are slightly more common at birth in boys than in girls. Some congenital heart defects are a characteristic of conditions, such as Turner syndrome (TS), that more commonly affect females.

Screening and Prevention

Almost all newborns in the United States are screened for congenital heart defects in the first few days after birth. However, if you are at high risk for having a baby with a congenital heart defect, your doctor may recommend screening before the baby is born or strategies to help prevent a congenital heart defect.

Screening during Pregnancy

It is sometimes possible to detect congenital heart defects before your baby is born.

Echocardiography is a painless test that uses sound waves to create moving pictures of the heart. Your doctor may recommend a fetal echocardiogram during pregnancy if the routine ultrasound shows any sign that the fetus may have a heart defect or if you have risk factors for congenital heart defects.

Fetal echocardiography is usually done at 18 to 22 weeks. If an echocardiogram is done before 16 weeks, your doctor may have to repeat the screening later to make sure any subtle heart defects are captured.

Newborn Screenings

Pulse oximetry determines whether a newborn has low levels of oxygen in the blood, which may be a symptom of critical congenital heart defects. This test is recommended for all newborns in the United States.

Pulse oximetry is done when the baby is more than 24 hours old or before the baby is sent home, if the baby is being sent home less than 24 hours after birth. The test involves attaching sensors to the baby's hands or feet to measure oxygen levels.

Low oxygen levels in the blood could be due to a congenital heart defect, or it could be a sign that something else is wrong. If your child has low oxygen levels, the doctor may have the test repeated or may have your child undergo more specific tests to diagnose a congenital heart defect.

Prevention Strategies

While you cannot always prevent a congenital heart defect, you can take steps to lower your and your baby's risk.

- Avoid certain medicines if you are trying to get pregnant or are pregnant. Talk to your doctor about what medicines you take and what is safe to take during pregnancy.

- Control existing conditions, such as diabetes and phenylketonuria, which increase your risk of having a baby with a congenital birth defect.

- Meet with a genetic counselor if you, your spouse, or one of your children have a congenital heart disease, and you are planning to have another child. A genetic counselor can answer questions about the risks and explain the choices that are available.

- Quit smoking and avoid secondhand smoke.

Signs, Symptoms, and Complications of Congenital Heart Defects

Some congenital heart defects cause few or no signs and symptoms. Since more children with congenital heart defects are living longer, we now know that complications can develop later in life. Signs, symptoms, and complications will vary based on the type of congenital heart defect that you or your child have.

Signs and Symptoms

Signs and symptoms may be different for newborns and adults. They also depend on the number, type, and severity of the heart defect. Some common signs and symptoms include:

- Cyanosis

- Fatigue

- Heart murmurs

- Poor blood circulation

- Rapid breathing

Congenital heart defects do not cause chest pain or other painful symptoms. Older children or adults may get tired easily or short of breath during physical activity.

Complications

Complications depend on the type of congenital heart defect you have. Some of the possible complications include:

- **Arrhythmia**

- **Blood clots**

- **Developmental disorders and delays.** Children with congenital heart defects are more likely to have problems with behavior. They are also more likely to have speech and attention deficit hyperactivity disorders (ADHD).

- **Emotional health issues.** Depression, anxiety, and posttraumatic stress disorder (PTSD) are common among people with congenital heart defects.

- **Endocarditis,** a type of heart inflammation

- **Endocrine disorders,** including thyroid problems, bone health issues, and diabetes. Problems with the hormones that deal with calcium can cause bone problems.

- **Heart failure.** Heart failure is the leading cause of death in adults with congenital heart defects. Some children with congenital heart defects develop heart failure.

- **Kidney disease**

- **Liver disease**

- **Pneumonia.** Pneumonia is a leading cause of death in adults with congenital heart disease.

- **Pregnancy complications.** Women with congenital heart defects have an increased risk of complications during pregnancy and childbirth.

- **Pulmonary hypertension**

- **Stroke**

Diagnosis of Congenital Heart Defects

Some congenital heart defects are diagnosed during pregnancy or soon after birth. Others may not be diagnosed until adulthood. Your or your child's doctor will perform a physical exam and order diagnostic tests and procedures based on what she or he finds in the physical exam.

Physical Exam

During a physical exam, your doctor will do the following:

- Listen to your or your child's heart and lungs with a stethoscope

- Look at your baby's general appearance. Some children with certain heart defects also have genetic syndromes that make them look a certain way.

- Look for signs of a heart defect, such as shortness of breath, rapid breathing, delayed growth, signs of heart failure, or cyanosis

Diagnostic Tests and Procedures

To diagnose a congenital heart defect, your doctor may have you or your baby undergo some of the following tests and procedures:

- **Echocardiography** to diagnose a heart defect or follow your or your child's progress over time. Fetal echocardiography can sometimes diagnose a congenital heart defect before birth.

- **Electrocardiogram (EKG or ECG)** to evaluate the rhythm of the heartbeat

- **Cardiac catheterization** to measure the pressure and oxygen level inside the heart chambers and blood vessels. This can help the doctor figure out whether blood is flowing from the left side of the heart into the right side of the heart, instead of going to the rest of the body.

- **Chest** X-ray to show whether the heart is enlarged. It can also show whether the lungs have extra blood flow or extra fluid, which is a sign of heart failure.

- **Genetic testing** to determine if particular genes or genetic syndromes, such as Down syndrome, are causing the congenital heart defect. Your doctor may refer you or your child to a specialist in genetic testing.

- **Cardiac magnetic resonance imaging (MRI)** to diagnose a heart defect or follow your or your child's progress over time

- **Pulse oximetry** to estimate how much oxygen is in the blood. A small sensor is attached to an infant's hand or foot or an older person's finger or toe.

Treatment of Congenital Heart Defects

Treatment will depend on which type of congenital heart defect you have. Treatments for congenital heart defects include medicines, surgery, and cardiac catheterization procedures. Many congenital heart defects do not require treatment at all. However, children with critical congenital heart defects will need surgery in the first year of life. Some people with congenital heart defects may need treatment, including repeated surgery, throughout their lives. All people with congenital heart defects should be followed by a cardiologist, a doctor who specializes in the heart, throughout their whole life.

Medicines

Your child's doctor may prescribe medicines to help close patent ductus arteriosus in premature infants.

- Indomethacin or ibuprofen triggers the patent ductus arteriosus to constrict or tighten, which closes the opening.

- Acetaminophen is sometimes used to close patent ductus arteriosus.

Procedures

Cardiac catheterization is a common procedure that is sometimes used to repair simple heart defects, such as atrial septal defect and patent ductus arteriosus, if they do not repair themselves. It may also be used to open up valves or blood vessels that are narrowed or have stenosis.

In this procedure, a thin, flexible tube called a "catheter" is put into a vein in the groin or neck. The tube is threaded to the heart. Possible complications include bleeding, infection, pain at the catheter insertion site, and damage to blood vessels.

Surgery

In heart surgery, a cardiac surgeon opens the chest to work directly on the heart.

Surgery may be done for these reasons:

- To repair a hole in the heart, such as a ventricular septal defect or an atrial septal defect

- To repair a patent ductus arteriosus

- To repair complex defects, such as problems with the location of blood vessels near the heart or how they are formed

- To repair or replace a valve

- To widen narrowed blood vessels

359

Surgeries that are sometimes needed to treat congenital heart defects include:

- **Heart transplant.** Children may receive a heart transplant if they have a complex congenital heart defect that cannot be repaired surgically or if the heart fails after surgery. Children may also receive a heart transplant if they are dependent on a ventilator or have severe symptoms of heart failure. Some adults with congenital heart defects may eventually need a heart transplant.

- **Palliative surgery.** Some babies with only one ventricle are too weak or too small to have heart surgery. They must have palliative surgery, or temporary surgery, first to improve oxygen levels in the blood. In this surgery, the surgeon installs a shunt, a tube that creates an additional pathway for blood to travel to the lungs to get oxygen. The surgeon removes the shunt when the baby's heart defects are fixed during the full repair.

- **Ventricular assist device (VAD).** For people with heart failure from a congenital heart defect, this device supports the heart until a transplant occurs. These devices can be difficult to use in people who have congenital heart defects because of the heart's abnormal structure.

- **Total artificial heart (TAH).** For some people with complex congenital heart defects, a total artificial heart may be needed instead of a ventricular assist device.

Living with Congenital Heart Defects

The outlook for children who have congenital heart defects is much better nowadays than it was in the past. Advances in diagnosis and treatment allow most of these children to survive to adulthood, which means that more and more adults are living with congenital heart disease. Even if your congenital heart defect was repaired in childhood, you need regular medical follow-up to maintain good health.

Receive Routine Follow-Up Care

- Having checkups with a pediatric cardiologist or an adult congenital heart specialist as directed

- Seeing your or your child's primary care doctor for routine exams

- Taking medicines as prescribed to prevent complications

- Going to the dentist for routine cleanings and brushing your teeth regularly

Adults should go to medical centers that have specialized programs for adults with congenital heart disease.

Heart-Healthy Lifestyle Changes

Your doctor will recommend that you adopt lifelong heart-healthy lifestyle changes.

- **Heart-healthy eating.** Following a heart-healthy eating pattern, which includes consuming plenty of vegetables, fruits, and whole grains, reduces the risk of high blood pressure and obesity.

- **Being physically active.** Most people with congenital heart defects can be physically active. Physical activity can improve physical fitness and lower many heart disease risk factors, including high blood pressure. The amount or type of physical activity you or your child can do depends on the type of congenital heart defect, the medicines you may be taking, and the devices that may be implanted. Some people with congenital heart defects may need to avoid competitive sports. Most people with congenital heart defects can participate in recreational sports, physical education classes, or general physical activity. Ask your doctor how much and what kinds of physical activity are safe for you or your child. Remember to ask the doctor for a note that describes any limits on your child's physical activities. Schools and other groups may need this information.

- **Aiming for a healthy weight.** After treatments and surgery, growth and development may improve. Children and adults with congenital heart defects are at risk for obesity, which can lead to high blood pressure and other conditions that can increase the risk for heart problems.

Developmental Disorders and Delays

Some babies and children who have congenital heart defects do not grow as fast as other children. They may not eat as much as they should and, as a result, may be smaller and thinner than other children.

361

Children with congenital heart defects may also start certain activities—such as rolling over, sitting, and walking—later than other children.

Children who have developmental problems as a result of their heart defects may need tutoring, special education, physical therapy, occupational therapy, or speech therapy.

Emotional Health

Congenital heart defects can lead to emotional-health issues for the person with the health problem and her or his close family.

- Adults may experience depression or anxiety because of their heart health. They may feel lonely or self-conscious about surgical scars. Psychotherapy may help.

- Children and teens who have serious conditions or illnesses may feel isolated if they need to be in the hospital a lot. Some may feel sad or frustrated if they have growth, development, or learning delays when compared to other children their age. If you have concerns about your child's emotional health, talk with your child and your child's doctor.

- Parents or caregivers may find it stressful caring for a child with a congenital heart defect. Your child's doctor may be able to help you find support.

Birth Control and Pregnancy

Adult women with congenital heart defects are at increased risk of pregnancy complications and have special health considerations for birth control and pregnancy. Talk to your doctor about the following:

- **Birth control.** Some women with congenital heart defects should avoid some methods of birth control. Talk to your doctor about the best method for you.

- **Medicines.** Some medicines prescribed to adults with congenital heart defects are not safe to take during pregnancy, as they may harm the fetus.

- **Tests to evaluate your heart.** During pregnancy, a woman's organ systems, including the heart and blood vessels, go through major changes to support the fetus. Your doctor may order extra tests before pregnancy to determine whether your heart can tolerate pregnancy. Most women with congenital heart defects can have normal pregnancies.

- **Genetic testing.** People who have congenital heart defects are at an increased risk for miscarriage and of having children with congenital heart defects. Your doctor may suggest that you speak with a genetic counselor or have genetic tests done. Your doctor may have you undergo fetal echocardiography, a test to look for congenital heart defects in the fetus.

Transition to Adult Care

The move from pediatric care to adult care is an important step in treatment.

Talk with your teen's healthcare team about creating a plan to help your teen transition to adult care. Start planning as soon as your teen is able and willing to fully take part in this process.

Following a transition plan has many benefits. It will help your teen with the following:

- Getting used to talking with healthcare providers

- Learning about the adult healthcare system

- Taking responsibility for her or his medical care

- Understanding the importance of having health insurance and learn what her or his insurance covers

A transition plan also can help your teen think about other important issues, such as future education and employment, birth control and pregnancy planning, and making healthy choices about heart-healthy eating, physical activity, and other heart-healthy lifestyle changes. Emotional health should also be part of the transition plan.

Older teens should start practicing going to the doctor without a parent.

For the transition plan, work with healthcare providers to compile a packet of medical records and information that covers all aspects of the heart defect, including:

- Diagnosis

- Health insurance

- Prescribed medicines

- Procedures or surgeries

- Recommendations about medical follow-up and how to prevent complications

Know Your Rights

Several laws protect the employment rights of people who have health conditions, such as congenital heart defects. The Americans with Disabilities Act (ADA) and the Work Incentives Improvement Act try to ensure fairness in hiring for all people, including those who have health conditions.

Monitor Your Condition

To monitor your or your child's condition, your doctor may recommend the following tests, depending on the type of congenital heart defect:

- Blood or urine tests to monitor the function of organs affected by a congenital heart defect.

- Spirometry to measure how well the lungs are working.

- Abdominal imaging by ultrasound, MRI, or computed tomography (CT) to look for liver disease.

Prevent and Control Complications over Your Lifetime

People with congenital heart defects, and their caregivers or family members, can take steps to help prevent complications of their condition or from surgical treatments of their congenital heart defect.

- **Antiarrhythmics.** These drugs control arrhythmia and may be used for patients whose congenital heart defect causes arrhythmia.

- **Antibiotics.** People with certain types of congenital heart defects may have an increased risk of infective endocarditis (IE). Your doctor may recommend antibiotics to reduce the risk of infective endocarditis before dental procedures or other procedures that run the risk of introducing bacteria to the bloodstream. Good oral health also decreases the risk of infective endocarditis.

- **Anticlotting medicines.** You may need to take anticoagulant, antiplatelet, and fibrinolytic medicines to treat blood clots or prevent blood clots from forming. These medicines are often prescribed long-term to people with artificial shunts and mechanical heart valves. Long-term use of warfarin, a common anticoagulant, may increase the risk of osteoporosis.

- **Blood pressure medicines.** These drugs help control blood pressure. Common types of blood pressure medicines include diuretics, beta-blockers, and angiotensin-converting enzyme (ACE) inhibitors.

- **Pacemaker.** Pacemakers can be given to both children and adults with congenital heart defects to help control abnormal heart rhythms, also known as "arrhythmias."

- **Routine vaccinations.** Routine vaccinations are especially important for children with congenital heart defects. Adults with ongoing heart or immune problems should have a pneumococcal vaccination to prevent pneumonia and complications, such as meningitis.

- **Special care during surgery.** Be sure your doctor is aware of your congenital heart defect before any surgery, not just heart surgery. People with congenital heart defects are at higher risk of problems during surgery.

- **Training for sudden cardiac arrest (SCA).** Caregivers and family members can train in cardiopulmonary resuscitation (CPR) and using a type of defibrillator called an "automated external defibrillator" (AED).

Section 30.2

Kawasaki Disease: A Disorder with Cardiovascular Implications

This section includes text excerpted from "Kawasaki Disease," Genetic and Rare Diseases Information Center (GARD), National Center for Advancing Translational Sciences (NCATS), September 3, 2017.

What Is Kawasaki Disease?

Kawasaki disease (KD) is a disease that involves inflammation of the blood vessels. It is typically diagnosed in young children, but older children and adults can also develop this condition. KD begins with a fever that lasts at least five days. Other classic symptoms may include red eyes, lips, and mouth; rash; swollen and red hands and feet; and swollen lymph nodes. Sometimes, the disease affects the coronary arteries which carry oxygen-rich blood to the heart, which can lead to serious heart problems. KD occurs most often in people of Asian and Pacific Island descent. The cause of KD is unknown. An infection along with genetic factors may be involved. Treatment includes intravenous gamma globulin (IVIg) and high doses of aspirin in a hospital setting. The prognosis is generally very good, but in cases of heart complications, it depends on the severity of the coronary disease.

What Causes Kawasaki Disease

The cause of KD is unknown. The disease results when cells move into the tissues and buildup there, leading to vascular damage, but what causes the cell buildup in the first place is unknown. The body's response to a virus or infection combined with genetic factors may cause the disease. However, no specific virus or infection has been identified, and the role of genetics is not well understood.

Genetic factors appear to be important to this disorder, as suggested by the increased frequency of the disease in Asian and Asian American populations and among family members of an affected child. A number of gene variants (polymorphisms) are associated with an increased risk of developing (susceptibility) KD, and some of these variants are also associated with coronary artery lesions and aneurysm formation.

Other theories suggest that the disease is caused by a response from the body's immune system.

Kawasaki disease is not contagious; it cannot be passed from one person to another. Other risk factors include being of male gender, being between six months and five years of age, and having a family history of KD.

How Is Kawasaki Disease Inherited?

A susceptibility to KD appears to be passed through generations in families, but the inheritance pattern is unknown. Children of parents who have had KD have twice the risk of developing the disease when compared to the general population. Children whose siblings have had KD are ten times more likely to develop KD than the general population, but it is still rare for more than one child in a family to develop the disease.

What Genes Are Related to Kawasaki Disease?

A variation in the *ITPKC* gene has been associated with an increased risk of developing KD. This gene provides instructions for making an enzyme called "inositol 1,4,5-triphosphate 3-kinase C" (ITPKC). This enzyme helps limit the activity of immune system cells called "T cells," which identify foreign substances and defend the body against infection. Reducing the activity of T cells, when appropriate, prevents the overproduction of immune proteins called "cytokines" that lead to inflammation and can, when present in large quantities, cause tissue damage. Researchers believe that variations in the ITPKC gene may interfere with the body's ability to reduce T cell activity, leading to inflammation that damages blood vessels and results in the symptoms of this disease. It is likely that other factors, including changes in additional genes, also influence the development of this complex disorder.

Is Your New Baby at Risk to Develop Kawasaki Disease?

Children of parents who have had KD have twice the risk of developing the disorder when compared to the general population. Children with affected siblings have a tenfold higher risk.

It is encouraged to discuss the specific risks for your family with your healthcare provider and/or genetics professional.

367

Can Kawasaki Disease Cause Behavioral Problems or Slow a Child's Development?

Both generalized and localized central nervous system (CNS) symptoms have been reported in KD. While neurologic complications or symptoms may occur in a small number of patients with KD, the vast majority escape serious CNS damage, and data suggests that milder CNS effects, in the form of cognitive and academic difficulties, are rare. In some cases, however, KD can be associated with significant behavioral symptoms.

A study conducted by WJ King found that cognitive development and academic performance were not significantly affected by KD. This study did find, however, that individuals who had previous KD experienced significantly more behavior problems than their healthy siblings. These problems were predominantly internalizing and reflected a cluster of specific difficulties including somatic complaints, anxious-depressed behavior, and social problems. These children were also rated as having significantly more attention difficulties than their healthy siblings. A large proportion of parents in this study also perceived that the episode of KD had a long-lasting effect on their child, although this perception was often vague and was not related to the increased risk of behavior problems.

The reported behavioral difficulties may be due to residual CNS effects of the disease process, the experience of acute illness and hospitalization, and/or continued family anxiety after the illness. Heightened parental anxieties about children who have completely recovered from an illness can lead to overprotective relationships that may contribute to difficulties in the psychological development of their children.

Can Kawasaki Disease Diagnosed in Childhood Have Later Effects on Adults?

Although KD is generally self-limiting, 10 to 15 percent of children may develop problems in their coronary arteries, even after being treated with aspirin and intravenous gamma globulin (purified antibodies—also known as "IVIG"). Inflammation of the heart muscle (myocardium), heart valves (endocardium), and/or sac surrounding the heart (pericardium) may occur acutely (at the onset of the disease) or many years later. The most common late complication is the persistence of coronary artery aneurysms (CAA), weakened areas of a blood vessel that balloons out. Such aneurysms can lead to a heart attack at a young age or later in life.

In addition, adults may present with ischemic heart disease (ischemic means that an organ, in this case, the heart muscle, has not received enough blood and oxygen) as a sequela (late effects) of unrecognized KD in childhood.

How Might Adults with a History of Kawasaki Disease in Childhood Be Managed?

Long-term follow-up in individuals with KD is recommended. The goal of long-term management is to prevent a block of blood flow to the heart, caused by a blood clot in the coronary artery (coronary thrombosis) and to treat any resulting reduction of blood flow and oxygen to the heart (myocardial ischemia). There are few studies that have been published to assist in creating guidelines for management. It has been suggested that management should vary, depending on the severity of coronary artery involvement.

In general, cardiac imaging—such as computerized tomographic angiography (CTA), magnetic resonance imaging (MRI), and echocardiogram—are recommended, with the use of CTA and MRI being utilized more frequently given evidence of more accurate imaging with age. Abnormalities of the coronary arteries may require ongoing medication, interventional catheterization, and/or cardiac surgery.

Is There a Method for Tracking Kawasaki Disease?

Cases of KD are tracked by the Centers for Disease Control and Prevention (CDC) using hospital discharge data, a surveillance system, and research studies. The Kawasaki syndrome (KS) surveillance system is based on voluntary reporting by healthcare providers and local and state health authorities.

Resources for Connecting with Other Parents Whose Child Has Developmental or Behavior Issues Following Kawasaki Disease

The Kawasaki Disease Foundation offers a program called "KDF Bridges," where families with children who have Kawasaki Disease are matched with trained volunteers who have either had children with KD or are adults who have recovered from KD. There are several families listed on their website who describe cognitive, behavioral, or developmental problems in their children and offer some suggestions for coping.

Section 30.3

Rheumatic Heart Disease Is More Common in Children than in Adults

"Rheumatic Heart Disease Is More Common in Children than in Adults" © 2016 Omnigraphics. Reviewed May 2019.

Symptoms

Rheumatic fever only occurs after a person has been infected by group A *streptococcus*. To prevent rheumatic fever, it is important to be aware of the symptoms of strep throat and treat the infection promptly with antibiotics. Experts recommend seeing a medical practitioner for a strep test if you notice the following symptoms:

- A sore throat, especially in the absence of cold symptoms

- Swollen or tender lymph nodes

- A fever of 101°F or above

- Inflamed tonsils, often with white patches

- A red rash

- Small red spots on the roof of the mouth

- A thick, bloody discharge from the nose

- Nausea or vomiting

- Headache

The symptoms of rheumatic fever typically appear two to four weeks after the initial strep infection. The symptoms may persist for several weeks or even months. Although the symptoms vary widely, they may include the following:

- Red, swollen, painful joints—especially the knees, ankles, elbows, and wrists

- Pain that migrates from one joint to another joint

- Nodules—or small, painless bumps—protruding under the skin of affected joints

- Fever

- A red, raised rash on the chest, abdomen, or back

- Weakness or shortness of breath

- Lethargy, fatigue, or a decreased attention span

- Chest pain

- Rapid fluttering or pounding heart palpitations

- Nosebleeds

- Stomach pain

- Vomiting

- Rapid, jerky, uncontrolled movements of the arms or legs, or twitching of the facial muscles (chorea)

- Inappropriate emotional outbursts, such as laughing or crying

Diagnosis and Treatment

To diagnose rheumatic fever, doctors will first perform blood tests to check for the presence of strep bacteria. Next, they will look for inflammation in the joints, nodules beneath the skin, and a skin rash. They may also perform movement tests to detect chorea, or nervous system dysfunction.

In patients diagnosed with rheumatic fever, the most serious potential long-term complication is damage to the heart valves. Doctors will typically listen to the heart through a stethoscope to check for abnormalities. They may also perform additional tests, such as an electrocardiogram to measure the electrical activity in the heart muscle, or an echocardiogram to produce sound wave images of the heart.

In more than half of all cases of rheumatic fever, the patient develops rheumatic heart disease. Damage to the heart valves forces the heart muscle to work harder to circulate blood through the body.

Eventually, the heart is unable to perform its vital function, leading to heart failure. Other heart conditions that may develop from rheumatic fever include valve stenosis, valve regurgitation, and atrial fibrillation.

The main treatment for rheumatic fever involves antibiotics to rid the body of group A *streptococcus*. Long-term antibiotic treatment may be prescribed to prevent the infection from taking hold again later. Other forms of treatment are generally used to control the symptoms of rheumatic fever and help patients feel more comfortable, including anti-inflammatory medications, to reduce swelling and pain; anticonvulsant medications, to reduce involuntary movements; and bed rest or restricted activity, to allow the heart to heal.

Prevention

The most effective methods of preventing rheumatic heart disease include avoiding strep infections, treating strep throat quickly and thoroughly with antibiotics, and being aware of risk factors for rheumatic fever.

Basic hygiene can help prevent strep infections. Experts suggest washing hands frequently, covering the mouth when coughing or sneezing, and avoiding contact with people who are sick. It is also important to recognize the symptoms of strep throat in children, seek medical attention promptly, and follow the recommended treatment— including completing the full course of antibiotics. It may also be a good idea to schedule a follow-up visit to ensure that the patient is no longer producing antibodies to strep bacteria.

Although rheumatic fever is rare, certain factors may increase a person's risk of developing it. These risk factors include a family history of the disease, the strain of strep bacteria that causes the initial infection, and poor sanitation and public health conditions often found in developing countries.

References

1.   Johnson, Shannon. "Rheumatic Fever," Healthline, 2016.

2.   "Understanding Rheumatic Fever—The Basics," WebMD, 2016

Chapter 31

Cardiovascular Disease in Women

Chapter Contents

Section 31.1

Women and Heart Disease: A Statistical Overview

This section contains text excerpted from the following sources: Text under the heading "Facts on Women and Heart Disease" is excerpted from "Women and Heart Disease Fact Sheet," Centers for Disease Control and Prevention (CDC), August 23, 2017; Text beginning with the heading "What Is Heart Disease?" is excerpted from "Heart Disease and Women," Office on Women's Health (OWH), U.S. Department of Health and Human Services (HHS), January 30, 2019.

Facts on Women and Heart Disease

Heart disease is the leading cause of death for women in the United States, killing 289,758 women in 2013—that is about 1 in every 4 female deaths. Although heart disease is sometimes thought of as a "man's disease," around the same number of women and men die each year of heart disease in the United States. Despite increases in awareness over the past decade, only 54 percent of women recognize that heart disease is their number 1 killer.

Heart disease is the leading cause of death for African American and White women in the United States. Among Hispanic women, heart disease and cancer cause roughly the same number of deaths each year. For American Indian or Alaska Native and Asian or Pacific Islander women, heart disease is second only to cancer. About 5.8 percent of all White women, 7.6 percent of Black women, and 5.6 percent of Mexican American women have coronary heart disease (CHD).

Almost two-thirds (64%) of women who die suddenly of CHD have no previous symptoms. Even if you have no symptoms, you may still be at risk for heart disease.

What Is Heart Disease?

"Heart disease" refers to several types of problems that affect the heart. The most common type of heart disease is coronary artery disease (CAD). Heart disease is also called "cardiovascular disease" (CVD). It includes diseases of the blood vessels, which carry blood to different parts of your body. These include CAD, vascular (peripheral artery) disease, and stroke.

What Is Coronary Artery Disease?

Coronary artery disease is also called "coronary heart disease." CAD is the most common type of heart disease. In CAD, plaque builds up on the walls of the arteries that carry blood to the heart muscle. Over time, this buildup causes the arteries to narrow and harden, a process called "atherosclerosis." Atherosclerosis prevents the heart from getting all the blood and oxygen it needs. This can lead to angina, or chest pain.

What Are Some Common Types of Heart Problems That Affect Women?

Atherosclerosis. This condition happens when plaque buildup in the arteries causing them to narrow and harden over time. When the plaque wears down or breaks open, a blood clot may develop. If the clot blocks blood flow to the heart, it can cause a heart attack.

- **Heart failure.** This happens when the heart is not able to pump blood through the body as well as it should. Heart failure is a serious medical problem because many organs, such as the lungs and kidneys, are no longer able to get the blood they need. Heart failure symptoms include:

  - Shortness of breath

  - Swelling in the feet, ankles, and legs

  - Extreme fatigue (tiredness)

- **Irregular heartbeat (arrhythmia).** Arrhythmias are problems with the rate or rhythm of your heartbeat. Your heart may beat too fast, too slow, or with an irregular rhythm. Changes in heartbeats are harmless for most people. As you get older, you are more likely to have arrhythmias, partly as a result of changing estrogen levels. It is normal to feel a few flutters or for your heart to race once in a while. **If you have flutters along with other symptoms of heart attack, such as dizziness or shortness of breath, call 911 right away.**

- **Atrial fibrillation (AF).** Atrial fibrillation is a type of arrhythmia. AF makes it easier for your blood to clot because your heart cannot pump as well as it should. This can lead to heart failure or stroke. The symptoms of AF include heart flutters and a fast heartbeat, as well as dizziness and shortness of breath.

- **Heart valve disease.** Heart valve disease affects the valves that control blood flow in and out of different parts of the heart. A birth defect, older age, or an infection can cause your heart valves to not open fully or close completely. This causes the heart to work harder to pump blood. Heart valve disease can lead to stroke, as well as heart failure, blood clots, or sudden cardiac arrest. Heart valve disease can cause problems during pregnancy, when your heart already has to work harder than usual to supply blood to the fetus. Your doctor can help you prevent problems during pregnancy if you know you have heart valve disease. But, some women do not find out that they have a heart valve problem until they get pregnant.

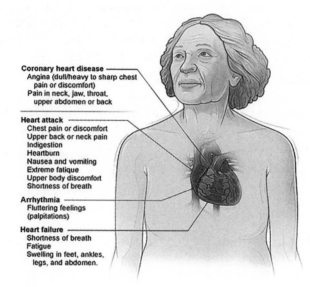

Coronary heart disease
Angina (dull/heavy to sharp chest pain or discomfort)
Pain in neck, jaw, throat, upper abdomen or back

Heart attack
Chest pain or discomfort
Upper back or neck pain
Indigestion
Heartburn
Nausea and vomiting
Extreme fatigue
Upper body discomfort
Shortness of breath

Arrhythmia
Fluttering feelings (palpitations)

Heart failure
Shortness of breath
Fatigue
Swelling in feet, ankles, legs, and abdomen.

Figure 31.1. *Major Symptoms of Heart Disease*

What Are Some Types of Heart Problems That Affect Women More than Men?

Certain types of heart problems affect women more than men.

Chest Pain (Angina)

About four million women in the United States suffer from angina (chest pain and discomfort). Angina also affects men, but women are more likely than men to get two specific types of angina: stable and variant (Prinzmetal's) angina.

- **Stable angina.** This is the most common type of angina. Women with stable angina may experience chest pain during physical activity or times of stress. The chest pain usually goes away with rest. But it can develop into unstable angina, the type of angina that happens most often while you are resting or sleeping. Unstable angina can lead to a heart attack or cardiac arrest.

- **Variant (Prinzmetal's) angina.** This type of unstable angina is rare. It is caused by a spasm in the coronary arteries, which carry blood to the heart muscle. Triggers for the spasm can include exposure to cold weather, stress, smoking, or cocaine use. The spasms can lead to painful attacks, often while you are resting or sleeping. This type of unstable angina rarely causes a heart attack and can be treated with medicine.

Cardiac Syndrome X

Cardiac syndrome X (CSX) is a health problem that happens when people with healthy, unblocked arteries have chest pain (angina) and coronary artery spasms. A spasm is when the artery pinches itself closed. The cause of CSX is not known. Some possible causes include:

- **Coronary microvascular disease (MVD).** In some women, CSX may be caused by MVD, a disease found in tiny arteries near the heart. These arteries are too small to see on an angiogram, a diagnostic test that takes X-ray pictures of the arteries. Women with CSX caused by MVD are often younger than 50 years of age and have a higher risk for heart attack. MVD affects about half of the women with CSX.

- **Hormonal changes.** Changes in estrogen levels after menopause could make women more likely to have heart problems. Most women with CSX are postmenopausal or are going through menopause.

Broken Heart Syndrome

Broken heart syndrome, also called "stress-induced cardiomyopathy" (or takotsubo cardiomyopathy), can happen even if you are healthy. Researchers do not know the exact cause of broken heart syndrome. Symptoms are often triggered by extreme stress, such as intense grief, anger, or surprise. Women are more likely than men to experience broken heart syndrome. Experts think that a surge of stress hormones stuns the heart, causing intense, short-lived symptoms that usually do not cause permanent damage to the heart.

Most women who experience broken heart syndrome are older, between 58 and 75 years of age. This is probably due to a drop in the estrogen levels after menopause.

Broken heart syndrome can be misdiagnosed as a heart attack. The symptoms and test results are similar, but there are no blocked heart arteries. Instead, a part of your heart temporarily enlarges while the rest of the heart works normally. Broken heart syndrome can lead to short-term heart failure, but it is usually easily treatable.

Section 31.2

Heart Attack and Women

This section includes text excerpted from "Heart Attack and Women," Office on Women's Health (OWH), U.S. Department of Health and Human Services (HHS), November 9, 2018.

A heart attack happens when blood flow in an artery to the heart is blocked by a blood clot or plaque, and the heart muscle begins to die. Women are more likely than men to die after a heart attack. But if you get help quickly, treatment can save your life and prevent permanent damage to your heart.

What Is a Heart Attack?

A heart attack happens when blood flow to your heart muscle is blocked, and the cells in your heart muscle begin to die. Many different health problems can cause a heart attack, but coronary artery disease (CAD) is the most common.

What Are the Symptoms of a Heart Attack in Women?

The most common symptoms of a heart attack for both women and men are pain and discomfort in the chest and upper body. Other symptoms, such as shortness of breath and nausea, are more common in women than men.

What Is the Difference between a Heart Attack and Cardiac Arrest?

A heart attack is not the same as cardiac arrest. In a heart attack, the heart keeps beating. The person has a pulse and usually stays conscious (awake). During cardiac arrest, the heart stops beating. The person has no pulse and is unconscious (not awake).

What Causes a Heart Attack

Coronary artery disease causes the most heart attacks. In people with CAD, plaque builds up on the walls of the arteries that supply blood to the heart. This is called "atherosclerosis."

Plaque can build up in fatty clumps or in a thin, smooth layer. Both types are dangerous. The plaque can break open or wear down, causing blood to clump together (clot) in that area. If a clot blocks blood flow to the heart, it can cause a heart attack.

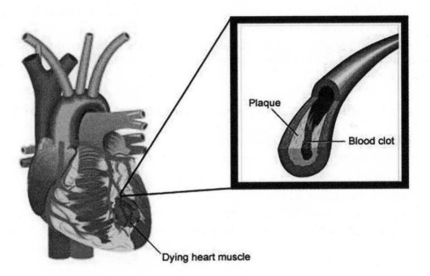

Figure 31.2. *Coronary Artery Disease and Heart Attack*

This picture shows how CAD causes a heart attack. Plaque builds up in an artery of the heart, and a blood clot forms. The clot blocks blood flow to part of the heart, and the heart muscle begins to die.

A heart attack can also happen if the artery pinches itself closed. This is called a "coronary spasm." Coronary spasms are rare. They happen more often in young women than in older women or men.

379

How Do You Know If You Are at Risk for a Heart Attack?

A heart attack can happen to anyone, woman or man, young or old. Some people are more at risk because of certain health problems, family health history, age, and habits. These are called "risk factors."

You cannot change some risk factors, such as your age, race or ethnicity, or family history. The good news is that you can change or control many risk factors, such as high blood pressure (HBP), diabetes, smoking, and unhealthy eating.

Do Women of Color Need to Worry about Heart Attack Risk?

Yes. All women need to be aware of their heart attack risk and take steps to prevent heart disease.

African American, Hispanic, and American Indian or Alaska Native women often have more heart attack risk factors than White women. These risk factors can include obesity, lack of physical activity, high blood pressure, and diabetes.

African American women are also more likely to have a heart attack and more likely to die from a heart attack when compared with White women.

Do Women Do Worse than Men after a Heart Attack?

Yes. In all age groups, women do worse than men after a heart attack. Researchers are not sure why this is, especially for younger women.

- **Women between 45 and 65 years of age** who have a heart attack are more likely than men of the same age to die within a year of a heart attack. However, heart attack is less common in younger women than in younger men. This is partly because the hormone estrogen protects against heart disease in younger women.

- **Women older than 65 years of age** are more likely than men of the same age to die within a few weeks of a heart attack. Women usually have heart attacks about 10 years later than men. The average age of a first heart attack for men is 64 years of age, but it is 72 years of age for women.

Many women who have had a heart attack go on to lead full, active lives. Know the symptoms of a heart attack and what to do if you have any symptoms. Take steps to recover after a heart attack and to prevent another heart attack.

How Is a Heart Attack Diagnosed?

To diagnose a heart attack, a doctor will ask you about your symptoms, your health, and your family health history. The doctor will also order tests.

Doctors often use these types of tests to diagnose a heart attack and choose the best treatment.

- **Blood tests.** During a heart attack, heart muscle cells die and burst open. This process releases proteins into your blood. Heart attack blood tests measure the amount of these protein "markers" of heart damage. Common heart attack blood tests include:

  - **Cardiac troponin.** This is the most common blood test. This marker is released from the injured heart muscle. It is not found in the blood of healthy people. Troponin levels go up three to six hours after your heart attack starts, so the test may not find a heart attack right away.

  - **Creatine Kinase-MB (CKMB).** The CKMB test measures the amount of damage to the heart because of blocked blood flow. The test can tell whether treatments to restore blood flow to the heart are working. CKMB levels rise about 4 to 6 hours after a heart attack starts and peak 24 hours later.

  - **Myoglobin.** This test helps diagnose a heart attack in the very early stages. After a heart attack, myoglobin levels rise within 1 to 4 hours but peak after 12 hours.

- **Coronary angiography,** or angiogram. This test takes pictures of a dye flowing through your blood vessels. By watching how smoothly the dye flows, doctors can locate narrowed or blocked coronary arteries that might need to be opened, or find other problems.

Women are more likely than men to have a less-common type of plaque that forms a smooth layer over the arteries instead of a few big lumps. Often, angiograms cannot see this thin, smooth plaque, but this type of plaque is still very dangerous. Other tests (such as those described above) might be needed for women who show signs or have symptoms of a heart attack but whose coronary angiography results do not show any problems.

- **Nuclear heart scan.** This test takes pictures to show areas of the heart that may be damaged because they are not getting enough blood. It can also show how well the heart is pumping. Tell your doctor if you are pregnant or breastfeeding. The test uses radioactive material that can harm your baby.

- **Electrocardiogram (ECG or EKG).** This test detects and records your heart's electrical activity. Certain changes in the electrical waves on an ECG can show whether you are having, or have had, a heart attack. An ECG can also be done during physical activity to monitor your heart when it is working hard.

How Is a Heart Attack Treated?

Heart attack is most often treated with medicine or nonsurgical procedures that break up blood clots and restore normal blood flow to the heart. Some treatments will start right away when the ambulance comes. You will get other treatments later in the hospital.

Getting treatment right away for a heart attack can help prevent or limit damage to your heart muscle. This is one reason why it is important to call 911 if you think you are having a heart attack, rather than driving yourself to the hospital.

What Medicines Do Treat a Heart Attack?

Medicines you might receive if you have a heart attack include:

- **Clot busters.** These drugs are also called "thrombolytics." They stop a heart attack by breaking up blood clots to open blocked arteries. For the best results, these medicines must be given as soon as possible after the start of heart attack symptoms. You might get them in the ambulance or in the hospital. If you get them soon after having a heart attack, you are more likely to survive, and your heart is more likely to recover.

- **Aspirin and blood thinners.** These medicines stop blood cells from clumping together and forming new clots. If you call 911 for a heart attack, the operator might tell you to chew up and swallow an aspirin while you wait for the ambulance. It can help reduce damage to your heart and your risk of dying by 25 percent. Once you arrive at the hospital, you might get a different blood thinner called an "anticoagulant" through an intravenous line (IV) that carries the medicine right into your bloodstream.

- **Nitrates.** Nitrates widen your arteries and increase blood flow to your heart. Once you arrive in the hospital, you may be treated with nitrates through an IV. One common nitrate is called "nitroglycerin."

- **Beta-blockers.** Beta-blockers lower your heart's workload. These medicines help relieve chest pain and discomfort and prevent repeat heart attacks. Beta-blockers may also be used to treat arrhythmias (irregular heartbeats), which often happen during a heart attack.

- **ACE inhibitors.** Angiotensin-converting enzyme (ACE) inhibitors lower blood pressure and strain on your heart. They also help slow down weakening of the heart muscle.

You may also be given other medicines to relieve pain or anxiety or to lower your cholesterol.

What Procedures Do Treat a Heart Attack?

The most common procedures to treat a heart attack include:

- **Angioplasty and stenting.** Angioplasty, also called "percutaneous coronary intervention" (PCI), is a nonsurgical procedure that opens blocked or narrowed coronary arteries. A thin, flexible tube with a medical balloon on the end is threaded through a blood vessel to the narrowed or blocked coronary artery. Once in place, the balloon is inflated to open the artery to allow blood flow to the heart. The balloon is then deflated and removed. A small mesh tube called a "stent" may be permanently placed in the artery. The stent helps prevent new blockages in the artery.

- **Coronary artery bypass grafting.** The surgeon uses a healthy blood vessel from another part of your body to reroute blood around the blockage in your artery. You may need this surgery if more than one artery is blocked, or if angioplasty and stenting did not work to restore blood flow to the heart.

After a heart attack, you may also need cardiac rehabilitation to recover from the damage the heart attack did to your heart.

How Can You Prevent a Heart Attack?

All women can make changes to help prevent a heart attack. These changes include making healthier food choices, being more physically active, and not smoking. Once you know your heart attack risk factors, you and your doctor can work together to lower your risk.

Even if you had a heart attack before, you can make changes to help prevent another heart attack.

Section 31.3

Stroke and Women

This section includes text excerpted from "Stroke and Women," Office on Women's Health (OWH), U.S. Department of Health and Human Services (HHS), December 7, 2018.

Stroke kills about twice as many women as breast cancer each year. In fact, stroke is the third leading cause of death for women. Stroke also kills more women than men each year. A stroke can leave you permanently disabled. But, many strokes are preventable and treatable. Every woman can take steps to prevent stroke by knowing her risk factors and making healthy changes.

What Is Stroke?

A stroke is sometimes called a "brain attack." Stroke happens when blood flow to a part of the brain stops or is blocked by a blood clot or plaque, and brain cells begin to die.

What Are the Different Types of Stroke?

There are two types of stroke:

- Stroke caused by a blockage of blood flow to the brain (ischemic stroke). This is the most common type of stroke. This type of stroke happens most often when an artery is clogged with plaque (atherosclerosis) or a blood clot.

384

- Stroke caused by bleeding into the brain (hemorrhagic stroke). This type of stroke happens when a blood vessel in the brain bursts, and blood bleeds into the brain. This type of stroke can be caused by an aneurysm, which is a thin or weak spot in an artery that can burst.

Both types of stroke can cause brain cells to die. Depending on which part of the brain the stroke affects, you may have problems with your speech, movement, balance, vision, or memory.

If you think you are having a stroke, call 911.

What Is a "Mini-Stroke"?

A "mini-stroke" is also called a "transient ischemic attack" (TIA). A TIA happens when, for a short time, less blood than normal gets to the brain. You may have some stroke symptoms, or you may not notice any symptoms.

A transient ischemic attack usually lasts only a few minutes, although it can last up to several hours. Many people do not even know they have had a stroke. A TIA can be a warning sign of a full stroke in the future, or you can have another mini-stroke at a later time.

What Are the Effects of Stroke?

How stroke affects you depends on:

- The type of stroke
- The area of the brain where the stroke happened
- The amount of brain injury

A mild stroke can cause little or no brain damage. A major stroke can cause severe brain damage and even death. Some effects of stroke may improve with time and rehabilitation.

A stroke can happen in different parts of the brain. The brain is divided into four main parts:

- The right hemisphere (or half)
- The left hemisphere (or half)
- The cerebellum, which controls balance and coordination
- The brain stem, which controls all of our body's functions that we do not think about, such as heart rate, blood pressure, sweating, or digestion

A stroke in the right half of the brain can cause:

- Problems moving the left side of your body

- Problems judging distances. You may misjudge distances and fall. Or you might not be able to guide your hands to pick something up.

- Impaired judgment and behavior. You may misjudge your ability to do things. You may also do things you would not normally do, such as leave your house without getting fully dressed.

- Short-term memory loss. You may be able to remember events from 30 years ago, but not how to get to the place where you work today.

A stroke in the left half of the brain can cause:

- Problems moving the right side of your body

- Speech and language problems. You may have trouble speaking or understanding others.

- Slow and cautious behavior. You may need a lot of help to complete everyday tasks.

- Memory problems. You may not remember what you did 10 minutes ago, or you may have a hard time learning new things.

A stroke in the cerebellum can cause:

- Stiffness and tightness in the upper body that can cause spasms or jerky movements

- Eye problems, such as blurry or double vision

- Balance problems

- Dizziness, nausea (feeling sick to your stomach), and vomiting

Strokes in the brain stem are very harmful. Since impulses that start in the brain must travel through the brain stem on their way to the arms and legs, patients with a brain stem stroke may also develop paralysis.

How Do You Know If You Are at Risk of Stroke?

A stroke can happen to anyone. Some women are more at risk because of certain health problems, family health history, age, and habits. These are called "risk factors."

You cannot change some risk factors, such as your age, race or ethnicity, or family history. The good news is that you can control many other stroke risk factors, such as high blood pressure, diabetes, smoking, and unhealthy eating.

How Do You Know If You Are Having a Stroke?

Strokes happen fast and are a medical emergency. If you think you or someone else may be having a stroke, use the F.A.S.T. test:

F—Face: Look in the mirror and smile, or ask the person to smile. Does one side of the face droop?

A—Arms: Raise both arms. Does one arm drift downward?

S—Speech: Repeat a simple phrase, such as "Hello, my name is ____." Is the speech slurred or strange?

T—Time: Act fast. If you see any of these signs, call 911 right away. Some treatments for stroke work only if given in the first three hours (or up to four and a half hours for some people) after symptoms appear.

Section 31.4

Menopause and Heart Disease

"Menopause and Heart Disease,"
© 2016 Omnigraphics. Reviewed May 2019.

Menopause is the point in the female life cycle that marks the end of menstruation and fertility. It is a natural part of the aging process that begins around the age of 50 for most women. Menopause involves a number of physical changes, such as declining production of estrogen—the hormones that are primarily responsible for female sexual and reproductive development.

Research has shown that some of the changes associated with menopause can increase a woman's risk of developing heart disease.

In fact, cardiovascular disease accounts for nearly half of the deaths of American women over the age of 50. For women who have experienced menopause, therefore, it is particularly important to make healthy diet and lifestyle choices to reduce the risk of heart disease.

Menopause and Heart Health

Researchers attribute at least some of the increase in heart disease risk after menopause to declining levels of estrogen in the bloodstream. Estrogen impacts the arteries by strengthening their walls and helping them to remain flexible. When estrogen levels decline, it may accelerate the process of atherosclerosis (hardening of the arteries), which is associated with coronary artery disease.

In addition to drops in estrogen levels, however, several other menopausal changes may increase heart disease risk. Women's blood pressure levels tend to rise during menopause, for instance, as do levels of triglycerides and low-density lipoprotein (LDL) cholesterol in the bloodstream. The negative effects of menopausal changes are compounded in women who have other heart disease risk factors, such as smoking, diabetes, obesity, an inactive lifestyle, or a family history of cardiovascular illness.

To reduce the risk of heart disease during and after menopause, doctors recommend that women redouble their efforts to adopt a healthy lifestyle. Some tips for promoting heart health include the following:

- Quit smoking and avoid secondhand smoke.

- Get regular medical checkups that include heart health screenings, such as cholesterol, blood glucose, blood pressure, waist circumference, and body mass index (BMI).

- Obtain treatment as needed to control such medical conditions as diabetes, high blood pressure, and high cholesterol.

- Maintain a healthy body weight.

- Follow a regular exercise routine that includes at least 150 minutes of activity per week.

- Eat a healthy diet that is low in saturated fat and high in fiber, whole grains, legumes, fruits, vegetables, and lean proteins.

- Pay attention to mood and mental health, as depression can occur after menopause and affect cardiovascular health.

Hormone Replacement Therapy and Heart Health

Hormone replacement therapy (HRT) was once used extensively to relieve the symptoms of menopause, such as hot flashes, vaginal dryness, loss of sex drive, insomnia, and mood swings. Doctors also believed that HRT would help reduce the risk of chronic health conditions related to decreasing estrogen levels, such as osteoporosis and heart disease. In the early 2000s, however, studies showed that HRT actually led to an increased the risk of breast cancer, stroke, blood clots, and heart disease. The negative effects of HRT appeared most strongly in women over the age of 60.

The U.S. Food and Drug Administration (FDA) responded by changing its guidelines regarding hormone replacement therapy. Doctors are now encouraged to prescribe estrogen at the lowest possible dose and for the shortest possible length of time to achieve treatment goals. Experts saw a significant drop in cases of heart disease and breast cancer in postmenopausal women over the age of 50 as soon as the new guidelines went into effect. As of 2016, only about 10 percent of women take HRT to treat severe menopausal symptoms, and it is no longer recommended as a method of reducing a woman's risk of heart disease.

References

1. "Menopause and Heart Disease," American Heart Association, 2016.

2. "Menopause and Heart Disease," WebMD, 2016.

Chapter 32

Cardiovascular Disease in Men

Chapter Contents

Section 32.1

Men and Heart Disease: A Statistical Overview

This section contains text excerpted from the following sources: Text in this section begins with excerpts from "Heart Disease and Men," Centers for Disease Control and Prevention (CDC), February 13, 2018; Text beginning with the heading "Heart Disease Facts in Men" is excerpted from "Men and Heart Disease Fact Sheet," Centers for Disease Control and Prevention (CDC), August 23, 2017.

Heart disease is a term that includes several more specific heart conditions. The most common heart disease in the United States is coronary artery disease (CAD). CAD occurs when the arteries that supply blood to the heart muscle harden and narrow due to the buildup of plaque. The narrowing and buildup of plaques is called "atherosclerosis." Plaques are a mixture of fatty and other substances, including cholesterol and other lipids. Blood flow to the heart is reduced, which reduces oxygen to the heart muscle. This can lead to a heart attack. Other heart conditions include angina, heart failure, and arrhythmias.

Heart Disease Facts in Men

Heart disease is the leading cause of death for men in the United States, killing 321,000 men in 2013—that is 1 in every 4 male deaths.

Heart disease is the leading cause of death for men of most racial/ethnic groups in the United States, including African Americans, American Indians or Alaska Natives, Hispanics, and Whites. For Asian American or Pacific Islander men, heart disease is second only to cancer.

About 8.5 percent of all White men, 7.9 percent of Black men, and 6.3 percent of Mexican American men have coronary heart disease.

Half of the men who die suddenly of coronary heart disease have no previous symptoms. Even if you have no symptoms, you may still be at risk for heart disease.

Between 70 to 89 percent of sudden cardiac events occur in men.

Risk Factors for Heart Disease

High blood pressure, high low-density lipoprotein (LDL) cholesterol, and smoking are key risk factors for heart disease. About half of Americans (49%) have at least one of these three risk factors.

Several other medical conditions and lifestyle choices can also put people at a higher risk for heart disease, including:

- Diabetes

- Being overweight or obese

- Poor diet

- Physical inactivity

- Excessive alcohol use

Section 32.2

Cardiovascular Implications of Erectile Dysfunction

Erectile dysfunction (ED)—also known as "impotence"—is the inability to achieve or sustain an erection as needed for sexual intercourse. It is believed to affect around 10 percent of adult men on a regular or long-term basis, while a much higher percentage of men experience occasional problems. ED affects up to 30 million men in the United States. Men who fail to achieve an erection more than half the time are considered to have a physical or psychological condition that requires treatment.

A key reason to seek treatment for erectile dysfunction is that it is often linked to cardiovascular health. Studies have shown that ED is a major risk factor for heart disease. For men younger than 50 years of age, in fact, it carries similar risks as smoking or having a family history of coronary artery disease. In addition, obtaining treatment for current heart disease and related conditions can improve erectile dysfunction.

Causes and Treatment

The ability to achieve an erection depends on three factors: adequate blood circulation in the penis, proper nerve function in the penis, and stimulus from the brain. Erectile dysfunction can result from various diseases, conditions, and medications that interfere with one or more of these factors. Some common causes of ED include the following:

- Vascular diseases, such as atherosclerosis (hardening of the arteries), hypertension (high blood pressure), and high cholesterol, which can restrict blood flow to the penis

- Diabetes, which can cause nerve and artery damage

- Kidney disease, which can affect circulation, nerve function, and libido (sex drive)

- Neurological diseases, such as stroke, Alzheimer's disease, multiple sclerosis (MS), and Parkinson's disease, which can interfere with nerve impulses between the brain and penis

- Treatments for prostate, bladder, or colon cancer

- More than 200 different types of prescription medications

- Tobacco, alcohol, or drug use, which can damage blood vessels and restrict blood flow to the penis

- Injury to the penis, brain, or spinal cord

- Chronic illness

- Psychological conditions, such as depression or performance anxiety

It is important to note that ED is not considered a normal part of the aging process. Although older men may require more stimulation to achieve an erection, they should be capable of sexual intercourse. There are several prescription drugs available to treat ED, including sildenafil (Viagra), vardenafil (Levitra), and tadalafil (Cialis). These drugs (phosphor-diesterase-5 inhibitor PDE5-1) work by relaxing the cavernosal smooth muscle in order to increase the blood flow to the penis.

Erectile Dysfunction and Cardiovascular Health

Erectile dysfunction is a major predictor of heart disease. In fact, most men who experience ED will develop symptoms of cardiovascular illness within 5 years. One study found that 64 percent of men who were hospitalized for a heart attack and 57 percent of men who underwent heart bypass surgery had experienced ED. Although ED does not always point to an underlying heart problem, experts recommend that men with ED that does not have an obvious cause should undergo a complete cardiovascular health screening.

Doctors are uncertain about the exact nature of the link between erectile dysfunction and heart problems. One possible explanation is that the buildup of plaques in the arteries—which often occurs in people with heart disease—might also reduce blood flow to the penis. Many doctors attribute the link to dysfunction of the endothelium that lines the blood vessels, which impairs blood flow to the heart, penis, and other organs.

The link between erectile dysfunction and cardiovascular health also extends to risk factors that are shared between the two conditions, such as:

- Smoking

- Drinking alcohol

- Diabetes

- High blood pressure

- High cholesterol

- Obesity

- Low testosterone

For men who have both erectile dysfunction and heart disease, adopting healthy lifestyle changes can lead to improvements in both conditions. Some suggested changes include quitting smoking, drinking alcohol in moderation if at all, exercising regularly, maintaining a healthy weight, and choosing a healthy diet that is low in saturated fats. It is also important to note that some medications—including nitrates—used to treat heart disease; high blood pressure; a benign prostate; and hypertrophy are not safe to use in conjunction with the drugs used to treat erectile dysfunction.

References

1. "Erectile Dysfunction: A Sign of Heart Disease?" Mayo Clinic, 2016.

2. "Heart Disease and Erectile Dysfunction." Cleveland Clinic, 2012.

Section 32.3

Stroke in Men

This section includes text excerpted from "Men and
Stroke," Centers for Disease Control and Prevention (CDC),
October 29, 2015. Reviewed May 2019.

Stroke is the fifth leading cause of death in men, killing almost
the same number of men each year as prostate cancer and Alzheimer
disease (AD) combined. Stroke is a leading cause of long-term disability among American men. In addition, men have strokes at younger
ages than women. These facts are alarming, but there is some good
news: up to 80 percent of strokes can be prevented. This means it is
important to know your risk of having a stroke and taking action to
reduce that risk.

What Is a Stroke?

A stroke, sometimes called a "brain attack," occurs when blood
flow to an area of the brain is cut off. When brain cells are starved of
oxygen, they die. A stroke is a medical emergency. It is important to
get treatment as soon as possible. A delay in treatment increases the
risk of permanent brain damage or death.

What Does Put Men at Risk of Stroke?

Some of the major risk factors are listed below.

- High blood pressure is a main risk factor for stroke, yet nearly
  one in three men with high blood pressure does not know he has
  it.

- Smoking damages blood vessels, which can cause a stroke. Men
  are more likely to be smokers than women.

- Being overweight or obese increases your risk of stroke. Almost
  three in four American men are in weight ranges that increase
  their risk for stroke.

- More men than women have been diagnosed with diabetes,
  which increases the risk of stroke because it can cause disease of
  blood vessels in the brain.

- Men are more likely than women to drink too much alcohol,
  increasing their risk for stroke.

Being inactive can increase the risk of stroke. Only 1 in 4 men gets enough physical activity, even though exercising only 30 minutes a day can decrease the risk of stroke.

How Can You Prevent Stroke?

Most strokes can be prevented by keeping medical conditions under control and making lifestyle changes. A good place to start is to know your ABCs of heart health:

- Aspirin. Aspirin may help reduce your risk for stroke. But, you should check with your doctor before taking aspirin because it can make some types of stroke worse. Before taking aspirin, talk with your doctor about whether aspirin is right for you.

- Blood Pressure. Control your blood pressure.

- Cholesterol. Manage your cholesterol.

- Smoking. Quit smoking, or do not start.

Make lifestyle changes:

- Eat healthy and stay active. Choose healthy foods most of the time, including foods with less salt, or sodium, to lower your blood pressure, and get regular exercise. Being overweight or obese raises your risk of stroke.

- Talk to your doctor about your risk factors for stroke, including your age and whether anyone in your family has had a stroke.

- Get other health conditions under control, such as diabetes or heart disease

If Stroke Happens, Act F.A.S.T.

Knowing your chances of having a stroke is only half the battle. Strokes come on suddenly and should be treated as medical emergencies. If you think you or someone else may be having a stroke, act F.A.S.T.

F—Face: Ask the person to smile. Does one side of the face droop?

A—Arms: Ask the person to raise both arms. Does one arm drift downward?

S—Speech: Ask the person to repeat a simple phrase. Is the speech slurred or strange?

T—Time: If you see any of these signs, call 911 right away.

Calling an ambulance is critical because emergency medical technicians, or EMTs, can take you to a hospital that can treat stroke patients, and in some cases, they can begin life-saving treatment on the way to the emergency room. Some treatments for stroke work only if given within the first three hours after symptoms start.

Chapter 33

Cardiovascular Disease in Minority Populations

Chapter Contents

Section 33.1

Cardiovascular Disease among U.S. Racial and Ethnic Minorities: Some Statistics

This section includes text excerpted from "Heart Disease
Facts," Centers for Disease Control and Prevention (CDC),
November 28, 2017

Heart Disease in the United States

About 610,000 people die of heart disease in the United States every
year—that is 1 in every 4 deaths. Heart disease is the leading cause
of death for both men and women. More than half of the deaths due
to heart disease in 2009 were in men.

Coronary heart disease (CHD) is the most common type of heart
disease, killing over 370,000 people annually.

Every year, about 735,000 Americans have a heart attack. Of these,
525,000 are a first heart attack and 210,000 happen in people who
have already had a heart attack.

Heart Disease Deaths Vary by Race and Ethnicity

Heart disease is the leading cause of death for people of most eth-
nicities in the United States, including African Americans, Hispanics,
and Whites. For American Indians or Alaska Natives and Asians or
Pacific Islanders, heart disease is second only to cancer. Below are
the percentages of all deaths caused by heart disease in 2008, listed
by ethnicity.

Table 33.1. Percentage for Race of Ethnic Group

Race of Ethnic Group	Percentage of Deaths
American Indians or Alaska Natives	18.4
Asians or Pacific Islanders	22.2
Non-Hispanic Blacks	23.8
Non-Hispanic Whites	23.8
All	23.5

Section 33.2

African Americans and Cardiovascular Disease

This section includes text excerpted from "Jackson Heart Study:
Largest Investigation of Heart Disease in African Americans
Promises to Pave Way to Better Health," National Heart,
Lung, and Blood Institute (NHLBI), February 15, 2017.

It is the most sweeping—and significant—study ever of cardio-vascular disease (CVD) in African Americans. Now, experts with the groundbreaking Jackson Heart Study (JHS) are taking stock of some of the many insights gleaned since the study began in 2000. They are insights researchers say will go a long way toward helping boost the long-term health of a group marked by a stubbornly high rate of heart disease compared to the rest of the population. Heart disease is the number one cause of death for all Americans, and almost half of African Americans have some form of cardiovascular disease (which includes heart disease, stroke, and high blood pressure (HBP)). Approximately one in four African American males and females dies of heart disease.

The 17-year-long observational study follows the health of about 5,300 African Americans in the Jackson, Mississippi metropolitan area. It is comparable in scope to the Massachusetts-based Framing-ham Heart study, started in 1948; however, those participants were mainly White. The National Heart, Lung, and Blood Institute (NHLBI) and the National Institute on Minority Health and Health Disparities (NIMHD), which fund Jackson Heart, are continuing to explore the reasons behind the troubling disparities in heart health. Here are some of the findings emerging from the JHS:

- A gene defect doubles the risk of heart disease. African Americans with a gene called *"APOL1"* carry a greater risk for kidney disease and have almost twice the risk of cardiovascular disease as people who do not carry this gene. The gene is present in 1 in 10 blacks and is uncommon in Whites and non-African populations. Scientists believe that this gene variant originated as a way to protect against sleeping sickness in Africa.

- Even small spikes in blood pressure can lead to a higher risk of death. A new analysis of data from the JHS found that for each 10 millimeters of mercury (mm Hg) increase in systolic blood pressure, there was a 12 percent higher risk of death for African

401

Americans and a 7 percent greater risk of hospitalization due to heart failure. The finding could help improve future guidelines for treating hypertension in this at-risk population, the researchers say.

- Preventing heart disease is highly possible. While there is no magic pill, researchers have found that there are concrete steps people can take to live a longer, more productive life—without heart disease. In a study of more than 4,700 JHS participants, researchers found that those who adopted certain health measures had a lower risk for heart disease. These measures, known as "Life's Simple 7," include managing blood pressure, controlling cholesterol, reducing blood sugar, getting more exercise, eating better, losing weight, and avoiding smoking.

In addition to these findings on heart disease, researchers have also made the following JHS discoveries, and more are anticipated:

- Sickle cell trait is linked to a higher risk of kidney disease. African Americans with sickle cell trait (SCT) have a nearly 60 percent higher risk of developing kidney disease than those without the trait. With the sickle cell trait, people carry only one copy of the sickle cell gene variant instead of two and tend to have fewer medical complications when compared to those with full-blown sickle cell disease (SCD). Researchers suggest that people with sickle cell trait may need closer monitoring for signs of kidney disease. The study could lead to new ways to prevent kidney disease in this population, they say.

- Target identified: Rare gene can lower the risk of diabetes. Some gene defects can help protect you against disease. In 2014, researchers conducted a genetic analysis of 150,000 people and discovered that rare mutations in a gene called "*SLC30A8*" lowered the risk of developing type 2 diabetes by 65 percent. The gene was found in multiple ethnic groups, including a small number of participants from the JHS. The identification of this target could lead to a way to prevent diabetes, researchers suggest.

Section 33.3

American Indian and Alaska Native Heart Disease and Stroke

This section includes text excerpted from "American Indian and Alaska Native Heart Disease and Stroke Fact Sheet," Centers for Disease Control and Prevention (CDC), June 16, 2016.

Heart disease is the leading cause of death among American Indians and Alaska Natives. In 2014, heart disease caused 3,288 deaths.

Stroke is the seventh leading cause of death among American Indians and Alaska Natives. In 2014, stroke caused 649 deaths among American Indians and Alaska Natives.

Heart disease and stroke are also major causes of disability and can decrease a person's quality of life (QOL).

The American Indian and Alaska Native Population

There are approximately 4.5 million American Indians and Alaska Natives in the United States, 1.5 percent of the population, including those of more than one race. The median age of American Indians and Alaska Natives is 30.7 years, which is younger than the 36.2 years of the total U.S. population.

California has the largest population of American Indians and Alaska Natives (696,600), followed by Oklahoma (401,100), and Arizona (334,700). Alaska has the highest proportion of American Indians and Alaska Natives in its populations (20%), followed by Oklahoma and New Mexico (11% each). Los Angeles County is the county with the most American Indians and Alaska Natives (154,000).

A language other than English is spoken at home by 25 percent of American Indians and Alaska Natives 5 years of age and older. A high-school diploma is held by 76 percent of American Indians and Alaska Natives over the age of 25; 14 percent have a bachelor's degree or higher. The poverty rate of people who report American Indian and Alaska Native race only is 25 percent. Approximately 177,000 American Indians and Alaska Natives are veterans.

American Indian and Alaska Native Heart Disease and Stroke Facts

Heart disease is the first and stroke the sixth leading cause of death Among American Indians and Alaska Natives. The heart disease death rate was 20 percent greater and the stroke death rate 14 percent greater among American Indians and Alaska Natives (1996–1998) than among all U.S. races (1997) after adjusting for misreporting of American Indian and Alaska Native race on state death certificates.

The highest heart disease death rates are located primarily in South Dakota and North Dakota, Wisconsin, and Michigan. Counties with the highest stroke death rates are primarily in Alaska, Washington, Idaho, Montana, Wyoming, South Dakota, Wisconsin, and Minnesota.

American Indians and Alaska Natives die from heart diseases at younger ages than other racial and ethnic groups in the United States. 36 percent of those who die of heart disease die before the age of 65.

Diabetes is an extremely important risk factor for cardiovascular disease (CVD) among American Indians. Cigarette smoking, a risk factor for heart disease and stroke, is highest in the Northern Plains (44.1%) and Alaska (39.0%) and lowest in the Southwest (21.2%) among American Indians and Alaska Natives.

Preventing Heart Disease and Stroke among American Indians and Alaska Natives
Prevent and Control High Blood Cholesterol

High blood cholesterol is a major risk factor for heart disease. Preventing and treating high blood cholesterol includes eating a diet low in saturated fat and cholesterol and high in fiber, keeping a healthy weight, and getting regular exercise. All adults should have their cholesterol levels checked once every five years. If yours is high, your doctor may prescribe medicines to help lower it.

Prevent and Control High Blood Pressure

Lifestyle actions, such as healthy diet, regular physical activity, not smoking, and healthy weight will help you to keep normal blood pressure levels. Blood pressure is easily checked, and all adults should have it checked on a regular basis. If your blood pressure is high, you can work with your doctor to treat it and bring it down to the normal range. A high blood pressure can usually be controlled with lifestyle changes and with medicines when needed.

Prevent and Control Diabetes

Diabetes has been shown to be a very important risk factor for heart disease among American Indians and Alaska Natives. People with diabetes have an increased risk for heart disease but can reduce their risk. Also, people can take steps to reduce their risk for diabetes in the first place through weight loss and regular physical activity.

No Tobacco

Chewing, dipping, and cigarette smoking are nontraditional uses of tobacco among American Indians and Alaska Natives. Smoking increases the risk of high blood pressure, heart disease, and stroke. Never smoking is one of the best things a person can do to lower their risk. And, quitting smoking will also help lower a person's risk of heart disease. A person's risk of heart attack decreases soon after quitting. If you smoke, your doctor can suggest programs to help you quit smoking.

Moderate Alcohol Use

Excessive alcohol use increases the risk of high blood pressure, heart attack, and stroke. People who drink should do so only in moderation and always responsibly.

Maintain a Healthy Weight

Healthy weight status in adults is usually assessed by using weight and height to compute a number called the "body mass index" (BMI). BMI usually indicates the amount of body fat on a person. An adult who has a BMI of 30 or higher is considered obese. Overweight is a BMI between 25 and 29.9. Normal weight is a BMI of 18 to 24.9. Proper diet and regular physical activity can help to maintain a healthy weight.

Regular Physical Activity

Adults should engage in moderate level physical activities for at least 30 minutes on most days of the week.

Diet and Nutrition

Along with healthy weight and regular physical activity, an overall healthy diet can help to lower blood pressure and cholesterol levels, and prevent obesity, diabetes, heart disease, and stroke. This includes eating lots of fresh fruits and vegetables, lowering or cutting out added salt or sodium, and eating less saturated fat and cholesterol to lower these risks.

Treat Atrial Fibrillation

Atrial fibrillation (AF) is an irregular beating of the heart. It can cause clots that can lead to stroke. A doctor can prescribe medications to help reduce the chance of clots.

Genetic Risk Factors

Stroke can run in families. Genes play a role in stroke risk factors, such as high blood pressure, heart disease, diabetes, and vascular conditions. It is also possible that an increased risk for stroke within a family is due to factors such as a common sedentary lifestyle or poor eating habits, rather than hereditary factors.

Section 33.4

Heart Disease in the Hispanic Population

This section includes text excerpted from "Heart Disease
and Hispanic Americans," Office of Minority Health (OMH),
U.S. Department of Health and Human Services (HHS),
January 28, 2016.

In general, Hispanic American adults are less likely to have coronary heart disease (CHD) than non-Hispanic White adults. They are also less likely to die from heart disease than non-Hispanic White adults.

In 2012, Hispanics were 10 percent less likely to have CHD than non-Hispanic Whites.

In 2013, Hispanic men and women were 30 percent less likely to die from heart disease than non-Hispanic Whites.

Table 33.2. Age-Adjusted Percentages of Coronary Heart Disease among Persons 18 Years of Age and Over, 2012

Hispanics/Latinos	5.3
Non-Hispanic White	6.2
Hispanic/Non-Hispanic White Ratio	0.9

(Source: Centers for Disease Control and Prevention (CDC), 2014. Summary Health Statistics for U.S. Adults: 2012.)

Table 33.3. Heart Disease and Hispanics

Age-adjusted percentage of adults aged 20 and over screened for cholesterol, 2011-2012			
	Hispanic	**Non-Hispanic White**	**Hispanic /Non- Hispanic White Ratio**
Men	54.6	70.6	0.8
Women	64.2	72.9	0.9
Total	59.3	71.8	0.8

(Source: Centers for Disease Control and Prevention (CDC), 2013. National Center for Health Statistics (NCHS) Data Brief, No. 132)

Treatment at a Glance—Death Rate

Table 33.4. Age-Adjusted Heart Disease Death Rates per 100,000 (2013)

	Hispanics/ Latinos	**Non-Hispanic White**	**Hispanic/Non-Hispanic White Ratio**
Men	151.1	217.9	0.7
Women	97	134.6	0.7
Total	121.2	171.8	0.7

(Source: Centers for Disease Control and Prevention (CDC), 2014. National Vital Statistic Report.)

Treatment at a Glance—Risk Factors

There are several risk factors related to diabetes. Some of these risk factors are:

- Overweight and obesity
- High Cholesterol
- Hypertension
- Cigarette Smoking

Table 33.5. Age-Adjusted Percentage of Persons 20 Years of Age and over Who Have High Blood Pressure, 2009–2012

	Mexican American	**Non-Hispanic White**	**Mexican/Non-Hispanic White Ratio**
Men	27.3	29.6	0.9
Women	29.3	27.5	1.1

(Source: Centers for Disease Control and Prevention (CDC) 2015. Health United States, 2014.)

Table 33.6. Age-Adjusted Percentage of Persons 18 Years of Age and over Who Have High Blood Pressure, 2012

Hispanics	Non-Hispanic White	Hispanic /Non-Hispanic White Ratio
20.9	23.4	0.9

(Source: Centers for Disease Control and Prevention (CDC), 2014. Summary Health Statistics for U.S. Adults: 2012.)

Table 33.7. Percent of Adults Age 18 and over with Hypertension Whose Blood Pressure Is Under Control, 2011–2012

Hispanic American	Non-Hispanic White	Hispanic American /Non-Hispanic White Ratio
45.9	53.9	0.9

(Source: Centers for Disease Control and Prevention (CDC), 2015. Health Indicators Warehouse.)

Table 33.8. Age-Adjusted Percentage of Persons 20 Years of Age and over Who Have High Cholesterol, 2009–2012

	Mexican American	Non-Hispanic White	Mexican/Non-Hispanic White Ratio
Men	27.2	28.1	1
Women	26.2	28.2	0.9

(Source: Centers for Disease Control and Prevention (CDC), 2015. Health United States, 2014.)

Table 33.9. Adults Who Received a Blood Cholesterol Measurement in the Last 5 Years, 2008

Hispanics	Non-Hispanic White	Hispanic/Non-Hispanic White Ratio
71.8	74.1	1

(Source: Agency for Healthcare Research and Quality (AHRQ), 2015. National Healthcare Quality and Disparities Reports.)

Table 33.10. Age-Adjusted Percentage of Persons 18 Years of Age and over Who Are Current Cigarette Smokers, 2011–2013

	Hispanic	Non-Hispanic White	Hispanic/Non-Hispanic White Ratio
Men	16.7	22.1	0.8
Women	7.5	19.2	0.4

(Source: Centers for Disease Control and Prevention (CDC), 2015. Health United States, 2014.)

Table 33.11. Percentage of Current Smokers Age 18 and over with a Checkup Who Reported Receiving Advice to Quit Smoking, 2009

	Hispanic	Non-Hispanic White	Hispanic/Non-Hispanic White Ratio
Men	50	66.3	0.8
Women	67.6	73.8	0.9
Total	56.6	70.5	0.8

(Source: 2012 National Healthcare Quality Report.)

At a Glance—Treatment

Table 33.12. Hospital Patients with Heart Attack Who Were Prescribed Ace Inhibitor or Arb at Discharge, United States, 2010

Hispanic	White	Hispanic/White Ratio
96.7	96.1	1

(Source: The Agency for Healthcare Research and Quality (AHRQ), 2015. National Healthcare Quality and Disparities Reports.)

Section 33.5

Heart Disease and Native Hawaiians/Pacific Islanders

This section includes text excerpted from "Heart Disease and Native Hawaiians/Pacific Islanders," Office of Minority Health (OMH), U.S. Department of Health and Human Services (HHS), August 15, 2017.

National data related to heart disease for Native Hawaiians/Pacific Islanders is not available at this time for many conditions and risk factors. Local data from states with high populations of Native Hawaiians/Pacific Islanders may be useful in illustrating disparities among certain populations. Heart-related health issues vary among various Asian and Pacific Islander subpopulations.

In Hawaii, Native Hawaiians are 1.7 times more likely (70 percent more likely) to die from heart disease than White individuals.

In 2014, Native Hawaiians/Pacific Islanders were 10 percent more likely to be diagnosed with coronary heart disease than non-Hispanic White adults.

At a Glance—Diagnosed Cases of Coronary Heart Disease

Table 33.13. Age-Adjusted Percentages of Coronary Heart Disease Among Persons 18 Years of Age and Over, 2014

Native Hawaiian/Pacific Islander	Non-Hispanic White	Native Hawaiian/Pacific Islander/Non-Hispanic White Ratio
6	5.7	1.1

(Source: Centers for Disease Control and Prevention (CDC), 2017. Selected Health Conditions Among Native Hawaiian and Pacific Islander Adults: United States, 2014.)

At a Glance—Death Rate

There is no national data available at this time.

A report from the state of Hawaii, a state with a high percentage of Native Hawaiian/Pacific Islander residents, reveals some relevant facts:

Table 33.14. Mortality Rate for Major Cardiovascular Diseases, Hawaii 2005

	Population	Population/White Ratio
White	180.9	--
Filipino	396.3	2.2
Japanese	180.3	1
Native Hawaiian	313.1	1.7

(Source: State of Hawaii, 2007. The Burden of Cardiovascular Disease in Hawaii 2007.)

Table 33.15. Prevalence of Adults Who Reported a History of Myocardial Infarction (MI), the Behavioral Risk Factor Surveillance System Hawaii, 2005

	Population	Population/White Ratio
White	4	--
Filipino	2.7	0.7
Japanese	3.5	0.9
Native Hawaiian	4.4	1.1

(Source: State of Hawaii, 2007. The Burden of Cardiovascular Disease in Hawaii 2007.)

At a Glance—Risk Factors

Table 33.16. Age-Adjusted Percentage of Persons 18 Years of Age and over Who Have High Blood Pressure, 2012

Native Hawaiian/Pacific Islander	Non-Hispanic White	Native Hawaiian/Pacific Islander/Non-Hispanic White Ratio
36.5	23.4	1.6

(Source: Centers for Disease Control and Prevention (CDC), 2014. Summary Health Statistics for U.S. Adults: 2012.)

Table 33.17. Age-adjusted percentage of persons 18 years of age and over who are current cigarette smokers, 2012

Native Hawaiian/Pacific Islander	Non-Hispanic White	Native Hawaiian/Pacific Islander/Non-Hispanic White Ratio
20.1*	20.6	1

(Source: Centers for Disease Control and Prevention (CDC), 2012. Summary Health Statistics for U.S. Adults: 2011.)

Table 33.18. Percentage of Adult Smoking, the Behavioral Risk Factor Surveillance System Hawaii 2011

	Population	Population/White Ratio
White	17.8	--
Filipino	12.4	0.7
Japanese	11.7	0.7
Native Hawaiian	26.8	1.8

(Source: State of Hawaii, 2015. Hawaii Health Data Warehouse.)

At a Glance—United States Territories

Table 33.19. Age-Adjusted Heart Disease Death Rates per 100,000 (2010)

	Territory	Non-Hispanic White (U.S. National)	Guam/Non-Hispanic White Ratio
Guam	176.5	171.8	1
American Samoa	62.1	171.8	0.4
Northern Marianas	74.3	171.8	0.4

(Source: Centers for Disease Control and Prevention (CDC), 2012. National Vital Statistics Report.)

Estimates are considered unreliable. Data shown have a relative standard error of greater than 30 percent.

Part Five

Diagnosing
Cardiovascular Disorders

Chapter 34

Recognizing Signs and Symptoms of Heart Disease

How would you react to a medical emergency? When it comes to life-threatening conditions, such as heart attack or stroke, every minute counts. Get to know the signs and symptoms of these health threats. If you think you or someone else might be having a heart attack or stroke, get medical help right away. Acting fast could save your life or someone else's.

Heart disease and stroke are 2 of the top killers among both women and men in the United States. Nationwide, someone dies from a heart attack about every 90 seconds, and stroke kills someone about every 4 minutes, according to the Centers for Disease Control (CDC) and Prevention. Quick medical help could prevent many of these deaths. Fast action can also limit permanent damage to the body.

Heart attack and stroke are caused by interruptions to the normal flow of blood to the heart or brain—the two organs that are essential to life. Without access to oxygen-rich blood and nutrients, heart or brain cells begin to malfunction and die. This cell death can set off a series of harmful effects throughout the body. The changes ultimately lead to the familiar symptoms of a heart or brain emergency.

You might know the most common symptoms of heart attack: sustained, crushing chest pain and difficulty breathing. A heart attack

This chapter includes text excerpted from "Can You Recognize a Heart Attack or Stroke?" *NIH News in Health,* National Institutes of Health (NIH), August 2014. Reviewed May 2019.

might also cause cold sweats, a racing heart, pain down the left arm, jaw stiffness, or shoulder pain.

Many people do not know that women often have different heart attack symptoms than men. For instance, instead of having chest pain during a heart attack, women may feel extremely exhausted and fatigued or have indigestion and nausea.

"Many women have a vague sense of gloom and doom, a sense of 'I just do not feel quite right and do not know why,'" says Dr. Patrice Desvigne-Nickens, an expert in heart health at the National Institutes of Health (NIH).

The symptoms of stroke include sudden difficulty with seeing, speaking, or walking, and feelings of weakness, numbness, dizziness, and confusion. "Some people get a severe headache that is immediate and strong, different from any kind you have ever had," says Dr. Salina Waddy, an NIH stroke expert.

At the first sign of any of these symptoms, fast action by you, someone you know, or a passerby can make a huge difference. There are medicines, procedures, and devices that can help limit heart and brain damage following an attack, as long as medical help arrives quickly. If the heart is starved for blood for too long—generally more than 20 minutes—heart muscle can be irreversibly damaged, Desvigne-Nickens says. "You need to be in the hospital because there is a risk of cardiac arrest (your heart stopping)," which could be deadly. At the hospital, doctors can administer clot-busting drugs and other emergency procedures.

With stroke, Waddy says, "The longer you wait, the more brain cells are dying," and the greater the chance for permanent damage or disability.

Emergency treatment for stroke depends on the kind of stroke. The most common type, ischemic stroke, is caused by a clot that clogs a blood vessel in the brain. The clot-dissolving drug tissue plasminogen activator (tPA) works best when given soon after symptoms begin. The NIH research shows that patients who received tPA within three hours of stroke onset were more likely to recover fully.

Other strokes are caused by a hemorrhage—when a blood vessel breaks and bleeds into the brain. "The patient can have a larger hemorrhage within the first three hours," Waddy says. A hospital medical team can help contain the bleeding, so every moment counts.

Even if you are unsure, do not feel embarrassed or hesitate to call 911 if you suspect a heart attack or stroke. "You should not go get your car keys. Your spouse should not be driving you to the hospital," advises Desvigne-Nickens. "The emergency crew is trained to treat these symptoms, and it could mean the difference between life and death."

Heart attack or stroke can happen to anyone, but your risk increases with age. A family or personal history of heart attack or stroke also raises your risk. But, some risk factors for heart attack and stroke are within your control. Treating them can dramatically reduce your risk.

"If you have high blood pressure, high cholesterol, or diabetes, work with your doctor to get these conditions under control," Waddy says. "Know your numbers (blood pressure, blood sugar, and cholesterol) and what they mean."

You can also prepare for a medical emergency, to some degree. A hospital may not have access to your medical records when you arrive. Keep important health information handy, such as the medicines you are taking, allergies, and emergency contacts. It would be important for the medical team to know, for example, if you have been taking anticoagulants to help prevent blood clots; these blood thinners put you at increased risk of bleeding. You might consider carrying an NIH wallet card that lists heart attack symptoms and has room for your personal medical information.

Researchers at the NIH are studying new drugs and procedures to help the heart and brain repair themselves and improve organ function. "But, there is absolutely nothing that will save both your time and health, as well as prevention," says Dr. Jeremy Brown, director of NIH's Office of Emergency Care Research (OECR). Studies show that making healthy lifestyle choices can help prevent these medical emergencies from happening in the first place. Eat a healthy diet rich in protein, whole grains, and fruits and vegetables, and low in saturated fat. Get regular physical activity and do not smoke.

"I think one of the most important things we can do is to take a basic cardiopulmonary resuscitation (CPR) and first aid course," recommends Brown. "We know the majority of cardiac arrests happen outside of hospitals and of that many, many can be saved if we get people with basic training on the scene quickly. An ambulance can never get there as quickly as a citizen passing by."

Whether or not you are trained to offer help, if you see someone having symptoms of a heart attack or stroke, call for help immediately.

"If you are even thinking about calling 911, you should call," Desvigne-Nickens says. "Yes, other conditions can mimic the signs and symptoms of a heart attack or stroke, but let the emergency physician figure that out in the emergency room."

Know the Symptoms for Heart Attack and Stroke

Do not hesitate to call 911 if you see these symptoms of heart attack or stroke. Every minute counts.

Heart Attack

- Chest pain or discomfort
- Pain, stiffness, or numbness in the neck, back, or one or both arms or shoulders
- Shortness of breath
- Cold sweat, nausea, dizziness

Stroke

- Sudden numbness or weakness of the face, arm, or leg, especially on one side of the body
- Sudden severe headache, dizziness, confusion
- Sudden difficulty with vision, balance, speech

Chapter 35

Cardiac Diagnostic Tests

Heart diseases are the number one killer in the United States. They are also a major cause of disability. If you do have a heart disease, it is important to find it early, when it is easier to treat. Blood tests and heart health tests can help find heart diseases or identify problems that can lead to heart diseases. There are several different types of heart health tests. Your doctor will decide which test or tests you need, based on your symptoms (if any), risk factors, and medical history.

Cardiac Catheterization

Cardiac catheterization is a medical procedure that is used to diagnose and treat some heart conditions. For the procedure, your doctor puts a catheter (a long, thin, flexible tube) into a blood vessel in your arm, groin, or neck, and threads it to your heart. The doctor can use the catheter to:

- Do a coronary angiography. This involves putting a special type of dye in the catheter, so the dye can flow through your bloodstream to your heart. Then your doctor takes X-rays of your heart. The dye allows your doctor to see your coronary arteries on the X-ray and check for coronary artery disease (CAD).

- Take samples of blood and heart muscle

This chapter includes text excerpted from "Heart Health Tests," MedlinePlus, National Institutes of Health (NIH), February 28, 2017.

- Do procedures, such as minor heart surgery or angioplasty, if your doctor finds that you need it

Cardiac Computed Tomography Scan

A cardiac computed tomography (CT) scan is a painless imaging test that uses X-rays to take detailed pictures of your heart and its blood vessels. Computers can combine these pictures to create a three-dimensional (3-D) model of the whole heart. This test can help doctors detect or evaluate

- Coronary artery disease
- Calcium buildup in the coronary arteries
- Problems with the aorta
- Problems with heart function and valves
- Pericardial diseases

Before you have the test, you receive an injection of contrast dye. The dye highlights your heart and blood vessels in the pictures. The CT scanner is a large, tunnel-like machine. You lie still on a table that slides you into the scanner, and the scanner takes the pictures for about 15 minutes.

Cardiac Magnetic Resonance Imaging

Cardiac magnetic resonance imaging (MRI) is a painless imaging test that uses radio waves, magnets, and a computer to create detailed pictures of your heart. It can help your doctor figure out whether you have heart disease, and if so, how severe it is. A cardiac MRI can also help your doctor decide the best way to treat heart problems, such as:

- Coronary artery disease
- Heart valve problems
- Pericarditis
- Cardiac tumors
- Damage from a heart attack

The MRI is a large, tunnel-like machine. You lie still on a table that slides you into the MRI machine. The machine makes loud noises as it takes pictures of your heart. It usually takes about 30 to 90 minutes.

Sometimes, before the test, you might receive an injection of contrast dye. The dye highlights your heart and blood vessels in the pictures.

Chest X-Ray

A chest X-ray creates pictures of the organs and structures inside your chest, such as your heart, lungs, and blood vessels. It can reveal signs of heart failure, as well as lung disorders and other causes of symptoms not related to heart disease.

Coronary Angiography

A coronary angiography (angiogram) is a procedure that uses contrast dye and X-ray pictures to look at the insides of your arteries. It can show whether plaque is blocking your arteries and how severe the blockage is. Doctors use this procedure to diagnose heart diseases after chest pain; sudden cardiac arrest (SCA); or abnormal results from other heart tests, such as an EKG or a stress test.

You usually have a cardiac catheterization to get the dye into your coronary arteries. Then special X-rays are taken while the dye is flowing through your coronary arteries. The dye lets your doctor study the flow of blood through your heart and blood vessels.

Echocardiography

An echocardiography, or echo, is a painless test that uses sound waves to create moving pictures of your heart. The pictures show the size and shape of your heart. They also show how well your heart's chambers and valves are working. Doctors use an echo to diagnose many different heart problems and to check how severe they are.

For the test, a technician applies gel to your chest. The gel helps sound waves reach your heart. The technician moves a transducer (wand-like device) around on your chest. The transducer connects to a computer. It transmits ultrasound waves into your chest, and the waves bounce (echo) back. The computer converts the echoes into pictures of your heart.

Electrocardiogram

An electrocardiogram, also called an "ECG" or "EKG," is a painless test that detects and records your heart's electrical activity. It shows how fast your heart is beating and whether its rhythm is steady or irregular.

An EKG may be part of a routine exam to screen for heart disease. Or you may get it to detect and study heart problems, such as heart attacks, arrhythmia, and heart failure.

For the test, you lie still on a table, and a nurse or technician attaches electrodes (patches that have sensors) to the skin on your chest, arms, and legs. Wires connect the electrodes to a machine that records your heart's electrical activity.

Stress Testing

Stress testing looks at how your heart works during physical stress. It can help to diagnose coronary artery disease and check how severe it is. It can also check for other problems, including heart valve disease and heart failure.

For the test, you exercise (or are given medicine if you are unable to exercise) to make your heart work hard and beat fast. While this is happening, you get an EKG and your blood pressure is monitored. Sometimes, you may also have an echocardiogram or other imaging tests, such as a nuclear scan. For the nuclear scan, you get an injection of a tracer (a radioactive substance), which travels to your heart. Special cameras detect the energy from the tracer to make pictures of your heart. You have pictures taken after you exercise, and then after you rest.

Chapter 36

Blood Tests Used to Diagnose Cardiovascular Disorders

Chapter Contents

Section 36.1

Blood Tests

This section includes text excerpted from "Blood Tests," National Heart, Lung, and Blood Institute (NHLBI), August 4, 2015. Reviewed May 2019.

What Are Blood Tests?

Blood tests help doctors check for certain diseases and conditions. They also help check the function of your organs and show how well treatments are working.

Specifically, blood tests can help doctors:

- Evaluate how well organs—such as the kidneys, liver, thyroid, and heart—are working

- Diagnose diseases and conditions, such as cancer, human immunodeficiency virus (HIV), acquired immunodeficiency syndrome (AIDS), diabetes, anemia, and coronary heart disease (CHD)

- Find out whether you have risk factors for heart disease

- Check whether medicines you are taking are working

- Assess how well your blood is clotting

Types of Blood Tests

Some of the most common blood tests are:

- A complete blood count (CBC)
- Blood chemistry tests
- Blood enzyme tests
- Blood tests to assess heart disease risk

Complete Blood Count

A complete blood count is one of the most common blood tests. It is often done as part of a routine checkup. The CBC can help detect blood diseases and disorders, such as anemia, infections, clotting problems, blood cancers, and immune system disorders. This test measures many different parts of your blood.

Red Blood Cells

Red blood cells (RBCs) carry oxygen from your lungs to the rest of your body. Abnormal RBC levels may be a sign of anemia, dehydration (too little fluid in the body), bleeding, or another disorder.

White Blood Cells

White blood cells (WBC) are part of your immune system, which fights infections and diseases. Abnormal WBC levels may be a sign of infection, blood cancer, or an immune system disorder.

A complete blood count measures the overall number of WBCs in your blood. A CBC with differential looks at the amounts of different types of WBCs in your blood.

Platelets

Platelets are blood cell fragments that help your blood clot. They stick together to seal cuts or breaks on blood vessel walls and stop bleeding.

Abnormal platelet levels may be a sign of a bleeding disorder (not enough clotting) or a thrombotic disorder (too much clotting).

Hemoglobin

Hemoglobin is an iron-rich protein in RBCs that carries oxygen. Abnormal hemoglobin levels may be a sign of anemia, sickle cell anemia (SCA), thalassemia, or other blood disorders.

If you have diabetes, excess glucose in your blood can attach to hemoglobin and raise the level of hemoglobin A1C.

Hematocrit

Hematocrit is a measure of how much space RBCs take up in your blood. A high hematocrit level might mean you are dehydrated. A low hematocrit level might mean you have anemia. Abnormal hematocrit levels also may be a sign of a blood or bone marrow disorder.

Mean Corpuscular Volume

Mean corpuscular volume (MCV) is a measure of the average size of your RBCs. Abnormal MCV levels may be a sign of anemia or thalassemia.

Blood Chemistry Tests / Basic Metabolic Panel

The basic metabolic panel (BMP) is a group of tests that measures different chemicals in the blood. These tests usually are done on the fluid (plasma) part of blood. The tests can give doctors information about your muscles (including the heart); bones; and organs, such as the kidneys and liver.

The BMP includes blood glucose, calcium, and electrolyte tests, as well as blood tests that measure kidney function. Some of these tests require you to fast (not eat any food) before the test, and others do not. Your doctor will tell you how to prepare for the test(s) you are having.

Blood Glucose

Glucose is a type of sugar that the body uses for energy. Abnormal glucose levels in your blood may be a sign of diabetes.

For some blood glucose tests, you have to fast before your blood is drawn. Other blood glucose tests are done after a meal or at any time with no preparation.

Calcium

Calcium is an important mineral in the body. Abnormal calcium levels in the blood may be a sign of kidney problems, bone disease, thyroid disease, cancer, malnutrition, or another disorder.

Electrolytes

Electrolytes are minerals that help maintain fluid levels and acid-base balance in the body. They include sodium, potassium, bicarbonate, and chloride.

Abnormal electrolyte levels may be a sign of dehydration, kidney disease, liver disease, heart failure, high blood pressure (HBP), or other disorders.

Kidneys

Blood tests for kidney function measure levels of blood urea nitrogen (BUN) and creatinine. Both of these are waste products that the kidneys filter out of the body. Abnormal BUN and creatinine levels may be signs of a kidney disease or disorder.

Blood Enzyme Tests

Enzymes are chemicals that help control chemical reactions in your body. There are many blood enzyme tests. This section focuses on blood enzyme tests used to check for heart attack. These include troponin and creatine kinase (CK) tests.

Troponin

Troponin is a muscle protein that helps your muscles contract. When muscle or heart cells are injured, troponin leaks out, and its levels in your blood rise.

For example, blood levels of troponin rise when you have a heart attack. For this reason, doctors often order troponin tests when patients have chest pain or other heart attack signs and symptoms.

Creatine Kinase

A blood product called "creatine kinase-muscle/brain" (CK-MB) is released when the heart muscle is damaged. High levels of CK-MB in the blood can mean that you have had a heart attack.

Blood Tests to Assess Heart Disease Risk

A lipoprotein panel is a blood test that can help show whether you are at risk for coronary heart disease. This test looks at substances in your blood that carry cholesterol.

A lipoprotein panel gives information about your:

- Total cholesterol

- Low-density lipoprotein cholesterol (LDL or "bad") cholesterol. This is the main source of cholesterol buildup and blockages in the arteries.

- High-density lipoprotein cholesterol (HDL or "good") cholesterol. This type of cholesterol helps decrease blockages in the arteries.

- Triglycerides. Triglycerides are a type of fat in your blood.

A lipoprotein panel measures the levels of LDL and HDL cholesterol and triglycerides in your blood. Abnormal cholesterol and triglyceride levels may be signs of increased risk for CHD.

Most people will need to fast for 9 to 12 hours before a lipoprotein panel.

Blood Clotting Tests

Blood clotting tests sometimes are called a "coagulation panel." These tests check proteins in your blood that affect the blood clotting process. Abnormal test results might suggest that you are at risk of bleeding or developing clots in your blood vessels.

Your doctor may recommend these tests if she or he thinks you have a disorder or disease related to blood clotting.

Blood clotting tests also are used to monitor people who are taking medicines to lower the risk of blood clots. Warfarin and heparin are two examples of such medicines.

What to Expect with Blood Tests
What to Expect before Blood Tests

Many blood tests do not require any special preparation and take only a few minutes.

Other blood tests require fasting (not eating any food) for 8 to 12 hours before the test. Your doctor will tell you how to prepare for your blood test(s).

What to Expect during Blood Tests

Blood usually is drawn from a vein in your arm or other parts of your body using a needle. It also can be drawn using a finger prick.

The person who draws your blood might tie a band around the upper part of your arm or ask you to make a fist. Doing this can make the veins in your arms stick out more, which makes it easier to insert the needle.

The needle that goes into your vein is attached to a small test tube. The person who draws your blood removes the tube when it is full, and the tube seals on its own. The needle is then removed from your vein. If you are getting a few blood tests, more than one test tube may be attached to the needle before it is withdrawn.

Some people get nervous about blood tests because they are afraid of needles. Others may not want to see blood leaving their bodies.

If you are nervous or scared, it can help to look away or talk to someone to distract yourself. You might feel a slight sting when the needle goes in or comes out.

Drawing blood usually takes less than three minutes.

What to Expect after Blood Tests

Once the needle is withdrawn, you will be asked to apply gentle pressure with a piece of gauze or bandage to the place where the needle was inserted. This helps stop bleeding. It also helps prevent swelling and bruising.

Most of the time, you can remove the pressure after a minute or two. You may want to keep a bandage on for a few hours.

Usually, you do not need to do anything else after a blood test. Results can take anywhere from a few minutes to a few weeks to come back. Your doctor should get the results. It is important that you follow up with your doctor to discuss your test results.

What Are the Risks of Blood Tests?

The main risks of blood tests are discomfort and bruising at the site where the needle goes in. These complications usually are minor and go away shortly after the tests are done.

What Do Blood Tests Show?

Blood tests show whether the levels of different substances in your blood fall within a normal range.

For many blood substances, the normal range is the range of levels seen in 95 percent of healthy people in a certain group. For many tests, normal ranges vary depending on your age, gender, race, and other factors.

Your blood test results may fall outside the normal range for many reasons. Abnormal results might be a sign of a disorder or disease. Other factors—such as diet, menstrual cycle, physical activity level, alcohol intake, and medicines (both prescription and over-the-counter (OTC))—also can cause abnormal results.

Your doctor should discuss any unusual or abnormal blood test results with you. These results may or may not suggest a health problem.

Many diseases and medical problems cannot be diagnosed with blood tests alone. However, blood tests can help you and your doctor learn more about your health. Blood tests also can help find potential problems early, when treatments or lifestyle changes may work best.

Result Ranges for Common Blood Tests

All values in this section are for adults only. They do not apply to children. Talk to your child's doctor about values on blood tests for children.

Complete Blood Count

The table below shows some normal ranges for different parts of the complete blood count test. Some of the normal ranges differ between men and women. Other factors, such as age and race, also may affect normal ranges.

Your doctor should discuss your results with you. She or he will advise you further if your results are outside the normal range for your group.

Table 36.1. Complete Blood Count

Test	Normal Range Results*
Red blood cell (RBC) (varies with altitude)	Male: 5 to 6 million cells/mcL
	Female: 4 to 5 million cells/mcL
White blood cell (WBC)	4,500 to 10,000 cells/mcL
Platelets	140,000 to 450,000 cells/mcL
Hemoglobin (varies with altitude)	Male: 14 to 17 gm/dL
	Female: 12 to 15 gm/dL
Hematocrit (varies with altitude)	Male: 41 to 50 percent
	Female: 36 to 44 percent
Mean corpuscular volume	80 to 95 femtoliter[†]

Cells/mcL = cells per microliter; gm/dL = grams per deciliter.
[†] *A femtoliter is a measure of volume.*

Blood Glucose

This table shows the ranges for blood glucose levels after 8 to 12 hours of fasting (not eating). It shows the normal range and the abnormal ranges that are a sign of prediabetes or diabetes.

Table 36.2. Blood Glucose

Plasma Glucose Results (mg/dL)*	Diagnosis
70 to 99	Normal
100 to 125	Prediabetes
126 and above	Diabetes[†]

mg/dL = milligrams per deciliter.
[†] *The test is repeated on another day to confirm the results.*

Lipoprotein Panel

The table below shows ranges for total cholesterol, LDL cholesterol, and HDL cholesterol levels after 9 to 12 hours of fasting. High blood cholesterol is a risk factor for coronary heart disease (CHD).

Your doctor should discuss your results with you. She or he will advise you further if your results are outside the desirable range.

Table 36.3. Total Cholesterol Level

Total Cholesterol Level	Total Cholesterol Category
Less than 200 mg/dL	Desirable
200 to 239 mg/dL	Borderline high
240 mg/dL and above	High

Table 36.4. LDL Cholesterol Level

LDL Cholesterol Level	LDL Cholesterol Category
Less than 100 mg/dL	Optimal
100 to129 mg/dL	Near optimal/above optimal
130 to 159 mg/dL	Borderline high
160 to189 mg/dL	High
190 mg/dL and above	Very high

Table 36.5. HDL Cholesterol Level

HDL Cholesterol Level	HDL Cholesterol Category
Less than 40 mg/dL	A major risk factor for heart disease
40 to 59 mg/dL	The higher, the better
60 mg/dL and above	Considered protective against heart disease

Section 36.2

C-Reactive Protein Test

This section includes text excerpted from "C-Reactive
Protein (CRP) Test," MedlinePlus, National Institutes of
Health (NIH), November 7, 2018.

What Is a C-Reactive Protein Test?

A C-reactive protein test measures the level of C-reactive protein
(CRP) in your blood. CRP is a protein made by your liver. It is sent into
your bloodstream in response to inflammation. Inflammation is your
body's way of protecting your tissues if you have been injured or have
an infection. It can cause pain, redness, and swelling in the injured or
affected area. Some autoimmune disorders and chronic diseases can
also cause inflammation.

Normally, you have low levels of C-reactive protein in your blood.
High levels may be a sign of a serious infection or other disorder.

What Is C-Reactive Protein Test Used For?

A CRP test may be used to find or monitor conditions that cause
inflammation. These include:

- Bacterial infections, such as sepsis, a severe and sometimes
  life-threatening condition

- A fungal infection

- Inflammatory bowel disease (IBD), a disorder that causes
  swelling and bleeding in the intestines

- An autoimmune disorder, such as lupus or rheumatoid arthritis
  (RA)

- An infection of the bone called "osteomyelitis"

Why Do You Need a C-Reactive Protein Test?

You may need this test if you have symptoms of a serious bacterial
infection. Symptoms include:

- Fever

- Chills

- Rapid breathing

- Rapid heart rate

- Nausea and vomiting

If you have already been diagnosed with an infection or have a chronic disease, this test may be used to monitor your treatment. CRP levels rise and fall depending on how much inflammation you have. If your CRP levels go down, it is a sign that your treatment for inflammation is working.

What Happens during a C-Reactive Protein Test?

A healthcare professional will take a blood sample from a vein in your arm, using a small needle. After the needle is inserted, a small amount of blood will be collected into a test tube or vial. You may feel a little sting when the needle goes in or out. This process usually takes less than five minutes.

Will You Need to Do Anything to Prepare for the C-Reactive Protein Test?

You do not need any special preparations for a CRP test.

Are There Any Risks to the Test?

There is very little risk of having a blood test. You may have slight pain or bruising at the spot where the needle was put in, but most symptoms go away quickly.

What Do the C-Reactive Protein Test Results Mean?

If your results show a high level of CRP, it probably means you have some type of inflammation in your body. A CRP test does not explain the cause or location of the inflammation. So, if your results are not normal, your healthcare provider may order more tests to figure out why you have inflammation.

A higher than normal CRP level does not necessarily mean you have a medical condition needing treatment. There are other factors that can raise your CRP levels. These include cigarette smoking, obesity, and a lack of exercise.

Is There Anything Else You Need to Know about a C-Reactive Protein Test?

A CRP test is sometimes confused with a high-sensitivity-(hs) CRP test. Although they both measure CRP, they are used to diagnose different conditions. An hs-CRP test measures much lower levels of CRP. It is used to check for risk of heart disease.

Section 36.3

Homocysteine Test

This section includes text excerpted from "Homocysteine Test," MedlinePlus, National Institutes of Health (NIH), July 27, 2018.

What Is a Homocysteine Test?

A homocysteine test measures the amount of homocysteine in your blood. Homocysteine is a type of amino acid, a chemical your body uses to make proteins. Normally, vitamin B12, vitamin B6, and folic acid break down homocysteine and change it into other substances your body needs. There should be very little homocysteine left in the bloodstream. If you have high levels of homocysteine in your blood, it may be a sign of a vitamin deficiency, heart disease, or a rare inherited disorder.

What Is Homocysteine Test Used For?

A homocysteine test may be used to:

- Find out if you have deficiency in vitamin B12, B6, or folic acid

- Help diagnose homocystinuria, a rare, inherited disorder that prevents the body from breaking down certain proteins. It can cause serious health problems and usually starts in early childhood. Most U.S. states require all infants to get a homocysteine blood test as part of routine newborn screening.

- Screen for heart disease in people at high risk for heart attack or stroke

- Monitor people who have heart disease

Why Do You Need a Homocysteine Test?

You may need this test if you have symptoms of a vitamin B or folic acid deficiency. These include:

- Dizziness

- Weakness

- Fatigue

- Pale skin

- Sore tongue and mouth

- Tingling in the hands, feet, arms, and/or legs (in vitamin B12 deficiency)

You may also need this test if you are at high risk for heart disease because of prior heart problems or a family history of heart disease. Excess levels of homocysteine can build up in the arteries, which may increase your risk of blood clots, heart attack, and stroke.

What Happens during a Homocysteine Test?

A healthcare professional will take a blood sample from a vein in your arm, using a small needle. After the needle is inserted, a small amount of blood will be collected into a test tube or vial. You may feel a little sting when the needle goes in or out. This usually takes less than five minutes.

Will You Need to Do Anything to Prepare for the Test?

You may need to fast (not eat or drink) for 8 to 12 hours before a homocysteine test.

Are There Any Risks to the Test?

There is very little risk to having a blood test. You may have slight pain or bruising at the spot where the needle was put in, but most symptoms go away quickly.

What Do the Results Mean?

If your results show high homocysteine levels, it may mean:

- You are not getting enough vitamin B12, B6, or folic acid in your diet.

- You are at a higher risk of heart disease.

- Homocystinuria. If high levels of homocysteine are found, more testing will be needed to rule out or confirm a diagnosis.

If your homocysteine levels were not normal, it does not necessarily mean you have a medical condition needing treatment. Other factors can affect your results, including:

- Your age. Homocysteine levels can get higher as you get older.

- Your gender. Men usually have higher homocysteine levels than women.

- Alcohol use

- Smoking

- Use of vitamin B supplements

If you have questions about your results, talk to your healthcare provider.

Is There Anything Else You Need to Know about a Homocysteine Blood Test?

If your healthcare provider thinks a vitamin deficiency is the reason for your high homocysteine levels, she or he may recommend dietary changes to address the problem. Eating a balanced diet should ensure you get the right amount of vitamins.

If your healthcare provider thinks your homocysteine levels put you at risk for heart disease, she or he will monitor your condition and may order more tests.

Chapter 37

Electrocardiogram (EKG)

What Is an Electrocardiogram Test?

An electrocardiogram (EKG) test is a simple, painless procedure that measures electrical signals in your heart. Each time your heart beats, an electrical signal travels through the heart. An EKG can show if your heart is beating at a normal rate and strength. It also helps show the size and position of your heart's chambers. An abnormal EKG can be a sign of heart disease or damage.

What Is an Electrocardiogram Test Used For?

An EKG test is used to find and/or monitor various heart disorders. These include:

- Irregular heartbeat (known as "arrhythmia")
- Blocked arteries
- Heart damage
- Heart failure
- Heart attack. EKGs are often used in the ambulance, emergency room, or other hospital rooms to diagnose a suspected heart attack.

This chapter includes text excerpted from "Electrocardiogram," MedlinePlus, National Institutes of Health (NIH), January 31, 2019.

An EKG test is sometimes included in a routine exam for middle-aged and older adults, as they have a higher risk of heart disease than younger people.

Why Do You Need an Electrocardiogram Test?

You may need an EKG test if you have symptoms of a heart disorder. These include:

- Chest pain

- Rapid heartbeat

- Arrhythmia (it may feel like your heart has skipped a beat or is fluttering)

- Shortness of breath

- Dizziness

- Fatigue

You may also need this test if you:

- Have had a heart attack or other heart problems in the past

- Have a family history of heart disease

- Are scheduled for surgery. Your healthcare provider may want to check your heart health before the procedure.

- Have a pacemaker. The EKG can show how well the device is working.

- Are taking medicine for heart disease. The EKG can show if your medicine is effective, or if you need to make changes in your treatment.

What Happens during an Electrocardiogram Test?

An EKG test may be done in a provider's office, outpatient clinic, or a hospital. During the procedure:

- You will lie on an exam table.

- A healthcare provider will place several electrodes (small sensors that stick to the skin) on your arms, legs, and chest. The provider may need to shave or trim excess hair before placing the electrodes.

- The electrodes are attached by wires to a computer that records your heart's electrical activity.

- The activity will be displayed on the computer's monitor and/or printed out on paper.

- The procedure only takes about three minutes.

Will You Need to Do Anything to Prepare for the Electrocardiogram Test?

You do not need any special preparations for an EKG test.

Are There Any Risks to the Test?

There is very little risk of having an EKG. You may feel a little discomfort or skin irritation after the electrodes are removed. There is no risk of electric shock. The EKG does not send any electricity to your body. It only records electricity.

What Do the Electrocardiogram Test Results Mean?

Your healthcare provider will check your EKG results for a consistent heartbeat and rhythm. If your results were not normal, it may mean you have one of the following disorders:

- Arrhythmia

- A heartbeat that is too fast or too slow

- Inadequate blood supply to the heart

- A bulge in the heart's walls. This bulge is known as an "aneurysm."

- Thickening of the heart's walls

- A heart attack (Results can show if you have had a heart attack in the past or if you are having an attack during the EKG.)

If you have questions about your results, talk to your healthcare provider.

Elektrokardiogramm versus Electrocardiogram

An electrocardiogram may be called an "EKG" or an "electrocardiogram" (ECG). Both are correct and commonly used. EKG is based on the German spelling, elektrokardiogramm. EKG may be preferred over ECG to avoid confusion with an EEG, a test that measures brain waves.

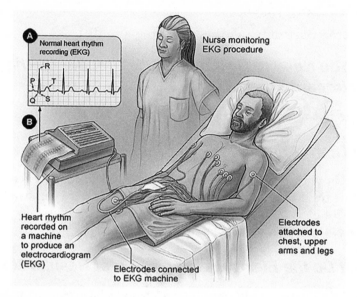

Figure 37.1. *Electrocardiogram*

The image shows the standard setup for an EKG. In figure A, a normal heart rhythm recording shows the electrical pattern of a regular heartbeat. In figure B, a patient lies in a bed with EKG electrodes attached to his chest, upper arms, and legs. A nurse monitors the painless procedure Content.

Chapter 38

Echocardiography

What Is Echocardiography?

Echocardiography, or echo, is a painless test that uses sound waves to create moving pictures of your heart. The pictures show the size and shape of your heart. They also show how well your heart's chambers and valves are working.

An echo also can pinpoint areas of heart muscle that are not contracting well because of poor blood flow or injury from a previous heart attack. A type of echo called "Doppler ultrasound" shows how well blood flows through your heart's chambers and valves.

An echo can detect possible blood clots inside the heart, fluid buildup in the pericardium (the sac around the heart), and problems with the aorta. The aorta is the main artery that carries oxygen-rich blood from your heart to your body.

Doctors also use echo to detect heart problems in infants and children.

Who Needs Echocardiography

Your doctor may recommend echocardiography if you have signs or symptoms of heart problems.

For example, shortness of breath and swelling in the legs are possible signs of heart failure. Heart failure is a condition in which your

This chapter includes text excerpted from "Echocardiography," National Heart, Lung, and Blood Institute (NHLBI), November 5, 2011. Reviewed May 2019.

heart cannot pump enough oxygen-rich blood to meet your body's needs. An echo can show how well your heart is pumping blood.

An echo also can help your doctor find the cause of abnormal heart sounds, such as heart murmurs. Heart murmurs are extra or unusual sounds heard during the heartbeat. Some heart murmurs are harmless, while others are signs of heart problems.

Your doctor also may use an echo to learn about:

- The size of your heart. An enlarged heart might be the result of high blood pressure (HBP), leaky heart valves, or heart failure. An echo also can detect the increased thickness of the ventricles (the heart's lower chambers). Increased thickness may be due to high blood pressure, heart valve disease, or congenital heart defects.

- Heart muscles that are weak and are not pumping well. Damage from a heart attack may cause weak areas of heart muscle. Weakening also might mean that the area is not getting enough blood supply, a sign of coronary heart disease (CHD).

- Heart valve problems. An echo can show whether any of your heart valves do not open normally or close tightly.

- Problems with your heart's structure. An echo can detect congenital heart defects, such as holes in the heart. Congenital heart defects are structural problems present at birth. Infants and children may have an echo to detect these heart defects.

- Blood clots or tumors. If you have had a stroke, you may have an echo to check for blood clots or tumors that could have caused the stroke.

Your doctor also might recommend an echo to see how well your heart responds to certain heart treatments, such as those used for heart failure.

Types

There are several types of echocardiography—all use sound waves to create moving pictures of your heart. This is the same technology that allows doctors to see a fetus.

Unlike X-rays and some other tests, an echo does not involve radiation.

Transthoracic Echocardiography

Transthoracic echo is the most common type of echocardiogram test. It is painless and noninvasive. "Noninvasive" means that no surgery is done and no instruments are inserted into your body.

This type of echo involves placing a device called a "transducer" on your chest. The device sends special sound waves, called "ultrasound," through your chest wall to your heart. The human ear cannot hear ultrasound waves.

As the ultrasound waves bounce off the structures of your heart, a computer in the echo machine converts them into pictures on a screen.

Stress Echocardiography

A stress echo is done as part of a stress test. During a stress test, you exercise or take medicine (given by your doctor) to make your heart work hard and beat fast. A technician will use echo to create pictures of your heart before you exercise and as soon as you finish.

Some heart problems, such as coronary heart disease, are easier to diagnose when the heart is working hard and beating fast.

Transesophageal Echocardiography

Your doctor may have a hard time seeing the aorta and other parts of your heart using a standard transthoracic echo. Thus, she or he may recommend transesophageal echo or TEE.

During this test, the transducer is attached to the end of a flexible tube. The tube is guided down your throat and into your esophagus (the passage leading from your mouth to your stomach). This allows your doctor to get more detailed pictures of your heart.

Fetal Echocardiography

Fetal echo is used to look at a fetus's heart. A doctor may recommend this test to check a baby for heart problems. When recommended, the test is commonly done at about 18 to 22 weeks of pregnancy. For this test, the transducer is moved over the pregnant woman's belly.

Three-Dimensional Echocardiography

A three-dimensional (3-D) echo creates 3-D images of your heart. These detailed images show how your heart looks and works.

During transthoracic echo, 3-D images can be taken as part of the process used to do these types of echo.

Doctors may use 3-D echo to diagnose heart problems in children. They also may use 3-D echo for planning and overseeing heart valve surgery.

Researchers continue to study new ways to use 3-D echo.

What to Expect before Echocardiography

Echocardiography is done in a doctor's office or a hospital. No special preparations are needed for most types of echo. You usually can eat, drink, and take any medicines as you normally would.

The exception is if you are having a transesophageal echo. This test usually requires that you do not eat or drink for eight hours prior to the test.

If you are having a stress echo, you may need to take steps to prepare for the stress test. Your doctor will let you know what steps you need to take.

What to Expect during Echocardiography

Echocardiography is painless; the test usually takes less than an hour to do. For some types of echo, your doctor will need to inject saline or a special dye into one of your veins. The substance makes your heart show up more clearly on the echo pictures.

The dye used for an echo is different from the dye used during angiography (a test used to examine the body's blood vessels).

For most types of echo, you will remove your clothing from the waist up. Women will be given a gown to wear during the test. You will lie on your back or left side on an exam table or stretcher.

Soft, sticky patches called "electrodes" will be attached to your chest to allow an electrocardiogram (EKG) to be done. An EKG is a test that records the heart's electrical activity.

A doctor or sonographer (a person specially trained to do ultrasounds) will apply gel to your chest. The gel helps the sound waves reach your heart. A transducer will then be moved around on your chest.

The transducer transmits ultrasound waves into your chest. A computer will convert echoes from the sound waves into pictures of your heart on a screen. During the test, the lights in the room will be dimmed so the computer screen is easier to see.

Echocardiography

The sonographer will record pictures of various parts of your heart. She or he will put the recordings on a computer disc for a cardiologist (heart specialist) to review.

During the test, you may be asked to change positions or hold your breath for a short time. This allows the sonographer to get better pictures of your heart.

At times, the sonographer may apply a bit of pressure to your chest with the transducer. You may find this pressure a little uncomfortable, but it helps get the best picture of your heart. You should let the sonographer know if you feel too uncomfortable.

The process described above is similar to the process for a fetal echo. For that test, however, the transducer is placed over the pregnant woman's belly at the location of the fetus's heart.

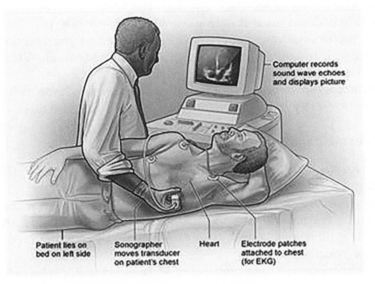

Figure 38.1. *Echocardiography*

The illustration shows a patient having echocardiography. The patient lies on his left side. A sonographer moves the transducer on the patient and chest, while viewing the echo pictures on a computer

Transesophageal Echocardiography

A transesophageal echo (TEE) is used if your doctor needs a more detailed view of your heart. For example, your doctor may use TEE to look for blood clots in your heart. A doctor, not a sonographer, will perform this type of echo.

A transesophageal echo uses the same technology as transthoracic echo, but the transducer is attached to the end of a flexible tube.

Your doctor will guide the tube down your throat and into your esophagus (the passage leading from your mouth to your stomach). From this angle, your doctor can get a more detailed image of the heart and major blood vessels leading to and from the heart.

For TEE, you will likely be given medicine to help you relax during the test. The medicine will be injected into one of your veins.

Your blood pressure, the oxygen content of your blood, and other vital signs will be checked during the test. You will be given oxygen through a tube in your nose. If you wear dentures or partials, you will have to remove them.

The back of your mouth will be numbed with gel or spray. Your doctor will gently place the tube with the transducer in your throat and guide it down until it is in place behind your heart.

The pictures of your heart are then recorded as your doctor moves the transducer around in your esophagus and stomach. You should not feel any discomfort as this happens.

Although the imaging usually takes less than an hour, you may be watched for a few hours at the doctor's office or hospital after the test.

Stress Echocardiography

A stress echo is a transthoracic echo that is combined with either an exercise or pharmacological stress test.

For an exercise stress test, you will walk or run on a treadmill or pedal a stationary bike to make your heart work hard and beat fast. For a pharmacological stress test, you will be given medicine to increase your heart rate.

A technician will take pictures of your heart using echo before you exercise and as soon as you finish.

What You May See and Hear during Echocardiography

As the doctor or sonographer moves the transducer around, you will see different views of your heart on the screen of the echo machine. The structures of your heart will appear as white objects, while any fluid or blood will appear black on the screen.

Doppler ultrasound often is used during echo tests. Doppler ultrasound is a special ultrasound that shows how blood is flowing through the blood vessels.

This test allows the sonographer to see blood flowing at different speeds and in different directions. The speed and direction of blood flow appear as different colors moving within the black and white images.

The human ear is unable to hear the sound waves used in echo. If you have a Doppler ultrasound, you may be able to hear "whooshing" sounds. Your doctor can use these sounds to learn about blood flow through your heart.

What to Expect after Echocardiography

You usually can go back to your normal activities right after having echocardiography.

If you have a transesophageal echo, you may be watched for a few hours at the doctor's office or hospital after the test. Your throat might be sore for a few hours after the test.

You also may not be able to drive for a short time after having TEE. Your doctor will let you know whether you need to arrange for a ride home.

What Does Echocardiography Show?

An echocardiography shows the size, structure, and movement of various parts of your heart. These parts include the heart valves, the septum (the wall separating the right and left heart chambers), and the walls of the heart chambers. Doppler ultrasound shows the movement of blood through your heart.

Your doctor may use echo to:

- Diagnose heart problems

- Guide or determine next steps for treatment

- Monitor changes and improvement

- Determine the need for more tests

An echo can detect many heart problems. Some might be minor and pose no risk to you. Others can be signs of serious heart disease or other heart conditions. Your doctor may use echo to learn about:

- The size of your heart. An enlarged heart might be the result of high blood pressure, leaky heart valves, or heart failure. An echo also can detect increased thickness of the ventricles (the heart's lower chambers). Increased thickness may be due to high blood pressure, heart valve disease, or congenital heart defects.

- Heart muscles that are weak and are not pumping well. Damage from a heart attack may cause weak areas of heart muscle. Weakening also might mean that the area is not getting enough blood supply, a sign of coronary heart disease.

- Heart valve problems. An echo can show whether any of your heart valves do not open normally or close tightly.

- Problems with your heart's structure. An echo can detect congenital heart defects, such as holes in the heart. Congenital heart defects are structural problems present at birth. Infants and children may have echo to detect these heart defects.

- Blood clots or tumors. If you have had a stroke, you may have echo to check for blood clots or tumors that could have caused the stroke.

What Are the Risks of Echocardiography?

Transthoracic and fetal echocardiography have no risks. These tests are safe for adults, children, and infants.

If you have a transesophageal echo, some risks are associated with the medicine given to help you relax. For example, you may have a bad reaction to medicine, problems breathing, and nausea (feeling sick to your stomach).

Your throat also might be sore for a few hours after the test. Rarely, the tube used during TEE causes minor throat injuries.

Stress echo has some risks, but they are related to the exercise or medicine used to raise your heart rate, not the echo. Serious complications from stress tests are very uncommon.

Chapter 39

Carotid Ultrasound

What Is Carotid Ultrasound?

Carotid ultrasound, also known as "carotid duplex," is a painless imaging test that uses high-frequency sound waves to create pictures of the inside of your carotid arteries. It uses an ultrasound machine, which includes a computer, a screen, and a transducer. The transducer is a handheld device that sends and receives sound waves. If combined with Doppler ultrasound, this test also can show how blood is moving through your arteries.

What Is Use of Carotid Ultrasound Test?

Carotid ultrasound is done to detect plaque buildup in one or both of the carotid arteries in the neck and to see whether the buildup is narrowing your carotid arteries and blocking blood flow to the brain. Test results will help your doctor plan treatment to remove the plaque and help prevent a stroke.

What Happens during Carotid Ultrasound Test

Carotid ultrasound usually is done in a doctor's office or hospital. You will lie on your back on an exam table for your test. The ultrasound technician will put gel on your neck where your carotid arteries are

This chapter includes text excerpted from "Carotid Ultrasound," National Heart, Lung, and Blood Institute (NHLBI), December 10, 2016.

located. The gel helps the sound waves reach your arteries. The technician will move the transducer against different areas on your neck. The transducer will detect the sound waves after they have bounced off your artery walls and blood cells. A computer will use the sound waves to create and record pictures of the inside of your carotid arteries and to show how blood is flowing in your carotid arteries.

Risks of Carotid Ultrasound

Carotid ultrasound has no risks because the test uses harmless sound waves. They are the same type of sound waves that doctors use to create and record pictures of a fetus.

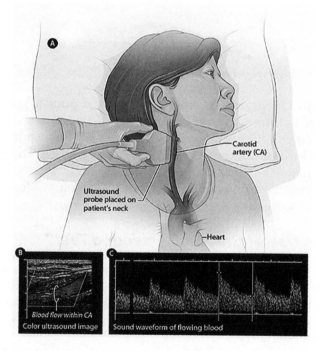

Figure 39.1. *Ultrasound Carotid Arteries* (Souce: "Ultrasound," National Institute of Biomedical Imaging and Bioengineering (NIBIB).)

The ultrasound probe (transducer) is placed over the carotid artery (top). A color ultrasound image (bottom, left) shows blood flow (the red color in the image) in the carotid artery. Waveform image (bottom right) shows the sound of flowing blood in the carotid artery.

Chapter 40

Holter and Event Monitors

What Are Holter and Event Monitors?

Holter and event monitors are small, portable electrocardiogram devices that record your heart's electrical activity for long periods of time while you do your normal activities. They are also known as "ambulatory electrocardiogram" (EKG/ECC), "continuous EKG" or "continuous or ECG," and "EKG event monitors."

What Is Holter and Event Monitors Used For?

These monitors can record how fast your heart is beating, whether the rhythm of your heartbeats is steady or irregular, and the strength and timing of the electrical impulses passing through each part of your heart. Information from these recordings helps doctors diagnose an arrhythmia, or irregular heartbeat, and check whether treatments for the irregular heartbeat are working.

Types of Holter and Event Monitors

There are many types of monitors, such as episodic monitors, auto detect recorders, 30-day event recorders, and transtelephonic event monitors.

This chapter includes text excerpted from "Holter and Event Monitors," National Heart, Lung, and Blood Institute (NHLBI), December 16, 2016.

Your doctor will decide which monitor is best for you. Most monitors have electrodes with sticky adhesive patches that attach to the skin on your chest. Some monitors and electrodes used for long-term recording may be implanted under your skin to make it easier for you to bathe and perform your daily activities. Your doctor will explain how to wear and use the monitor and tell you whether you need to adjust your activity during the testing period. You should avoid magnets, metal detectors, microwave ovens, electric blankets, electric toothbrushes, and electric razors while using your monitor. Usually, you will be instructed to keep electronic devices, such as cell phones, MP3 players, and tablets away from the monitor. After you are finished using the monitor, you will return it to your doctor's office or the place where you picked it up. If you were using an implantable recorder, your doctor will remove it from your chest.

Risks to Consider

There is a small risk that the sticky patches that attach the electrodes to your chest can irritate your skin. You may have an allergic reaction to the electrode adhesive, but the reaction will go away once the electrodes are removed. If you are using an implantable recorder, you may get an infection or have pain where the device was placed under your skin. Your doctor can prescribe medicine to treat these problems.

Chapter 41

Stress Testing

Stress tests show how well your heart handles physical activity. Your heart pumps harder and faster when you exercise. Some heart disorders are easier to find when your heart is hard at work. During a stress test, your heart will be checked while you exercise on a treadmill or stationary bicycle. If you are not healthy enough to exercise, you will be given a medicine that makes your heart beat faster and harder, as if you were actually exercising.

If you have trouble completing the stress test in a specified period of time, it may mean there is reduced blood flow to your heart. Reduced blood flow can be caused by several different heart conditions, some of which are very serious.

What Are They Used For?

Stress tests are most often used to:

- Diagnose coronary artery disease (CAD), a condition that causes a waxy substance called "plaque" to build up in the arteries. It can cause dangerous blockages in blood flow to the heart.

- Diagnose arrhythmia, a condition that causes an irregular heartbeat

- Find out what level of exercise is safe for you

This chapter includes text excerpted from "Stress Tests," MedlinePlus, National Institutes of Health (NIH), January 31, 2019.

- Find out how well your treatment is working if you have already been diagnosed with heart disease

- Show if you are at risk for a heart attack or other serious heart condition

Why Do You Need a Stress Test?

You may need a stress test if you have symptoms of limited blood flow to your heart. These include:

- Angina, a type of chest pain or discomfort caused by poor blood flow to the heart

- Shortness of breath

- Rapid heartbeat

- Irregular heartbeat (arrhythmia). This may feel like a fluttering in your chest.

You may also need a stress test to check your heart health if you:

- Are planning to start an exercise program

- Have had recent heart surgery

- Are being treated for heart disease. The test can show how well your treatment is working.

- Have had a heart attack in the past

- Are at a higher risk for heart disease due to health problems, such as diabetes, family history of heart disease, and/or previous heart problems

What Happens during a Stress Test

There are three main types of stress tests: exercise stress tests, nuclear stress tests, and stress echocardiograms. All types of stress tests may be done in a healthcare provider's office, outpatient clinic, or hospital.

During an exercise stress test:

- A healthcare provider will place several electrodes (small sensors that stick to the skin) on your arms, legs, and chest. The provider may need to shave excess hair before placing the electrodes.

- The electrodes are attached by wires to an electrocardiogram (EKG) machine, which records your heart's electrical activity.

- You will then walk on a treadmill or ride a stationary bicycle, starting slowly.

- Then, you will walk or pedal faster, with the incline and resistance increasing as you go.

- You will continue walking or riding until you reach a target heart rate set by your provider. You may need to stop sooner if you develop symptoms, such as chest pain, shortness of breath, dizziness, or fatigue. The test may also be stopped if the EKG shows a problem with your heart.

- After the test, you will be monitored for 10 to 15 minutes or until your heart rate returns to normal.

Both nuclear stress tests and stress echocardiograms are imaging tests. That means that pictures will be taken of your heart during testing.

During a nuclear stress test:

- You will lie down on an exam table.

- A healthcare provider will insert an intravenous (IV) line into your arm. The IV contains a radioactive dye. The dye makes it possible for the healthcare provider to view images of your heart. It takes between 15 to 40 minutes for the heart to absorb the dye.

- A special camera will scan your heart to create the images, which show your heart at rest.

- The rest of the test is the same as an exercise stress test. You will be hooked up to an EKG machine, then walk on a treadmill or ride a stationary bicycle.

- If you are not healthy enough to exercise, you will get a medicine that makes your heart beat faster and harder.

- When your heart is working at its hardest, you will get another injection of the radioactive dye.

- You will wait for about 15 to 40 minutes for your heart to absorb the dye.

- You will resume exercising and the special camera will take more pictures of your heart.

455

- Your provider will compare the two sets of images: one of your heart at rest; the other while hard at work.

- After the test, you will be monitored for 10 to 15 minutes or until your heart rate returns to normal.

- The radioactive dye will naturally leave your body through your urine. Drinking lots of water will help remove it faster.

During a stress echocardiogram:

- You will lie on an exam table.

- The provider will rub a special gel on a wand-like device called a "transducer." She or he will hold the transducer against your chest.

- This device makes sound waves, which create moving pictures of your heart.

- After these images are taken, you will exercise on a treadmill or bicycle, as in the other types of stress tests.

- If you are not healthy enough to exercise, you will get a medicine that makes your heart beat faster and harder.

- More images will be taken when your heart rate is increasing or when it is working at its hardest.

- Your provider will compare the two sets of images; one of your heart at rest; the other while hard at work.

- After the test, you will be monitored for 10 to 15 minutes or until your heart rate returns to normal.

Will You Need to Do Anything to Prepare for the Test?

You should wear comfortable shoes and loose clothing to make it easier to exercise. Your provider may ask you to not eat or drink for several hours before the test. If you have questions about how to prepare, talk to your healthcare provider.

Are There Any Risks to the Test?

Stress tests are usually safe. Sometimes, exercise or the medicine that increases your heart rate can cause symptoms, such as chest pain, dizziness, or nausea. You will be monitored closely throughout the test to reduce your risk of complications or to quickly treat any health problems. The radioactive dye used in a nuclear stress test is safe for most people. In rare cases, it may cause an allergic reaction.

Also, a nuclear stress test is not recommended for pregnant women, as the dye might be harmful to the fetus.

What Do the Results Mean?

A normal test result means no blood flow problems were found. If your test result was not normal, it can mean that there is reduced blood flow to your heart. Reasons for reduced blood flow include:

- Coronary artery disease

- Scarring from a previous heart attack

- Your current heart treatment is not working well

- Poor physical fitness

If your exercise stress test results were not normal, your healthcare provider may order a nuclear stress test or a stress echocardiogram. These tests are more accurate than exercise stress tests, but also more expensive. If these imaging tests show a problem with your heart, your provider may recommend more tests and/or treatment.

If you have questions about your results, talk to your healthcare provider.

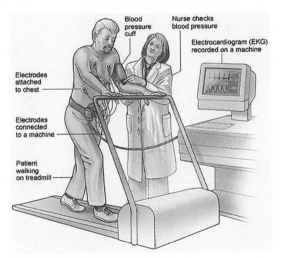

Figure 41.1. *Exercise Stress Test*

The image shows a patient having a stress test. Electrodes are attached to the patient's chest and connected to an EKG machine. The EKG records the heart's electrical activity. A blood pressure cuff is used to record the patient's blood pressure while he walks on a treadmill.

Chapter 42

Tilt-Table Testing

Tilt-table testing is one of the many procedures that is used to assess syncope (fainting). The person undergoing the test lies on a special table, which changes from a horizontal to a vertical position, inducing syncope and enabling measurement of how the body reacts to the force of gravity. A nurse or technician keeps track of the patient's heart rate and blood pressure during the test to monitor response to the position changes.

Why Is It Needed?

A tilt-table test will be required if there are recurring episodes of fainting and when other causes of syncope have been eliminated through previous tests. A tilt-table test will analyze what makes you feel light-headed or, in some instances, pass out completely. Typically, fainting may be caused by a number of factors, such as:

- Abnormal heart rhythm (arrhythmia)

- A very slow heart rate (bradycardia)

- Vasovagal syndrome (or, neurocardiogenic syncope), a sudden drop in blood pressure due to overstimulation of the vagus nerve

- Changes in the structure of the heart muscle or valves causing the heart to malfunction

"Tilt-Table Testing," © 2016 Omnigraphics. Reviewed May 2019.

- Damage to the heart muscle (or heart attack) caused by poor blood supply

- Ventricular dysfunction, or complications in the functioning of ventricles

- Reaction to certain medication

- Severe dehydration

- Low blood sugar (hypoglycemia)

- An extended period of bed-rest

Preparing for the Procedure

Before the test, the doctor will explain the procedure and will ask you to sign a consent form. It is important to let the doctor and technician know if:

- You have allergies

- You are sensitive to latex

- You are on medication (over-the-counter (OTC) and prescription) or other supplements

- You are, or you think you may be, pregnant

- You have a pacemaker

The doctor will give instructions regarding fasting for this procedure. If you are diabetic, ask the doctor to adjust dosage of your regular medication for the day of the test. The doctor might request other specific preparation depending on your medical condition.

How Is It Performed?

The tilt-table test is performed by a trained nurse or a technician in a hospital or an electrophysiology (EP) lab. The test, which has two parts, is designed to trigger symptoms of syncope to analyze what causes it. The first part alone lasts for about 30 to 40 minutes, while both together take about 90 minutes.

The first part of the test is performed to analyze how the body reacts to position changes:

- You lie on your back on a special table. Straps at your knees and waist will help you stay in place.

- An intravenous (IV) line is placed in your arm to administer medicine and IV fluids when needed, and electrocardiograph electrodes are attached to your chest to track heartbeat. A blood pressure cuff is placed on your arm and attached to a monitor.

- You will be asked to remain quiet and still until the end of the procedure, but you need to inform the nurse or technician if you feel uncomfortable.

- The table is tilted upward so that your head is slightly (30 degrees) above the rest of your body. Blood pressure and heart rate are checked by the nurse.

- A few minutes later, the table is further raised to almost vertical. Monitoring for symptoms, such as fainting, low blood pressure, low heart rate, and/or dizziness, will continue for up to 45 minutes.

- If there is a drop-in blood pressure during this time, the table will be lowered and the test will be stopped. The second part of the test will not be required.

- If no symptoms occur, the table will be lowered and the second part of the test will be performed.

The second part of the tilt-table test measures the heart's response to a medication given to speed up the heart rate:

- You will be given a medicine, such as isoproterenol, through the IV tube to induce a faster heartbeat and, thereby, increase sensitivity to the tilt-table test.

- The table is tilted upward again, to an angle of 60 degrees, to determine whether any of the symptoms of syncope occur.

- If there is a drop-in blood pressure within 15 minutes, the nurse will lower the table, stop the medicine, and end the test.

- If none of the symptoms occur, the test will be stopped once the nurse has all the necessary information. You will be allowed to rest for a while in a flat position while your heart rate and blood pressure continue to be monitored.

What Happens after the Test

It is possible to feel a little tired or sick after the test. You may be asked to stay for 30 to 60 minutes in order for the nurse to keep track of your heart rate and blood pressure. Most people can drive home and get back to their normal routines right after the test; however, those who lose consciousness during the test will need more testing and observation. It is advisable not to drive if you have fainted during the procedure.

What about the Results

The result is either "negative" or "positive," and you are most likely to know the result right after the test. If there is no drop-in blood pressure during the test, and if there are no other symptoms, the result is negative (normal). If there is a change in blood pressure, along with symptoms, such as dizziness or feeling faint, the test is positive. In such a case, the doctor may prescribe further tests or a change in medication. If the fainting was induced by bradycardia, you may need a pacemaker.

What Are the Risks?

Some of the possible risks of a tilt-table test include:

- Headache

- Dizziness

- Nausea

- Episodes of fainting

- Low or high blood pressure

- Heart palpitations

- Other risks, depending on already existing medical conditions

References

1. "Tilt-Table Test," American Heart Association, July 2015.

2. "Tilt-Table Procedure," Johns Hopkins Medicine, n.d.

Chapter 43

Coronary Angiography

What Is Coronary Angiography?

Coronary angiography is a procedure that uses contrast dye, usually containing iodine, and X-ray pictures to detect blockages in the coronary arteries that are caused by plaque buildup.

Blockages prevent your heart from getting oxygen and important nutrients. Coronary angiography is used to diagnose ischemic heart disease after chest pain; sudden cardiac arrest (SCA); or abnormal results from tests, such as an electrocardiogram (EKG) of the heart or an exercise stress test. It is important to detect blockages because over time they can cause chest pain, especially with physical activity or stress, or a heart attack. If you are having a heart attack, coronary angiography can help your doctors plan your treatment.

What Happens during Coronary Angiography

Cardiologists, or doctors who specialize in the heart, will perform coronary angiography in a hospital or specialized laboratory. You will stay awake so you can follow your doctor's instructions, but you will get medicine to relax you during the procedure. You will lie on your back on a movable table. Often, coronary angiography is done with a cardiac catheterization procedure. For this, your doctor will clean and numb an area on the arm, groin or upper thigh, or neck before making

This chapter includes text excerpted from "Coronary Angiography," National Heart, Lung, and Blood Institute (NHLBI), January 31, 2013. Reviewed May 2019.

a small hole in a blood vessel. Your doctor will insert a catheter tube into your blood vessel. Your doctor will take X-ray pictures to help place the catheter in your coronary artery. After the catheter is in place, your doctor will inject the contrast dye through the catheter to highlight blockages and take X-ray pictures of your heart. If blockages are detected, your doctor may use percutaneous coronary intervention (PCI), also known as "coronary angioplasty," to improve blood flow to your heart.

What Happens after Coronary Angiography

After coronary angiography, your doctor will remove the catheter; possibly use a closure device to close the blood vessel; and close and bandage the opening on your arm, groin, or neck. You may develop a bruise and soreness where the catheter was inserted. You will stay in the hospital for a few hours or overnight. During this time, your heart rate and blood pressure will be monitored. Your movement will be limited to prevent bleeding from the hole where the catheter was inserted. You will need a ride home after the procedure because of the medicines or anesthesia you received.

Complications Associated with Coronary Angiography

Coronary angiography is a common procedure that rarely causes serious problems. Possible complications may include bleeding, allergic reactions to the contrast dye, infection, blood vessel damage, arrhythmias, blood clots that can trigger a heart attack or stroke, kidney damage, and fluid buildup around the heart. The risk of complications is higher in people who are older or who have certain conditions, such as chronic kidney disease (CKD) or diabetes. An imaging test called "coronary computed tomography angiography," or "coronary CTA," may be preferred over coronary angiography to detect blockages in the heart. Even though coronary CTA still uses contrast dye, it does not require the invasive cardiac catheterization procedure that causes many of the complications of coronary angiography.

Chapter 44

Cardiac Computed Tomography (CT)

What Is Cardiac Computed Tomography?

A cardiac computed tomography (CT) scan is a painless imaging test that uses X-rays to take many detailed pictures of your heart and its blood vessels. Computers can combine pictures from a cardiac CT scan to create a three-dimensional (3-D) model of the whole heart. This imaging test can help doctors detect or evaluate ischemic heart disease, calcium buildup in the coronary arteries, problems with the aorta, problems with heart function and valves, and pericardial disease. This test also may be used to monitor the results of coronary artery bypass grafting or to follow-up on abnormal findings from earlier chest X-rays. Different CT scanners are used for different purposes. A multidetector CT is a very fast type of CT scanner that can produce high-quality pictures of the beating heart and can detect calcium or blockages in the coronary arteries. An electron beam CT scanner also can show calcium in coronary arteries.

How Is Cardiac Computed Tomography Performed?

Your cardiac CT scan may be performed in a medical imaging facility or hospital. The scan usually takes about 15 minutes to complete,

This chapter includes text excerpted from "Cardiac CT Scan," National Heart, Lung, and Blood Institute (NHLBI), January 31, 2013. Reviewed May 2019.

but it can take more than an hour including preparation time and, if needed, the time to take medicines, such as beta-blockers to slow your heart rate. Before the test, a contrast dye, often iodine, may be injected into a vein in your arm. This contrast dye highlights your blood vessels and creates clearer pictures. You may feel some discomfort from the needle or, after the contrast dye is injected, you may feel warm briefly or have a temporary metallic taste in your mouth.

The CT scanner is a large, tunnel-like machine that has a table. You will lie still on the table, and the table will slide into the scanner. Talk to your doctor if you are uncomfortable in tight or closed spaces to see if you need medicine to relax you during the test. During the scan, the technician will monitor your heart rate with an electrocardiogram (EKG). You will hear soft buzzing, clicking, or whirring sounds when you are inside the scanner while the scanner is taking pictures. You will be able to hear from and talk to the technician performing the test while you are inside the scanner. The technician may ask you to hold your breath for a few seconds during the test.

Risks of Cardiac Computed Tomography

Cardiac CT scans have some risks. In rare instances, some people may have an allergic reaction to the contrast dye. There is a slight risk of cancer, particularly in people younger than 40 years of age, because the test uses radiation. Even though, the amount of radiation from one test is similar to the amount of radiation you are naturally exposed to over one to five years, patients should not receive more CT scans than the number that clinical guidelines recommend. Another risk is that CT scans may detect an incidental finding, which is something that does not cause symptoms now but may require more tests after being found.

Talk to your doctor and the technicians performing the test about whether you are or could be pregnant. If the test is not urgent, they may have you wait to do the test until after your pregnancy. If it is urgent, the technicians will take extra steps to protect the fetus during this test. Let your doctor know if you are breastfeeding because contrast dye can pass into your breast milk. If you must have contrast dye injected, you may want to pump and save enough breast milk for one to two days after your test, or you may bottle-feed your baby for that time. People with asthma, chronic obstructive pulmonary disorder (COPD), or heart failure may have breathing problems during cardiac CT scans if they are given beta-blockers to slow their heart rates for this imaging test.

Chapter 45

Cardiac Magnetic Resonance Imaging

What Is Cardiac Magnetic Resonance Imaging?

Cardiac magnetic resonance imaging (MRI) is a painless imaging test that uses radio waves, magnets, and a computer to create detailed pictures of your heart. Cardiac MRI can provide detailed information on the type and severity of heart disease to help your doctor decide the best way to treat heart problems, such as coronary heart disease (CHD); heart valve problems; pericarditis; cardiac tumors; or damage from a heart attack. Cardiac MRI can help explain results from other imaging tests, such as chest X-rays and chest computed tomography (CT) scans.

How Is Cardiac Magnetic Resonance Imaging Done?

Cardiac MRI may be done in a medical imaging facility or hospital. Before your procedure, a contrast dye to highlight your heart and blood vessels may be injected into a vein in your arm. You may feel discomfort from the needle or a cool feeling as the contrast dye is injected. The MRI machine is a large, tunnel-like machine that has a table. You will lie still on the table and the table will slide into the machine. You

This chapter includes text excerpted from "Cardiac MRI," National Heart, Lung, and Blood Institute (NHLBI), April 26, 2013. Reviewed May 2019.

will hear loud humming, tapping, and buzzing sounds when you are inside the machine as pictures of your heart are being taken. You will be able to hear from and talk to the technician performing the test while you are inside the machine. The technician may ask you to hold your breath for a few seconds during the test.

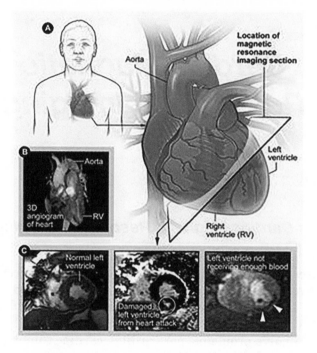

Figure 45.1. *3—Panel Image of Heart* (Source: National Heart, Lung, and Blood Institute (NHLBI).)

Panel A: An illustration showing how MRI can take cross-sectional images at any angle through the body. Panel B: A 3-D angiogram examining blood vessels coming off the aorta, the artery that connects the output of the heart to the rest of the body. Panel C: Three MRIs of the heart of a patient with a small heart attack, and who has much more heart muscle at risk.

Risks of Cardiac Magnetic Resonance Imaging

Cardiac MRI has few risks. In rare instances, the contrast dye may harm people who have kidney or liver disease, or it may cause an allergic reaction. Researchers are studying whether multiple contrast dye injections, defined as four or more, may cause other adverse effects. Talk to your doctor and the technicians performing the test about whether you are or could be pregnant. Let your doctor know if you are breastfeeding because the contrast dye can pass into your breast milk. If you must have the contrast dye injected, you may want to pump and save enough breast milk for one to two days after your test or you may bottle-feed your baby for that time. Tell your doctor if you have:

- A pacemaker or other implanted device because the MRI machine can damage these devices.

- Metal inside your body from previous surgeries because it can interfere with the MRI machine.

- Metal on your body from piercings, jewelry, or some transdermal skin patches because they can interfere with the MRI machine or cause skin burns. Tattoos may cause a problem because older tattoo inks may contain small amounts of metal.

Chapter 46

Nuclear Heart Scan

What Is Nuclear Heart Scan?

A nuclear heart scan is an imaging test that uses special cameras and a radioactive substance called a "tracer" to create pictures of your heart. The tracer is injected into your blood and travels to your heart. Nuclear heart scans use single photon emission computed tomography (SPECT) or cardiac positron emission tomography (PET) to detect the energy from the tracer to make pictures of your heart. This imaging test can detect if blood is not flowing to parts of the heart and can diagnose coronary heart disease (CHD). It also can check for damaged or dead heart muscle tissue, possibly from a previous heart attack, and assess how well your heart pumps blood to your body. Compared to single-photon emission computed tomography (SPECT), PET takes clearer pictures; however, either option may be used.

How Is Nuclear Heart Scan Performed?

A nuclear heart scan may be performed in a medical imaging facility or hospital. Your heart will be monitored during this test with an electrocardiogram (EKG). 2 sets of pictures will be taken, each taking 15 to 30 minutes. The first set of pictures is taken right after an exercise or medicine stress test because some problems can be detected only when the heart is working hard or beating fast. If you are not

This chapter includes text excerpted from "Nuclear Heart Scan," National Heart, Lung, and Blood Institute (NHLBI), December 10, 2016.

able to exercise, your doctor may give you medicine to increase your heart rate. Shortly after the stress test, the tracer will be injected into a vein in your arm. You may bruise at the injection site. You will lie still on a table that slides through a tunnel-like machine as the first set of pictures is taken. The second set of pictures will be taken on either the same day or the next day, after your heartbeat has returned to a normal rate.

Risks of Nuclear Heart Scans

Nuclear heart scans have few risks. The amount of radiation in this test is small. In rare instances, some people have a treatable allergic reaction to the tracer. If you have coronary heart disease (CHD), you may have chest pain during the stress test. Medicine can help relieve your chest pain. Talk to your doctor and the technicians performing the test about whether you are or could be pregnant. If the test is not urgent, they may have you wait to do the test until after your pregnancy. Let your doctor know if you are breastfeeding because radiation can pass into your breast milk. If the test is urgent, you may want to pump and save enough breast milk for one to two days after your test, or you may bottle-feed your baby for that time.

Chapter 47

Heart Biopsy

A biopsy is a procedure in which a small piece of tissue is removed from the body for examination. A heart biopsy, also known as a "cardiac biopsy" or "myocardial biopsy," is performed to detect heart disease. A small catheter called a "bioptome" is used to collect a sample of the heart-muscle tissue, which is then sent to a laboratory for analysis.

Why Is It Needed?

A doctor will request a heart biopsy to diagnose:

- Myocarditis or other heart disorders, such as cardiac amyloidosis or cardiomyopathy

- A rejection of a transplanted heart by identifying tissue damage caused by the immune system

Preparing for the Procedure

A heart biopsy is conducted in a hospital as an outpatient procedure; although, in rare circumstances, you could be required to enter the hospital the night before the procedure. The doctor will give instructions on what food can be consumed before the biopsy. Generally, you should restrict intake of food and liquids six to eight hours before the test.

"Heart Biopsy," © 2016 Omnigraphics. Reviewed May 2019.

The doctor should be made aware of any current medication or supplements and their dosages, as well as allergies, if any. If you are diabetic, ask the doctor to adjust your medication dosage for the day of the test. Make sure that someone is available to drive you home after the test because the sedatives given during the procedure may make you feel groggy.

How Is It Performed?

A healthcare provider will first explain the procedure, including the risks involved. You will be given a hospital gown to wear for the procedure and asked to lie flat on your back on a special table with a large camera above it and several TV monitors nearby. An intravenous (IV) line will be started in your arm to transfer fluids to keep you hydrated during the procedure and administer medication to regulate heartbeat or blood pressure if needed.

Depending on which region of the heart will be biopsied, as well as other factors, the doctor will make an incision either on your neck, arm, or groin. It will most likely be the neck if you are not having another surgery at this time. You will be awake during the procedure, and a local anesthetic will be given to numb the incision site. A plastic introducer sheath (a short, hollow tube) will be inserted into the blood vessel to hold the incision open, which may cause some discomfort.

Once the tube is placed, a bioptome will be inserted into the blood vessel and threaded to the heart. Fluoroscopy, which is a special type of X-ray, will be used to guide the bioptome. When the device reaches the correct position, a jaw-like structure at its end will obtain a sample of the muscle tissue. Each sample is roughly the size of the head of a pin. The bioptome and the sheath are then removed and pressure is applied on the insertion site to stop bleeding. The whole procedure generally takes between 30 and 60 minutes and is constantly monitored by medical staff.

After the procedure, you will be instructed on how to care for the wound site and when you can go back to regular activities. The doctor will discuss the results of the test when they are available. If they are negative, it indicates that the analyzed tissues are normal.

A positive result may confirm a number of conditions, including:

- Inflammation caused by an infection (myocarditis)

- Disorders, such as cardiac amyloidosis (a condition in which amyloid protein builds up in the heart)

- Different types of cardiomyopathy (diseased heart muscle)

- Damage to the heart due to alcohol abuse

- The presence of rejection cells after heart transplant surgery

What Are the Risks?

Before the procedure, the possible risks involved will be explained, and you will be asked to sign a consent form. However, complications are rare when the biopsy is performed by an experienced doctor.

Some of the possible risks include:

- Bleeding

- Blood clots

- Irregular heartbeat or aggravation of existing arrhythmia

- Damage to the vein in which the bioptome is inserted

- Damage to the recurrent laryngeal nerve, which controls speech

- Infection

- Collapsed lung

- In extremely rare cases, rupture of the heart

References

1. Herndon, Jaime. "Myocardial Biopsy," Healthline, January 20, 2016.

2. Beckerman, James. "Heart Disease and the Heart Biopsy," WebMD, February 16, 2016.

Part Six

Treating Cardiovascular Disorders

Chapter 48

Medications for Treating Cardiovascular Disorders

Cardiovascular disease (CVD) is the leading cause of death for Americans. A variety of medications have been developed to help alleviate symptoms of heart disease and extend patients' lives. Although medications can be very helpful when used as prescribed, lifestyle modifications are also important in avoiding the serious health consequences of heart disease, such as arrhythmias, heart attacks, and heart failure. The following are some of the medications most commonly prescribed to treat cardiovascular disorders.

Angiotensin-Converting Enzyme Inhibitors

Angiotensin-converting enzyme (ACE) inhibitors are typically prescribed to help lower blood pressure, which makes it easier for the heart to pump blood through the body. They work by reducing the levels of angiotensin, a hormone that constricts blood vessels. When the blood vessels dilate or expand, blood flows through them more easily and blood pressure decreases. ACE inhibitors, such as benazepril (Lotensin), ramipril (Altace), and captopril (Capoten), are usually prescribed for patients with high blood pressure, heart failure, or recent heart attacks to ease the workload on the heart muscle.

"Medications for Treating Cardiovascular Disorders," © 2016 Omnigraphics. Reviewed May 2019.

Angiotensin II Receptor Blockers

Angiotensin II receptor blockers (ARBs) are similar to ACE inhibitors in that they reduce blood pressure and allow blood to flow more freely through the body. They work by completely blocking the effects of the hormone angiotensin II. ARBs, such as losartan (Cozaar) and valsartan (Diovan), are commonly prescribed to treat high blood pressure, congestive heart failure, or a recent heart attack. The medication has also been shown to slow the progression of kidney disease in patients with type 2 diabetes.

Anticoagulants

Anticoagulants, such as enoxaparin (Lovenox), heparin, and warfarin (Coumadin), help prevent blood clots from forming. Plaques in the arteries of people with coronary artery disease (CAD) can rupture and create blood clots, which are associated with serious health risks, such as heart attacks and strokes. Although anticoagulants cannot dissolve existing blood clots, they can help prevent new clots from forming.

Antiplatelet Agents

Antiplatelet medications are similar to anticoagulants because they help thin the blood and prevent blood clots from forming. Antiplatelet medications, such as aspirin, clopidogrel (Plavix), and prasugrel (Effient), are often prescribed to prevent heart attacks in people with CAD. They may also be prescribed for people who face an increased risk of blood clots due to abnormal heart rhythms, such as atrial fibrillation (AF).

Beta-Blockers

Beta-blockers are a broad category of medications used to control and reduce the heart rate. They work by blocking the effects of adrenaline (epinephrine), a hormone produced in response to stress. Beta-blockers, such as metoprolol (Lopressor), labetalol (Trandate), and propranolol (Inderal) are often prescribed to treat arrhythmias, heart failure, chest pain, and high blood pressure. They may also help prevent heart attacks.

Calcium Channel Blockers

Since calcium triggers heart contractions, calcium channel blockers can slow the heart rate, relax the blood vessels, and increase the supply of oxygen to the heart. Medications, such as amlodipine (Norvasc), dilti-azem (Cardizem), and nifedipine (Procardia), are commonly prescribed to treat high blood pressure, angina (chest pain), and arrhythmias.

Cholesterol-Lowering Medications

Cholesterol plays an important role in helping the body create new cells, lubricate nerves, and produce hormones. Yet, cholesterol buildup in the blood vessels can create plaques that block arteries or rupture to form dangerous blood clots, increasing the risk of heart attack and stroke.

Although adopting a healthier diet may help some patients lower their cholesterol levels, others may need medications to reduce their risk of CAD. Some of the main cholesterol-lowering medications include statins, such as atorvastatin (Lipitor), pravastatin sodium (Pravachol), and simvastatin (Zocor); bile acid resins, such as chole-styramine (Questran); cholesterol absorption inhibitors, such as eze-timibe (Zetia); fibric acid derivatives, such as fenofibrate (Tricor); and niacin (Niacor, Nicolar). Patients whose high cholesterol levels do not respond to statins may benefit from proprotein convertase subtilisin kexin type 9 (PCSK9) inhibitors, a new class of cholesterol-lowering drugs that block the action of a liver enzyme that prevents the removal of harmful cholesterol from the bloodstream.

Digitalis Medications

Digitalis medications, such as digoxin (Lanoxin), are used to increase the strength and efficiency of heart contractions. They are prescribed to treat patients with heart failure, irregular heartbeats, and poor circulation who may not experience benefits from ACE inhib-itors and diuretics.

Diuretics

Diuretics trigger the kidneys to get rid of excess fluid from the tissues and bloodstream by excreting it as urine. Since excess fluid makes it more difficult for the heart to pump blood through the body, diuretics can help protect the heart. Commonly known as "water pills," they are used to treat high blood pressure and to reduce the swelling and water retention caused by heart failure. Aldosterone inhibitors are a type of diuretic that works by blocking aldosterone, a chemical in the body that causes fluid retention and salt buildup. Aldosterone inhibitors, such as eplerenone (Inspra) and spironolactone (Aldactone), may be prescribed for patients with severe heart failure that does not respond to other medications.

Inotropic Therapy

Inotropic therapy is another pharmacological approach for treating end-stage heart failure. It involves using intravenous medications to increase the force of the heart muscle's contractions and relax the blood vessels to allow blood to flow more smoothly. It is generally used to relieve symptoms of heart failure when other medications are no longer effective.

Potassium and Magnesium

Low levels of these minerals can cause abnormal heart rhythms, so potassium and magnesium are sometimes prescribed as supplements for patients with arrhythmias.

Vasodilators

Vasodilators relax the blood vessels to allow blood to flow more easily. They are generally prescribed to treat heart failure and control blood pressure in patients who cannot tolerate ACE inhibitors.

References

1. "Common Heart Disease Drugs," WebMD, 2016.

2. Donovan, Robin. "Drugs to Treat Heart Disease," Healthline, 2016.

Chapter 49

Procedures to Treat Narrowed or Blocked Arteries

Chapter Contents

Section 49.1

Cardiac Catheterization

This section includes text excerpted from "Cardiac Catheterization," National Heart, Lung, and Blood Institute (NHLBI), October 31, 2016.

What Is Cardiac Catheterization?

Cardiac catheterization is a medical procedure used to diagnose and treat some heart conditions. It lets doctors take a close look at the heart to identify problems and perform other tests or procedures on your heart.

Your doctor may recommend cardiac catheterization to find out the cause of symptoms, such as chest pain or irregular heartbeat, or to find out whether you have ischemic heart disease due to blockages in the coronary arteries. Before the procedure, your doctor may need to do diagnostic tests, such as blood tests, heart imaging tests, or a stress test, to determine how well your heart is working and to help guide the procedure.

During cardiac catheterization, a long, thin, flexible tube called a "catheter" is put into a blood vessel in your arm, groin or upper thigh, or neck. The catheter is then threaded to your heart. Your doctor may use it to examine your heart valves or take samples of blood or heart muscle. Your doctor also may use ultrasound or inject a dye into your coronary arteries to see whether your arteries are narrowed or blocked. Cardiac catheterization may also be used instead of some heart surgeries to repair heart defects and replace heart valves.

Cardiac catheterization is safe for most people. Complications are rare but can include bleeding and blood clots. Your doctor will monitor your condition and may recommend medicines to prevent blood clots.

Who Needs Cardiac Catheterization

Your doctor may recommend cardiac catheterization to find out what is causing signs or symptoms of a heart problem or to treat or repair a heart problem. Cardiac catheterization is safe for most people.

When Is Cardiac Catheterization Recommended?

Your doctor may recommend cardiac catheterization to help with diagnoses or to plan treatment. It can be useful when your doctor wants to do any of the following:

- Better understand the results from other tests and procedures, such as echocardiography (echo), cardiac magnetic resonance imaging (MRI), and cardiac computed tomography (CT) scan, especially if other studies could not define the problem or if the results from other studies differ from what your doctor finds when examining you.

- Diagnose the cause of your chest pain, arrhythmia, or other signs and symptoms of a heart problem or evaluate you during an emergency, such as a heart attack. The procedure may help your doctor diagnose heart conditions, such as pulmonary hypertension (PH); cardiomyopathy; ischemic heart disease; and heart valve diseases, such as aortic stenosis and mitral regurgitation.

- Evaluate you before a possible heart transplant.

- Look at the pulmonary arteries for conditions, including pulmonary embolism, that can occur as a result of venous thromboembolism. The pulmonary arteries are the blood vessels that carry blood from your heart to your lungs, where the blood receives oxygen.

- Measure oxygen levels and pressures of the blood in your heart, such as in your ventricles, atria, and pulmonary arteries.

Your doctor may perform additional procedures to diagnose or treat your condition during cardiac catheterization. Some of these procedures include:

- **Biopsies** to take small samples of the heart tissue for further laboratory testing. Biopsies can be used for genetic testing or to check for myocarditis, a type of heart inflammation, or transplant rejection.

- **Coronary angiography** to look at the heart or blood vessels by injecting dye through the catheter.

- **Minor heart surgery** to treat congenital heart defects and replace or widen narrowed heart valves.

- **Percutaneous coronary intervention (PCI)** to open narrowed or blocked areas of the coronary arteries. PCI may include balloon dilation, or angioplasty, or stent placement. Most people who have heart attacks or underlying ischemic heart diseases have narrowed or blocked coronary arteries.

Who Should Not Have Cardiac Catheterization?

Your doctor may wait to do the procedure or recommend that you do not have cardiac catheterization if you have one of the following conditions:

- Abnormal electrolyte levels in your blood

- Acute gastrointestinal bleeding

- Acute kidney failure, or severe kidney disease that is not being treated with dialysis

- Acute stroke

- Blood that is too thin from medicines, such as warfarin, or other causes

- High blood levels of a heart medicine called "digoxin"

- Previous severe allergic reaction to the dye that is used during cardiac catheterization

- Severe anemia, which is a lower-than-normal red blood cell (RBC) count or hemoglobin

- Unexplained fever

- Untreated infection

What to Expect before Cardiac Catheterization

Before cardiac catheterization, you will meet with your cardiologist, a doctor who specializes in the heart. The doctor will ask you about your medical history, including what medicines you are taking and any allergies you may have, and do a physical exam. Your doctor will also give you instructions on how to prepare for the procedure.

Diagnostic Tests and Procedures

You may have some of the following tests before your catheterization procedure:

- Electrocardiogram (ECG or EKG) to look at your heart's rhythm and other electrical activity of your heart. It can show arrhythmias, heart attacks, and other problems with the heart.

- A chest X-ray to look at your lungs, your heart, your major blood vessels, and other structures in the chest.

- An echocardiogram (echo) to look at the structure and function of your heart.

- A stress test to look at how well your heart works during physical stress. The stress may be physical exercise, such as walking on a treadmill, or it may be a medicine given to have the same effect.

- Cardiac CT scan to look for narrowing of your heart's blood vessels, and problems with the heart, larger blood vessels, and heart valves. These pictures also may help your doctor plan for procedures to open the coronary arteries.

- Cardiac MRI to provide information on the structure and function of your heart, as well as the type and severity of heart disease.

- Blood tests, including a complete blood count (CBC), to check your hemoglobin and platelet levels; blood chemistry tests to check how well your liver and kidneys are working; and tests to check your blood's ability to clot.

Preparing for the Procedure

Talk to your doctor about your medical history, including any medicines you take; other surgical procedures you have had; and any medical conditions you have, such as diabetes or kidney disease.

Your doctor will talk to you about how to prepare for the procedure, including:

- When to arrive at the hospital and where to go

- When you should stop eating or drinking

- If and when you should start or stop taking medicines

- How long you should expect to stay

- What happens during the procedure

- What to expect after the procedure, including potential complications, such as bleeding or soreness

- Instructions to follow after the procedure, including what medicines to take

What to Expect during Cardiac Catheterization

Cardiac catheterization takes place in a catheterization laboratory, or cath lab, which is similar to a small operating room. The procedure is often done in a hospital, but you may be able to have the procedure in a catheterization laboratory located in a medical clinic, depending on the reason you are having the procedure and the risk for complications.

How Is Cardiac Catheterization Done?

Before cardiac catheterization, an intravenous line (IV) will be placed in a vein in your arm. Through this IV, you will get a medicine to either help you relax or make you sleep during the procedure.

You will get numbing medicine, or local anesthesia, at the site where the doctor will insert the catheter. This site is called the "access site" and may be in the upper thigh, arm, neck, or under the collarbone. The doctor places a needle into a blood vessel at the access site. A guidewire is inserted into the needle, and the needle is taken out. Then the doctor places a small tube called a "sheath" in the blood vessel around the guidewire. The guidewire is removed. The catheter is then inserted through the sheath. Your doctor watches X-ray images to see where to place the tip of the catheter.

Once the catheter is in place, your doctor may use it to perform tests or treatments on your heart. For example, she or he may inject a dye into the catheter to look at blood flow in the heart. The dye will enter your blood vessels and make your coronary arteries visible in X-ray pictures.

Possible Risks and Complications

Cardiac catheterization is a relatively safe procedure, and complications are rare. Possible complications include the following:

- Allergic reaction to the dye used. This reaction may be hives or a more serious reaction.

- Arrhythmias

- Bleeding at the access site or inside your abdomen

- Blood clot formation at the access site, inside your abdomen, in a blood vessel, or in your heart

- Collapsed lung, called "pneumothorax," resulting in air in the space between your lung and chest wall

- Damage to blood vessels, heart valves, or your heart

- Heart attack

- Hypothermia, especially in small children

- Infection
- Low blood pressure from bleeding or as a reaction to the procedure
- Need for blood transfusion
- Need for emergency surgery to repair a tear in the aorta or coronary artery and restore blood flow to the heart. This may be done using a coronary artery bypass graft (CABG).
- Side effects of general anesthesia, if used. These can include nausea, vomiting, confusion, or an allergic reaction.
- Stroke

Although not an immediate risk, repeated radiation exposure from X-rays used to place the catheter in the heart, especially with children, may increase the risk of cancer and leukemia, damage to skin, and cataracts later in life.

What to Expect after Cardiac Catheterization

After the procedure, your doctor will remove the catheters, sheath, and guidewire. A dressing, accompanied by pressure, is applied to the site where the catheter was inserted to stop the bleeding. The pressure may be held by hand or with a sandbag or other device. You will be moved to a recovery room, where you will lie in bed. Your heartbeat and blood pressure will be monitored.

Depending on your health before the cardiac catheterization and what additional procedures were done during the cardiac catheterization, you may have to spend the night in the hospital. You should follow your doctor's instructions on what medicines to take and when to resume activity.

What Are the Risks of Cardiac Catheterization?

If you have had cardiac catheterization, it is important that you receive follow-up care, know about the possible complications that may occur after the procedure, and follow the treatment plan that your doctor recommends for your condition.

Receive Follow-Up Care

It is important to get routine follow-up care after you have cardiac catheterization. Talk with your doctor about how often you should schedule office visits.

- Adopt a heart-healthy lifestyle, especially if your cardiac catheterization was needed because of ischemic heart disease or heart attack.

- Follow any instructions for when to resume physical activity and lifting and at what levels.

- Follow instructions on how to care for the site where the doctor accessed your blood vessel, including when you can take a bath or swim.

- Keep any follow-up appointments or tests.

- Take any medicines as directed by your doctor.

- Talk to your doctor about any blood tests you may need if you were placed on blood thinners after your procedure.

Learn the Warning Signs of Complications and Have a Plan

Complications from cardiac catheterization are rare but can be serious. A small bruise and tenderness at the access site is normal. Call your doctor immediately if you experience any of the following, as they may be signs of serious complications.

- Bleeding from the access site that cannot be stopped with firm pressure

- Chest pain or shortness of breath

- Dizziness

- Fever

- Increased pain, redness, or bruising at the access site

- Irregular, very slow, or fast heartbeat

- Swelling at the access site

- Yellow or green discharge draining from the access site

- Your leg or arm that was used for access becoming numb or weak or any part of it turning cold or blue

Other serious complications after catheterization, although rare, include heart attack and stroke. If you think that you are or someone else is having the following symptoms, call 911 immediately.

Heart attack signs and symptoms include:

- Chest pain or discomfort in the center of the chest or upper abdomen that lasts for more than a few minutes or goes away and comes back. It can feel like pressure, squeezing, fullness, heartburn, or indigestion.

- Nausea, vomiting, light-headedness or fainting, or breaking out in a cold sweat. These symptoms of a heart attack are more common in women.

- Shortness of breath, which may occur with or before chest discomfort.

- Upper body discomfort in one or both arms or the back, neck, jaw, or upper part of the stomach

If you think someone may be having a stroke, act F.A.S.T. and perform the following simple test.

- **F—Face:** Ask the person to smile. Does one side of the face droop?

- **A—Arms:** Ask the person to raise both arms. Does one arm drift downward?

- **S—Speech:** Ask the person to repeat a simple phrase. Is their speech slurred or strange?

- **T—Time:** If you observe any of these signs, call for help immediately. Early treatment is essential.

Section 49.2

Carotid Endarterectomy

This section includes text excerpted from "Questions and Answers
about Carotid Endarterectomy," National Institute of Neurological
Disorders and Stroke (NINDS), July 6, 2018.

What Is a Carotid Endarterectomy?

A carotid endarterectomy is a surgical procedure in which a doctor
removes fatty deposits blocking one of the two carotid arteries, the
main supply of blood for the brain. Carotid artery problems become
more common as people age. The disease process that causes the
buildup of fat and other material inside the artery walls is called
"atherosclerosis," popularly known as "hardening of the arteries." The
fatty deposit is called "plaque;" the narrowing of the artery is called
"stenosis." The degree of stenosis is usually expressed as a percentage
of the normal diameter of the opening.

Why Is Surgery Performed?

Carotid endarterectomy is performed to prevent stroke. Two large
clinical trials supported by the National Institute of Neurological Disorders and Stroke (NINDS) have identified specific individuals for
whom the surgery is beneficial when performed by surgeons and in
institutions that can match the standards set in those studies. The
surgery has been found highly beneficial for persons who have already
had a stroke or experienced the symptoms of a stroke and have a
severe stenosis of 70 to 99 percent. In this group, surgery reduces the
estimated 2-year risk of stroke or death by more than 80 percent, from
greater than 1 in 4 to less than 1 in 10.

For patients who have already had transient or mild stroke symptoms due to moderate carotid stenosis (50% to 69%), surgery reduces
the 5-year risk of stroke or death by 6.5 percent. The failure rate for
ipsilateral stroke or death for the medical group is 22.2 percent, and
for the surgery group is 15.7 percent, from greater than 1 in 4 to less
than 1 in 7. Individuals who have already had stroke symptoms, and
who have carotid stenosis greater than 50 percent, may wish to consider surgery to prevent future stroke. Based on findings of the North
American Symptomatic Carotid Endarterectomy Trial (NASCET) trial,
patients with moderate (50% to 69%) stenosis are now better able to
make more informed decisions.

In another trial (Asymptomatic Carotid Atherosclerosis Study, or ACAS), the procedure has also been found highly beneficial for persons who are symptom-free but have a carotid stenosis of 60 to 99 percent. In this group, the surgery reduces the estimated 5-year risk of stroke by more than one-half, from about 1 in 10 to less than 1 in 20.

The Carotid Revascularization Endarterectomy vs. Stenting Trial (CREST) compared carotid endarterectomy surgery to carotid artery stenting and found no significance between the procedures regarding the 4-year rate of stroke or death in patients with or without a previous stroke. The pivotal differences were the lower rate of stroke following surgery and the lower rate of heart attack following stenting. The study also found that the age of the patient made a difference with a larger benefit for stenting, the younger the age of the patient. At 69 years of age and younger, stenting results were slightly better. Conversely, for patients older than 70 years of age, surgical benefits were slightly superior to stenting, with a larger benefit for surgery, the older the patient.

How Many Carotid Endarterectomies Are Performed Each Year?

An estimated 140,000 carotid endarterectomies were performed in the United States in 2009, according to the National Hospital Discharge Survey. The procedure was first described in the mid-1950s. It began to be used increasingly as a stroke prevention measure in the 1960s and 1970s. Its use peaked in the mid-1980s when more than 100,000 operations were performed each year. At that time, several authorities began to question the trend and the risk-benefit ratio for some groups, and the use of the procedure dropped precipitously. The NINDS-supported NASCET and ACAS trials were launched in the mid-1980s to identify the specific groups of people with carotid artery disease who would clearly benefit from the procedure.

What Are the Risk Factors and How Risky Is the Surgery?

Important risk factors in addition to the degree of stenosis include, gender, diabetes, the type of stroke symptoms, and blockage of the carotid artery on the opposite side. Without other complicating illnesses, age alone is not a worrisome risk factor. Risk factors can affect patients in two ways. They can, particularly in combination, greatly increase a person's risk of having a stroke. In addition, these risk factors can increase the likelihood of surgical complications.

Section 49.3

Coronary Angioplasty

This section includes text excerpted from "Percutaneous Coronary Intervention," National Heart, Lung, and Blood Institute (NHLBI), November 14, 2011. Reviewed May 2019.

What Is Coronary Angioplasty?

Percutaneous coronary intervention (PCI), also known as "coronary angioplasty," is a nonsurgical procedure that improves blood flow to your heart. It requires cardiac catheterization, which is the insertion of a catheter tube and injection of contrast dye, usually iodine-based, into your coronary arteries. Doctors use PCI to open coronary arteries that are narrowed or blocked by the buildup of atherosclerotic plaque. PCI may be used to relieve symptoms of coronary heart disease or to reduce heart damage during or after a heart attack.

How Is Coronary Angioplasty Performed?

A cardiologist, or doctor who specializes in the heart, will perform PCI in a hospital cardiac catheterization laboratory. You will stay awake, but you will be given medicine to relax you. Before your procedure, you will receive medicines through an intravenous (IV) line in your arm to prevent blood clots. Your doctor will clean and numb an area on the wrist or groin where they will then make a small hole and insert the catheter into your blood vessel. Live X-rays will help your doctor guide the catheter into your heart to inject special contrast dye that will highlight the blockage. To open a blocked artery, your doctor will insert another catheter over a guidewire and inflate a balloon at the tip of that catheter. Your doctor may put a small mesh tube called a "stent" in your artery to help keep the artery open.

What Happens After

After PCI, your doctor will remove the catheters and close and bandage the opening on your wrist or groin. You may develop a bruise and soreness where the catheters were inserted. It also is common to have discomfort or bleeding where the catheters were inserted. You will recover in a special unit of the hospital for a few hours or overnight. You will get instructions on how much activity you can do and what medicines to take. You will need a ride home because of the medicines or anesthesia you received. Your doctor will check your progress during a follow-up visit. If a stent is implanted, you will have to take special anticlotting medicines exactly as prescribed, usually for at least 3 to 12 months.

Complications and Risks

Serious complications from PCI do not occur often, but they can happen. These complications may include bleeding, blood vessel damage, a treatable allergic reaction to the contrast dye, the need for emergency coronary artery bypass grafting during the procedure, arrhythmias, damaged arteries, kidney damage, heart attack, stroke, or blood clots. Sometimes, chest pain can occur during PCI because the balloon briefly blocks blood supply to the heart. Restenosis, or tissue regrowth in the treated portion of the artery, may occur in the following months and cause the artery to become narrow or blocked again. The risk of complications is higher if you are older, have chronic kidney disease (CKD), are experiencing heart failure at the time of the procedure, or have extensive heart disease and multiple blockages in your coronary arteries.

Section 49.4

Coronary Artery Bypass Grafting

This section contains text excerpted from the following sources:
Text in this section begins with excerpts from "Coronary Artery
Bypass Surgery," MedlinePlus, National Institutes of Health
(NIH), February 8, 2019; Text beginning with the heading "What
Is Coronary Artery Bypass Grafting?" is excerpted from "Coronary
Artery Bypass Grafting," National Heart, Lung, and Blood
Institute (NHLBI), November 18, 2014. Reviewed May 2019.

In coronary artery disease (CAD), the arteries that supply blood
and oxygen to your heart muscle grow hardened and narrowed. You
may try treatments—such as lifestyle changes; medicines; and angioplasty, a procedure to open the arteries—to help the condition. If these
treatments do not help, you may need coronary artery bypass surgery.

The surgery creates a new path for blood to flow to the heart. The
surgeon takes a healthy piece of vein from the leg or artery from the
chest or wrist. Then the surgeon attaches it to the coronary artery, just
above and below the narrowed area or blockage. This allows blood to
bypass (get around) the blockage. Sometimes, people need more than
one bypass.

The results of the surgery usually are excellent. Many people
remain symptom-free for many years. You may need surgery again if
blockages form in the grafted arteries or veins or in arteries that were
not blocked before. Lifestyle changes and medicines may help prevent
arteries from becoming clogged again.

What Is Coronary Artery Bypass Grafting?

Coronary artery bypass grafting (CABG) is a type of surgery that
improves blood flow to the heart. Surgeons use CABG to treat people
who have severe coronary heart disease (CHD).

Coronary heart disease is a disease in which a waxy substance
called "plaque" builds up inside the coronary arteries. These arteries
supply oxygen-rich blood to your heart.

Over time, plaque can harden or rupture (break open). Hardened plaque narrows the coronary arteries and reduces the flow of
oxygen-rich blood to the heart. This can cause chest pain or discomfort,
called "angina."

If the plaque ruptures, a blood clot can form on its surface. A large
blood clot can mostly or completely block blood flow through a coronary

artery. This is the most common cause of a heart attack. Over time, ruptured plaque also hardens and narrows the coronary arteries.

Coronary artery bypass grafting is one treatment for CHD. During CABG, a healthy artery or vein from the body is connected, or grafted, to the blocked coronary artery. The grafted artery or vein bypasses (that is, goes around) the blocked portion of the coronary artery. This creates a new path for oxygen-rich blood to flow to the heart muscle.

Surgeons can bypass multiple coronary arteries during one surgery.

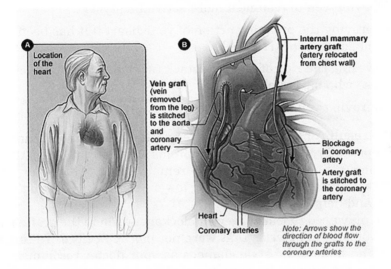

Figure 49.1. *Coronary Artery Bypass Grafting*

Figure A shows the location of the heart. Figure B shows how vein and artery bypass grafts are attached to the heart.

Coronary artery bypass grafting is the most common type of open-heart surgery in the United States. Doctors called "cardiothoracic surgeons" do this surgery.

However, coronary artery bypass grafting is not the only treatment for CHD. Other treatment options include lifestyle changes, medicines, and a procedure called "percutaneous coronary intervention (PCI)," also known as "coronary angioplasty."

Percutaneous coronary intervention is a nonsurgical procedure that opens blocked or narrowed coronary arteries. During PCI, a stent might be placed in a coronary artery to help keep it open. A stent is a small mesh tube that supports the inner artery wall.

Coronary artery bypass grafting or percutaneous coronary intervention may be options if you have severe blockages in your large

497

coronary arteries, especially if your heart's pumping action has already grown weak.

Coronary artery bypass grafting also may be an option if you have blockages in the heart that cannot be treated with PCI. In this situation, CABG may work better than other types of treatment.

The goals of CABG may include:

- Improving your quality of life and reducing angina and other CHD symptoms

- Allowing you to resume a more active lifestyle

- Improving the pumping action of your heart if it has been damaged by a heart attack

- Lowering the risk of a heart attack (in some patients, such as those who have diabetes)

- Improving your chance of survival

The results of CABG usually are excellent. The surgery improves or completely relieves angina symptoms in most patients. Although symptoms can recur, many people remain symptom-free for as long as 10 to 15 years. CABG also may lower your risk of having a heart attack and help you live longer.

You may need repeat surgery if blockages form in the grafted arteries or veins or in arteries that were not blocked before. Taking medicines and making lifestyle changes as your doctor recommends can lower the risk of a graft becoming blocked.

Types of Coronary Artery Bypass Grafting

There are several types of CABG. Your doctor will recommend the best option for you based on your needs.

Traditional Coronary Artery Bypass Grafting

Traditional CABG is used when at least one major artery needs to be bypassed. During the surgery, the chest bone is opened to access the heart.

Medicines are given to stop the heart; a heart-lung bypass machine keeps blood and oxygen moving throughout the body during surgery. This allows the surgeon to operate on a still heart.

After surgery, blood flow to the heart is restored. Usually, the heart starts beating again on its own. Sometimes, mild electric shocks are used to restart the heart.

Off-Pump Coronary Artery Bypass Grafting

This type of CABG is similar to traditional CABG because the chest bone is opened to access the heart. However, the heart is not stopped, and a heart-lung bypass machine is not used. Off-pump CABG sometimes is called "beating heart bypass grafting."

Minimally Invasive Direct Coronary Artery Bypass Grafting

This type of surgery differs from traditional CABG because the chest bone is not opened to reach the heart. Instead, several small cuts are made on the left side of the chest between the ribs. This type of surgery mainly is used to bypass blood vessels at the front of the heart.

Minimally invasive bypass grafting is a fairly new procedure. It is not right for everyone, especially if more than one or two coronary arteries need to be bypassed.

Who Needs Coronary Artery Bypass Grafting

Coronary artery bypass grafting is used to treat people who have severe CHD that could lead to a heart attack. CABG also might be used during or after a heart attack to treat blocked arteries.

Your doctor may recommend CABG if other treatments, such as lifestyle changes or medicines, have not worked. She or he also may recommend CABG if you have severe blockages in your large coronary (heart) arteries, especially if your heart's pumping action has already grown weak.

Coronary artery bypass grafting also might be a treatment option if you have blockages in your coronary arteries that cannot be treated with PCI.

Your doctor will decide whether you are a candidate for CABG based on factors, such as:

- The presence and severity of CHD symptoms

- The severity and location of blockages in your coronary arteries

- Your response to other treatments

- Your quality of life

- Any other medical problems you have

Physical Exam and Diagnostic Tests

To find out whether you are a candidate for CABG, your doctor will give you a physical exam. She or he will check your heart, lungs, and pulse.

Your doctor also may ask you about any symptoms you have, such as chest pain or shortness of breath. She or he will want to know how often and for how long your symptoms occur, as well as how severe they are.

Your doctor will recommend tests to find out which arteries are clogged, how much they are clogged, and whether you have any heart damage.

Electrocardiogram

An electrocardiogram (EKG) is a simple test that detects and records your heart's electrical activity. The test shows how fast the heart is beating and its rhythm (steady or irregular). An EKG also records the strength and timing of electrical signals as they pass through each part of the heart.

An EKG can show signs of heart damage due to CHD and signs of a previous or current heart attack.

Echocardiography

Echocardiography (echo) uses sound waves to create a moving picture of your heart. The test shows the size and shape of your heart and how well your heart chambers and valves are working.

An echo also can show areas of poor blood flow to the heart, areas of heart muscle that are not contracting normally, and previous injury to the heart muscle caused by poor blood flow.

There are several types of echo, including stress echo. This test is done both before and after a stress test. A stress echo usually is done to find out whether you have decreased blood flow to your heart, a sign of CHD.

Stress Test

Some heart problems are easier to diagnose when your heart is working hard and beating fast.

During stress testing, you exercise to make your heart work hard and beat fast while heart tests are done. If you cannot exercise, you may be given medicine to raise your heart rate.

The heart tests done during stress testing may include nuclear heart scanning, echo, and positron emission tomography (PET) scanning of the heart.

Coronary Angiography and Cardiac Catheterization

Coronary angiography is a test that uses dye and special X-rays to show the insides of your coronary arteries. To get the dye into your coronary arteries, your doctor will use a procedure called "cardiac catheterization."

A thin, flexible tube called a "catheter" is put into a blood vessel in your arm, groin (upper thigh), or neck. The tube is threaded into your coronary arteries, and the dye is released into your bloodstream.

Special X-rays are taken while the dye is flowing through the coronary arteries. The dye lets your doctor study blood flow through the heart and blood vessels. This helps your doctor find blockages that can cause a heart attack.

Other Considerations

When deciding whether you are a candidate for CABG, your doctor also will consider your:

- History and past treatment of heart disease, including surgeries, procedures, and medicines

- History of other diseases and conditions

- Age and general health

- Family history of CHD, heart attack, or other heart diseases

Your doctor may recommend medicines and other medical procedures before CABG. For example, she or he may prescribe medicines to lower your cholesterol and blood pressure and improve blood flow through your coronary arteries.

Percutaneous coronary intervention also might be tried. During this procedure, a thin, flexible tube with a balloon at its tip is threaded through a blood vessel to the narrow or blocked coronary artery.

Once in place, the balloon is inflated, pushing plaque against the artery wall. This creates a wider path for blood to flow to the heart. Sometimes, a stent is placed in the artery during PCI. A stent is a small mesh tube that supports the inner artery wall.

What to Expect before Coronary Artery Bypass Grafting

You may have tests to prepare you for CABG. For example, you may have blood tests, an EKG, echocardiography, a chest X-ray, cardiac catheterization, and coronary angiography.

Your doctor will tell you how to prepare for CABG surgery. She or he will advise you about what you can eat or drink, which medicines to take, and which activities to stop (such as smoking). You will likely be admitted to the hospital on the same day as the surgery.

If tests for coronary heart disease show that you have severe blockages in your coronary (heart) arteries, your doctor may admit you to the hospital right away. You may have CABG that day or the day after.

What to Expect during Coronary Artery Bypass Grafting

Coronary artery bypass grafting requires a team of experts. A cardiothoracic surgeon will do the surgery with support from an anesthesiologist, perfusionist (heart-lung bypass machine specialist), other surgeons, and nurses.

There are several types of CABG. They range from traditional surgery to newer, less-invasive methods.

Traditional Coronary Artery Bypass Grafting

This type of surgery usually lasts anywhere from three to six hours, depending on the number of arteries being bypassed. Many steps take place during traditional CABG.

You will be under general anesthesia for the surgery. The term "anesthesia" refers to a loss of feeling and awareness. General anesthesia temporarily puts you to sleep.

During the surgery, the anesthesiologist will check your heartbeat, blood pressure, oxygen levels, and breathing. A breathing tube will be placed in your lungs through your throat. The tube will connect to a ventilator (a machine that supports breathing).

The surgeon will make an incision (cut) down the center of your chest. She or he will cut your chest bone and open your rib cage to reach your heart.

You will receive medicines to stop your heart. This allows the surgeon to operate on your heart while it is not beating. You will also receive medicines to protect your heart function during the time that it is not beating.

A heart-lung bypass machine will keep oxygen-rich blood moving throughout your body during the surgery.

The surgeon will take an artery or vein from your body—for example, from your chest or leg—to use as the bypass graft. For surgeries with several bypasses, both artery and vein grafts are commonly used.

- **Artery grafts.** These grafts are much less likely than vein grafts to become blocked over time. The left internal mammary artery most often is used for an artery graft. This artery is located inside the chest, close to the heart. Arteries from the arm or other places in the body also are used.

- **Vein grafts.** Although veins are commonly used as grafts, they are more likely than artery grafts to become blocked over time. The saphenous vein—a long vein running along the inner side of the leg—typically is used.

When the surgeon finishes the grafting, she or he will restore blood flow to your heart. Usually, the heart starts beating again on its own. Sometimes, mild electric shocks are used to restart the heart.

You will be disconnected from the heart-lung bypass machine. Then, tubes will be inserted into your chest to drain fluid.

The surgeon will use wire to close your chest bone (much like how a broken bone is repaired). The wire will stay in your body permanently. After your chest bone heals, it will be as strong as it was before the surgery.

Stitches or staples will be used to close the skin incision. The breathing tube will be removed when you are able to breathe without it.

Nontraditional Coronary Artery Bypass Grafting

Nontraditional CABG includes off-pump CABG and minimally invasive CABG.

Off-Pump Coronary Artery Bypass Grafting

Surgeons can use off-pump CABG to bypass any of the coronary arteries. Off-pump CABG is similar to traditional CABG because the chest bone is opened to access the heart. However, the heart is not stopped and a heart-lung bypass machine is not used. Instead, the surgeon steadies the heart with a mechanical device.

503

Off-pump CABG sometimes is called "beating heart bypass grafting."

Minimally Invasive Direct Coronary Artery Bypass Grafting

There are several types of minimally invasive direct coronary artery bypass (MIDCAB) grafting. These types of surgery differ from traditional bypass surgery because the chest bone is not opened to reach the heart. Also, a heart-lung bypass machine is not always used for these procedures.

MIDCAB procedure. This type of surgery mainly is used to bypass blood vessels at the front of the heart. Small incisions are made between your ribs on the left side of your chest, directly over the artery that needs to be bypassed.

The incisions usually are about three inches long. (The incision made in traditional CABG is at least six to eight inches long.) The left internal mammary artery most often is used for the graft in this procedure. A heart-lung bypass machine is not used during MIDCAB grafting.

Port-access coronary artery bypass procedure. The surgeon does this procedure through small incisions (ports) made in your chest. Artery or vein grafts are used. A heart-lung bypass machine is used during this procedure.

Robot-assisted technique. This type of procedure allows for even smaller, keyhole-sized incisions. A small video camera is inserted in one incision to show the heart, while the surgeon uses remote-controlled surgical instruments to do the surgery. A heart-lung bypass machine sometimes is used during this procedure.

What to Expect after Coronary Artery Bypass Grafting
Recovery in the Hospital

After surgery, you will typically spend one or two days in an intensive care unit (ICU). Your heart rate, blood pressure, and oxygen levels will be checked regularly during this time.

An intravenous line (IV) will likely be inserted into a vein in your arm. Through the IV line, you may get medicines to control blood circulation and blood pressure. You also will likely have a tube in your bladder to drain urine and a tube to drain fluid from your chest.

You may receive oxygen therapy (oxygen given through nasal prongs or a mask) and a temporary pacemaker while in the ICU. A pacemaker is a small device that is placed in the chest or abdomen to help control abnormal heart rhythms.

Your doctor may recommend that you wear compression stockings on your legs as well. These stockings are tight at the ankle and become looser as they go up the leg. This creates gentle pressure up the leg. The pressure keeps blood from pooling and clotting.

While in the ICU, you will also have bandages on your chest incision and on the areas where an artery or vein was removed for grafting.

After you leave the ICU, you will be moved to a less intensive care area of the hospital for three to five days before going home.

Recovery at Home

Your doctor will give you specific instructions for recovering at home, especially concerning:

- How to care for your healing incisions

- How to recognize signs of infection or other complications

- When to call the doctor right away

- When to make follow-up appointments

You also may get instructions on how to deal with common side effects from surgery. Side effects often go away within four to six weeks after surgery, but may include:

- Discomfort or itching from healing incisions

- Swelling of the area where an artery or vein was removed for grafting

- Muscle pain or tightness in the shoulders and upper back

- Fatigue (tiredness), mood swings, or depression

- Problems sleeping or loss of appetite

- Constipation

- Chest pain around the site of the chest bone incision (more frequent with traditional CABG)

Full recovery from traditional CABG may take 6 to 12 weeks or more. Less recovery time is needed for nontraditional CABG.

Your doctor will tell you when you can start physical activity again. It varies from person to person, but there are some typical time frames.

Most people can resume sexual activity within about four weeks and driving after three to eight weeks.

Returning to work after six weeks is common, unless your job involves specific and demanding physical activity. Some people may need to find less physically demanding types of work or work a reduced schedule at first.

Ongoing Care

Care after surgery may include periodic checkups with doctors. During these visits, tests may be done to see how your heart is working. Tests may include an EKG, stress testing, echocardiography, and cardiac CT.

Coronary artery bypass grafting is not a cure for coronary heart disease. You and your doctor may develop a treatment plan that includes lifestyle changes to help you stay healthy and reduce the chance of CHD getting worse.

Lifestyle changes may include making changes to your diet, quitting smoking, doing physical activity regularly, and lowering and managing stress.

Your doctor also may refer you to cardiac rehabilitation (rehab). Cardiac rehab is a medically supervised program that helps improve the health and well-being of people who have heart problems.

Rehab programs include exercise training, education on heart healthy living, and counseling to reduce stress and help you return to an active life. Doctors supervise these programs, which may be offered in hospitals and other community facilities. Talk to your doctor about whether cardiac rehab might benefit you.

Taking medicines as prescribed also is an important part of care after surgery. Your doctor may prescribe medicines to manage pain during recovery, lower cholesterol and blood pressure, reduce the risk of blood clots forming, manage diabetes, or treat depression.

Section 49.5

Stents to Keep Coronary Arteries Open

This section includes text excerpted from "Stents,"
National Heart, Lung, and Blood Institute (NHLBI),
November 4, 2012. Reviewed May 2019.

What Is a Stent?

A stent is a small mesh tube that is used to treat narrow or weak arteries. Arteries are blood vessels that carry blood away from your heart to other parts of your body.

A stent is placed in an artery as part of a procedure called "percutaneous coronary intervention" (PCI), also known as "coronary angioplasty." PCI restores blood flow through narrow or blocked arteries. A stent helps support the inner wall of the artery in the months or years after PCI.

Doctors also may place stents in weak arteries to improve blood flow and help prevent the arteries from bursting.

Stents usually are made of metal mesh, but sometimes they are made of fabric. Fabric stents, also called "stent grafts," are used in larger arteries.

Some stents are coated with medicine that is slowly and continuously released into the artery. These stents are called "drug-eluting stents." The medicine helps prevent the artery from becoming blocked again.

How Are Stents Used?
For the Coronary Arteries

Doctors may use stents to treat coronary heart disease (CHD). CHD is a disease in which a waxy substance called "plaque" builds up inside the coronary arteries. These arteries supply your heart muscle with oxygen-rich blood.

When plaque builds up in the arteries, the condition is called "atherosclerosis."

Plaque narrows the coronary arteries, reducing the flow of oxygen-rich blood to your heart. This can lead to chest pain or discomfort called "angina."

The buildup of plaque also makes it more likely that blood clots will form in your coronary arteries. If blood clots block a coronary artery, a heart attack will occur.

Doctors may use percutaneous coronary intervention and stents to treat CHD. During PCI, a thin, flexible tube with a balloon or other device on the end is threaded through a blood vessel to the narrow or blocked coronary artery.

Once in place, the balloon is inflated to compress the plaque against the wall of the artery. This restores blood flow through the artery, which reduces angina and other CHD symptoms.

Unless an artery is too small, a stent usually is placed in the treated portion of the artery during PCI. The stent supports the artery's inner wall. It also reduces the chance that the artery will become narrow or blocked again. A stent also can support an artery that was torn or injured during PCI.

Even with a stent, there is about a 10 to 20 percent chance that an artery will become narrow or blocked again in the first year after PCI. When a stent is not used, the risk can be as much as 10 times as high. Research has shown that as time goes by, people who have coronary artery stents are in less danger of risks from the surgery but more prone to the risks of chronic diseases, such as type 2 diabetes and renal failure.

For the Carotid Arteries

Doctors also may use stents to treat carotid artery disease. This is a disease in which plaque builds up in the arteries that run along each side of your neck. These arteries, called "carotid arteries," supply oxygen-rich blood to your brain.

The buildup of plaque in the carotid arteries limits blood flow to your brain and puts you at risk for a stroke.

Doctors use stents to help support the carotid arteries after they are widened with PCI. Researchers continue to explore the risks and benefits of carotid artery stenting.

For Other Arteries

Plaque also can narrow other arteries, such as those in the kidneys and limbs. Narrow kidney arteries can affect kidney function and lead to severe high blood pressure.

Narrow arteries in the limbs, a condition called "peripheral artery disease" (PAD), can cause pain and cramping in the affected arm or leg. Severe narrowing can completely cut off blood flow to a limb, which could require surgery.

To relieve these problems, doctors may do PCI on a narrow kidney, arm, or leg artery. They often will place a stent in the affected artery during the procedure. The stent helps support the artery and keep it open.

For the Aorta in the Abdomen or Chest

The aorta is a major artery that carries oxygen-rich blood from the left side of the heart to the body. This artery runs through the chest and down into the abdomen.

Over time, some areas of the aorta's walls can weaken. These weak areas can cause a bulge in the artery called an "aneurysm." An aneurysm in the aorta can burst, leading to serious internal bleeding. When aneurysms occur, they are usually in the abdominal aorta.

To help avoid a burst, doctors may place a fabric stent in the weak area of the abdominal aorta. The stent creates a stronger inner lining for the artery.

Aneurysms also can develop in the part of the aorta that runs through the chest. Doctors also use stents to treat these aneurysms. How well the stents work over the long term still is not known.

To Close off Aortic Tears

Another problem that can occur in the aorta is a tear in its inner wall. If blood is forced into the tear, it will widen.

The tear can reduce blood flow to the tissues that the aorta serves. Over time, the tear can block blood flow through the artery or burst. If this happens, it usually occurs in the chest portion of the aorta.

Researchers are developing and testing new kinds of stents that will prevent blood from flowing into aortic tears. A stent placed within the torn area of the aorta might help restore normal blood flow and reduce the risk of a burst aorta.

How Are Stents Placed?

Doctors place stents in arteries as part of percutaneous coronary intervention. To place a stent, your doctor will make a small opening in a blood vessel in your groin (upper thigh), arm, or neck.

Through this opening, your doctor will thread a thin, flexible tube called a "catheter." The catheter will have a deflated balloon at its tip.

A stent is placed around the deflated balloon. Your doctor will move the tip of the catheter to the narrow section of the artery or to the aneurysm or aortic tear site.

Special X-ray movies will be taken of the tube as it is threaded through your blood vessel. These movies will help your doctor position the catheter.

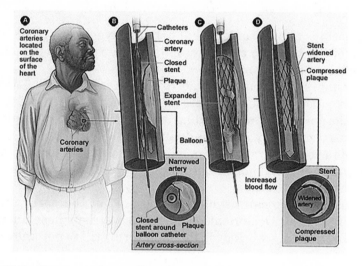

Figure 49.2. *Coronary Artery Stent Placement*

Figure A shows the location of the heart and coronary arteries. Figure B shows the deflated balloon catheter and closed stent inserted into the narrow coronary artery. The inset image shows a cross-section of the artery with the inserted balloon catheter and closed stent. In figure C, the balloon is inflated, expanding the stent and compressing plaque against the artery wall. Figure D shows the stent-widened artery. The inset image shows a cross-section of the compressed plaque and stent-widened artery

For Arteries Narrowed by Plaque

Your doctor will use special dye to help show narrow or blocked areas in the artery. She or he will then move the catheter to the area and inflate the balloon.

As the balloon inflates, it pushes plaque against the artery wall. This widens the artery and helps restore blood flow. The fully extended balloon also expands the stent, pushing it into place in the artery.

The balloon is deflated and pulled out along with the catheter. The stent remains in your artery. Over time, cells in your artery grow to cover the mesh of the stent. They create an inner layer that looks similar to the inside of a normal blood vessel.

A very narrow artery, or one that is hard to reach with a catheter, may require more steps to place a stent. At first, your doctor may use a small balloon to expand the artery. She or he then removes the balloon.

The small balloon is replaced with a larger balloon that has a collapsed stent around it. At this point, your doctor can follow the standard process of compressing the plaque and placing the stent.

Doctors use a special filter device when doing PCI and stent placement on the carotid arteries. The filter helps keep blood clots and loose pieces of plaque from traveling to the brain during the procedure.

For Aortic Aneurysms

The procedure to place a stent in an artery with an aneurysm is very similar to the one described above. However, the stent used to treat an aneurysm is different. It is made out of pleated fabric instead of metal mesh, and it often has one or more tiny hooks.

The stent is expanded to fit tight against the artery wall. The hooks latch on to the wall of the artery, holding the stent in place.

The stent creates a new inner lining for that portion of the artery. Over time, cells in the artery grow to cover the fabric. They create an inner layer that looks similar to the inside of a normal blood vessel.

What to Expect before a Stent Procedure

Most stent procedures require an overnight stay in a hospital and someone to take you home. Talk with your doctor about:

- When to stop eating and drinking before coming to the hospital

- What medicines you should or should not take on the day of the procedure

- When to come to the hospital and where to go

If you have diabetes, kidney disease, or other conditions, ask your doctor whether you need to take any extra steps during or after the procedure to avoid complications.

Before the procedure, your doctor may talk to you about medicines you will likely need to take after the stent is placed. These medicines help prevent blood clots from forming in the stent.

You will need to know how long you should take these medicines and why they are important.

What to Expect during a Stent Procedure
For Arteries Narrowed by Plaque

This procedure usually takes about an hour. It might take longer if stents are inserted into more than one artery during the procedure.

Before the procedure starts, you will get medicine to help you relax. You will be on your back and awake during the procedure. This allows you to follow your doctor's instructions.

Your doctor will numb the area where the catheter will be inserted. You will not feel the doctor threading the catheter, balloon, or stent inside the artery. You may feel some pain when the balloon is expanded to push the stent into place.

For Aortic Aneurysms

Although this procedure takes only a few hours, it often requires a two- to three-day hospital stay.

Before the procedure, you will be given medicine to help you relax. If your doctor is placing the stent in your abdominal aorta, you may receive medicine to numb your stomach area. However, you will be awake during the procedure.

If your doctor is placing the stent in the chest portion of your aorta, you will likely receive medicine to make you sleep during the procedure.

Once you are numb or asleep, your doctor will make a small cut in your groin (upper thigh). She or he will insert a catheter into the blood vessel through this cut.

Sometimes two cuts (one in the groin area of each leg) are needed to place fabric stents that come in two parts. You will not feel the doctor threading the catheter, balloon, or stent into the artery.

What to Expect after a Stent Procedure
Recovery

After either type of stent procedure (for arteries narrowed by plaque or aortic aneurysms), your doctor will remove the catheter from your artery. The site where the catheter was inserted will be bandaged.

A small sandbag or other type of weight may be put on top of the bandage to apply pressure and help prevent bleeding. You will recover in a special care area, where your movement will be limited.

While you are in recovery, a nurse will check your heart rate and blood pressure regularly. The nurse also will look to see whether you are bleeding from the insertion site. Eventually, a small bruise and sometimes a small, hard "knot" will appear at the insertion site. This area may feel sore or tender for about a week.

You should let your doctor know if:

- You have a constant or large amount of bleeding at the insertion site that cannot be stopped with a small bandage.

- You have any unusual pain, swelling, redness, or other signs of infection at or near the insertion site.

Common Precautions after a Stent Procedure

Blood Clotting Precautions

After a stent procedure, your doctor will likely recommend that you take aspirin and another anticlotting medicine. These medicines help prevent blood clots from forming in the stent. A blood clot can lead to a heart attack, stroke, or other serious problems.

If you have a metal stent, your doctor may recommend aspirin and another anticlotting medicine for at least 1 month. If your stent is coated with medicine, your doctor may recommend aspirin and another anticlotting medicine for 12 months or more. Your doctor will work with you to decide the best course of treatment.

Your risk of blood clots significantly increases if you stop taking the anticlotting medicine too early. Taking these medicines for as long as your doctor recommends is important. She or he may recommend lifelong treatment with aspirin.

If you are considering surgery for some other reason while you are on these medicines, talk to your doctor about whether it can wait until after you have stopped the medicine.

Also, anticlotting medicines can cause side effects, such as an allergic rash. Talk to your doctor about how to reduce the risk of these side effects.

Other Precautions

You should avoid vigorous exercise and heavy lifting for a short time after the stent procedure. Your doctor will let you know when you can go back to your normal activities.

Metal detectors used in airports and other screening areas do not affect stents. Your stent should not cause metal detectors to go off.

If you have an aortic fabric stent, your doctor will likely recommend follow-up imaging tests (for example, chest X-ray) within the first year of having the procedure. After the first year, she or he may recommend yearly imaging tests.

Lifestyle Changes

Stents help prevent arteries from becoming narrow or blocked again in the months or years after PCI. However, stents are not a cure for atherosclerosis or its risk factors.

Making lifestyle changes can help prevent plaque from building up in your arteries again. Talk with your doctor about your risk factors for atherosclerosis and the lifestyle changes you will need to make.

Lifestyle changes may include changing your diet, quitting smoking, being physically active, losing weight, and reducing stress. You also should take all medicines as your doctor prescribes. Your doctor may suggest taking statins, which are medicines that lower blood cholesterol levels.

What Are the Risks of Having a Stent?

Risks Related to Percutaneous Coronary Intervention

Percutaneous coronary intervention, the procedure used to place stents, is a medical procedure that carries a small risk of serious complications, such as:

- Bleeding from the site where the catheter was inserted into the skin

- Damage to the blood vessel from the catheter

- Arrhythmias (irregular heartbeats)

- Damage to the kidneys caused by the dye used during the procedure

- An allergic reaction to the dye used during the procedure

- Infection

Another problem that can occur after PCI is too much tissue growth within the treated portion of the artery. This can cause the artery to become narrow or blocked again. When this happens, it is called "restenosis."

Using drug-eluting stents can help prevent this problem. These stents are coated with medicine to stop excess tissue growth.

Treating the tissue around the stent with radiation also can delay tissue growth. For this procedure, the doctor threads a wire through a catheter to the stent. The wire releases radiation and stops cells around the stent from growing and blocking the artery.

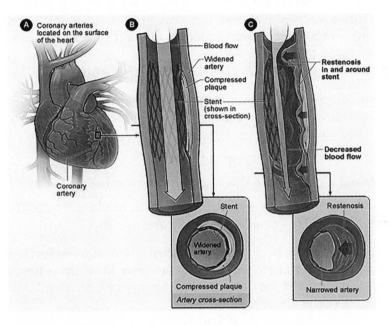

Figure 49.3. *Restenosis of a Stent-Widened Coronary Artery*

Figure A shows the coronary arteries located on the surface of the heart. Figure B shows a stent-widened artery with normal blood flow. The inset image shows a cross-section of the stent-widened artery. In figure C, tissue grows through and around the stent over time. This causes a partial blockage of the artery and abnormal blood flow. The inset image shows a cross-section of the tissue growth around the stent

Risks Related to Stents

About one to two percent of people who have stented arteries develop a blood clot at the stent site. Blood clots can cause a heart attack, stroke, or other serious problems. The risk of blood clots is greatest during the first few months after the stent is placed in the artery.

Your doctor will likely recommend that you take aspirin and another anticlotting medicine, such as clopidogrel, for at least one month or up to a year or more after having a stent procedure. These medicines help prevent blood clots.

The length of time you need to take anticlotting medicines depends on the type of stent you have. Your doctor may recommend lifelong treatment with aspirin.

Stents coated with medicine may raise your risk of dangerous blood clots. (These stents often are used to keep clogged heart arteries open.) However, research has not proven that these stents increase the chances of having a heart attack or dying if used as recommended.

Risks Related to Aortic Stents in the Abdomen

Although rare, a few serious problems can occur when surgery or a fabric stent is used to repair an aneurysm in the abdominal aorta. These problems include:

- A burst artery (aneurysm rupture)

- Blocked blood flow to the stomach or lower body

- Paralysis in the legs due to interruption of blood flow to the spinal cord. This problem is very rare.

Another possible problem is the fabric stent moving further down the aorta. This sometimes happens years after the stent is first placed. The stent movement may require a doctor to place another fabric stent in the area of the aneurysm.

Chapter 50

Procedures to Treat Heart Rhythm Disorders

Chapter Contents

517

Section 50.1

The Cardioversion Procedure

"Cardioversion," © 2016 Omnigraphics.
Reviewed May 2019.

Cardioversion is a medical procedure in which an electrical shock is administered to the heart in order to restore a normal heart rhythm. Although cardioversion is usually performed by placing electrodes on the patient's chest to send electric shocks to the heart, it is sometimes done with medications. Cardioversion is used to treat certain types of arrhythmias, such as atrial fibrillation (AF) or atrial flutter (AFL). It restores a normal sinus rhythm in around 90 percent of patients.

Ordinarily, a heartbeat begins with an electrical signal generated by the sinus node, a group of specialized cells located in the upper right atrium chamber of the heart. This signal travels through the heart to the lower chambers or ventricles, causing the heart muscle to contract and pump blood through the body. When the conduction of the electrical current occurs in a smooth, organized way, it results in a perfectly timed, rhythmic heartbeat. In people with atrial fibrillation, however, the electrical signal travels through the upper chambers in a chaotic, disorganized way. This improper conduction causes the atria to fibrillate or quiver, resulting in an irregular heartbeat.

Cardioversion should not be confused with defibrillation, which is an emergency procedure that delivers much more powerful electrical shocks to the heart. Cardioversion is performed when the heart is beating ineffectively to correct its rhythm. Defibrillation is usually performed when the heart stops beating to restore a heartbeat.

The Procedure

Electrical cardioversion is usually performed in a hospital on an outpatient basis. The patient is placed under anesthesia, so they feel no pain from the procedure. Electrodes are attached to the skin of the patient's chest and back. These patches or paddles are connected to a defibrillator machine, which administers a synchronized electrical shock to the patient's heart. The shock disrupts the abnormal electrical conduction for a split second, which allows the sinus node to reset the heartbeat to a normal rhythm. The procedure only takes a few minutes, although the patient will spend a few hours recovering from the anesthesia and being monitored for complications before going home. Repeat procedures are sometimes needed if the irregular heartbeat recurs.

The main complication associated with electrical cardioversion involves blood clots. When the upper chambers of the heart fibrillate irregularly for more than 48 hours, there is a possibility that blood clots may form in the heart. Cardioversion can cause a blood clot to dislodge from the heart and move through the bloodstream to other parts of the body, which can result in a stroke or other dangerous health complications.

To reduce this risk, patients who have experienced symptoms of AF or AFL for more than 48 hours generally must take blood-thinning medications called "anticoagulants" for 4 weeks before undergoing cardioversion. Common anticoagulants include aspirin, heparin, and warfarin. As an alternative, patients may undergo a procedure called a "transesophageal echocardiogram" (TEE) to check for blood clots prior to cardioversion. During a TEE, a probe is inserted into the patient's esophagus and fed into the chest, enabling the doctor to examine the atria. If no blood clots are found, the cardioversion can proceed.

In chemical cardioversion, the patient receives antiarrhythmic medications to alter the flow of electricity through the heart and restore a normal rhythm. This procedure is sometimes done on an outpatient basis, but it may be performed in the hospital under monitoring in patients with underlying heart disease or severe symptoms. Many patients are prescribed medications to help maintain a normal heart rhythm following cardioversion, as well as blood-thinning medications to prevent new blood clots from forming.

References

1. "Cardioversion," Heart Rhythm Society, 2016.

2. "Cardioversion." Mayo Clinic, 2016.

Section 50.2

Catheter Ablation

Catheter ablation is a medical procedure in which a narrow, flexible tube is inserted into the heart through a vein or artery to diagnose and treat heart rhythm disorders. Catheter ablation can be used to locate and correct the short circuits in the heart's electrical system that cause several different types of arrhythmias.

Ordinarily, a heartbeat begins with an electrical signal generated by the sinus node, a group of specialized cells located in the upper right atrium chamber of the heart. This signal travels downward to the atrioventricular node, an electrical relay station located between the heart's upper and lower chambers. Finally, the current passes through special fibers into the lower chambers or ventricles. The smooth, constant flow of signals through the heart's electrical system causes the upper and lower chambers of the heart to alternately contract and relax in a perfectly timed rhythm in order to pump blood through the body. If the current is disrupted along the heart's electrical pathway, however, it can create an irregular heartbeat known as an "arrhythmia." In a cardiac ablation, energy is delivered to the heart muscle through a catheter to remove the disruption and restore a normal heart rhythm.

When Catheter Ablation Is Used

Catheter ablation can be used to treat many different types of arrhythmias, often taking the place of open-heart surgery. It is particularly helpful for patients whose arrhythmias cannot be controlled with medication, or those who cannot tolerate medications designed to control arrhythmias. Some of the conditions catheter ablation can treat successfully include:

- Supraventricular tachycardia (SVT), a rapid heartbeat that originates with improper electrical activity above the atrioventricular (AV) node

- Ventricular tachycardia (VT), a rapid, potentially life-threatening heartbeat that originates from electrical impulses in the ventricles

- Atrial fibrillation (AF) and atrial flutter (AFL), ineffective, quivering heartbeats that originate with extra signals in the atria

- Accessory pathway, a condition in which extra electrical pathways present from birth relay the signals back from the ventricles to the atria

- AV nodal reentrant tachycardia (AVNRT), a condition in which an extra pathway near the AV node allows signals to travel in a circle

How Catheter Ablation Works

A catheter ablation is performed by a specialist called an "electrophysiologist" in a hospital setting. Before undergoing the procedure, patients should inquire about whether they should continue taking medications. Those on blood thinners, such as warfarin (Coumadin), and certain other drugs might need to stop taking them or adjust the dosage. Since patients will be receiving anesthesia, they should also avoid eating or drinking anything after midnight the night before the procedure.

After arriving at the hospital, patients will receive an IV to deliver medications to make them drowsy. They will also be connected to monitors for heart rhythm, blood pressure, blood oxygen level, and other vital signs. The insertion site for the catheters—which may be the neck, upper thigh, or arm—will be sterilized and shaved. Then the doctor will numb the insertion site and insert several catheters into a vein or artery through a small incision.

The catheters will be fed through the blood vessels until they reach the heart. A transducer will then be inserted through one of the catheters to allow the doctor to view the heart's internal structures using an intracardiac ultrasound. Next, electrodes at the tip of the catheters will send electrical impulses to enable the doctor to pinpoint the location of the short circuit in the heart's electrical system. Finally, the doctor will send energy through the catheters to either block damaged electrical pathways to prevent faulty signals from getting through or destroy short circuits to allow electrical signals to flow properly. The energy can take the form of hot (radio frequency waves) or freezing cold (cryoablation).

Once the ablation is complete, the electrophysiologist will observe the electrical signals in the patient's heart to ensure that the arrhythmia was corrected. The entire procedure is likely to last between four and eight hours. Afterward, the catheters will be removed, and the patient will remain in bed for several hours to prevent bleeding. Some patients are allowed to return home at this point, while others must remain in the hospital overnight for monitoring.

References

1. "Catheter Ablation." Cleveland Clinic, 2016.

2. "Catheter Ablation." Heart Rhythm Society, 2016.

Section 50.3

Pacemaker

This section includes text excerpted from "Pacemakers,"
National Heart, Lung, and Blood Institute (NHLBI),
January 24, 2014. Reviewed May 2019.

What Is a Pacemaker?

A pacemaker is a small device that is placed in the chest or abdomen to help control abnormal heart rhythms. This device uses electrical pulses to prompt the heart to beat at a normal rate.

Pacemakers are used to treat arrhythmias. Arrhythmias are problems with the rate or rhythm of the heartbeat. During an arrhythmia, the heart can beat too fast, too slow, or with an irregular rhythm.

A heartbeat that is too fast is called "tachycardia." A heartbeat that is too slow is called "bradycardia."

During an arrhythmia, the heart may not be able to pump enough blood to the body. This can cause symptoms, such as fatigue (tiredness), shortness of breath, or fainting. Severe arrhythmias can damage the body's vital organs and may even cause loss of consciousness or death.

A pacemaker can relieve some arrhythmia symptoms, such as fatigue and fainting. A pacemaker also can help a person who has abnormal heart rhythms resume a more active lifestyle.

Understanding the Heart's Electrical System

Your heart has its own internal electrical system that controls the rate and rhythm of your heartbeat. With each heartbeat, an electrical signal spreads from the top of your heart to the bottom. As the signal travels, it causes the heart to contract and pump blood.

Each electrical signal normally begins in a group of cells called the "sinus node or "sinoatrial (SA) node." As the signal spreads from the top of the heart to the bottom, it coordinates the timing of heart cell activity.

First, the heart's two upper chambers, the atria, contract. This contraction pumps blood into the heart's two lower chambers, the ventricles. The ventricles then contract and pump blood to the rest of the body. The combined contraction of the atria and ventricles is a heartbeat.

Who Needs a Pacemaker?

Doctors recommend pacemakers for many reasons. The most common reasons are bradycardia and heart block.

Bradycardia is a heartbeat that is slower than normal. Heart block is a disorder that occurs if an electrical signal is slowed or disrupted as it moves through the heart.

Heart block can happen as a result of aging, damage to the heart from a heart attack, or other conditions that disrupt the heart's electrical activity. Some nerve and muscle disorders also can cause heart block, including muscular dystrophy (MD).

Your doctor also may recommend a pacemaker if:

- Aging or heart disease damages your sinus node's ability to set the correct pace for your heartbeat. Such damage can cause slower than normal heartbeats or long pauses between heartbeats. The damage also can cause your heart to switch between slow and fast rhythms. This condition is called "sick sinus syndrome" (SSS).

- You have had a medical procedure to treat an arrhythmia called "atrial fibrillation" (AF). A pacemaker can help regulate your heartbeat after the procedure.

- You need to take certain heart medicines, such as beta-blockers. These medicines can slow your heartbeat too much.

- You faint or have other symptoms of a slow heartbeat. For example, this may happen if the main artery in your neck that

523

supplies your brain with blood is sensitive to pressure. Just quickly turning your neck can cause your heart to beat slower than normal. As a result, your brain might not get enough blood flow, causing you to feel faint or to collapse.

- You have heart muscle problems that cause electrical signals to travel too slowly through your heart muscle. Your pacemaker may provide cardiac resynchronization therapy (CRT) for this problem. CRT devices coordinate electrical signaling between the heart's lower chambers.

- You have long QT syndrome, which puts you at risk for dangerous arrhythmias.

Doctors also may recommend pacemakers for people who have certain types of congenital heart disease (CHD) or for people who have had heart transplants. Children, teens, and adults can use pacemakers.

Before recommending a pacemaker, your doctor will consider any arrhythmia symptoms you have, such as dizziness, unexplained fainting, or shortness of breath. She or he also will consider whether you have a history of heart disease, what medicines you are currently taking, and the results of heart tests.

Diagnostic Tests

Many tests are used to detect arrhythmias. You may have one or more of the following tests.

Electrocardiogram

An electrocardiogram (EKG) is a simple, painless test that detects and records the heart's electrical activity. The test shows how fast your heart is beating and its rhythm (steady or irregular).

An electrocardiogram also records the strength and timing of electrical signals as they pass through your heart. The test can help diagnose bradycardia and heart block (the most common reasons for needing a pacemaker).

A standard EKG only records the heartbeat for a few seconds. It will not detect arrhythmias that do not happen during the test.

To diagnose heart rhythm problems that come and go, your doctor may have you wear a portable EKG monitor. The two most common types of portable EKGs are Holter and event monitors.

Holter and Event Monitors

A Holter monitor records the heart's electrical activity for a full 24- or 48-hour period. You wear one while you do your normal daily activities. This allows the monitor to record your heart for a longer time than a standard EKG.

An event monitor is similar to a Holter monitor. You wear an event monitor while doing your normal activities. However, an event monitor only records your heart's electrical activity at certain times while you are wearing it.

For many event monitors, you push a button to start the monitor when you feel symptoms. Other event monitors start automatically when they sense abnormal heart rhythms.

You can wear an event monitor for weeks or until symptoms occur.

Echocardiography

Echocardiography (echo) uses sound waves to create a moving picture of your heart. The test shows the size and shape of your heart and how well your heart chambers and valves are working.

An echo also can show areas of poor blood flow to the heart, areas of heart muscle that are not contracting normally, and injury to the heart muscle caused by poor blood flow.

Electrophysiology Study

For this test, a thin, flexible wire is passed through a vein in your groin (upper thigh) or arm to your heart. The wire records the heart's electrical signals.

Your doctor uses the wire to electrically stimulate your heart. This allows her or him to see how your heart's electrical system responds. This test helps pinpoint where the heart's electrical system is damaged.

Stress Test

Some heart problems are easier to diagnose when your heart is working hard and beating fast.

During stress testing, you exercise to make your heart work hard and beat fast while heart tests, such as an EKG or echo, are done. If you cannot exercise, you may be given medicine to raise your heart rate.

How Does a Pacemaker Work?

A pacemaker consists of a battery, a computerized generator, and wires with sensors at their tips. (The sensors are called "electrodes.") The battery powers the generator, and both are surrounded by a thin metal box. The wires connect the generator to the heart.

A pacemaker can recognize a problem with your heart's rhythm and send out its own electrical pulse to make your heart beat regularly and on time. The pulse it generates is sent through special wires called leads, normally placed inside the heart. The leads also help the Pacemaker sense the heart's rhythm.

A pacemaker helps monitor and control your heartbeat. The electrodes detect your heart's electrical activity and send data through the wires to the computer in the generator.

If your heart rhythm is abnormal, the computer will direct the generator to send electrical pulses to your heart. The pulses travel through the wires to reach your heart.

Newer pacemakers can monitor your blood temperature, breathing, and other factors. They also can adjust your heart rate to changes in your activity.

The pacemaker's computer also records your heart's electrical activity and heart rhythm. Your doctor will use these recordings to adjust your pacemaker so it works better for you.

Your doctor can program the pacemaker's computer with an external device. She or he does not have to use needles or have direct contact with the pacemaker.

Pacemakers have one to three wires that are each placed in different chambers of the heart.

- The wires in a single-chamber pacemaker usually carry pulses from the generator to the right ventricle (the lower right chamber of your heart).

- The wires in a dual-chamber pacemaker carry pulses from the generator to the right atrium (the upper right chamber of your heart) and the right ventricle. The pulses help coordinate the timing of these two chambers' contractions.

- The wires in a biventricular pacemaker carry pulses from the generator to an atrium and both ventricles. The pulses help coordinate electrical signaling between the two ventricles. This type of pacemaker also is called a "cardiac resynchronization therapy" device.

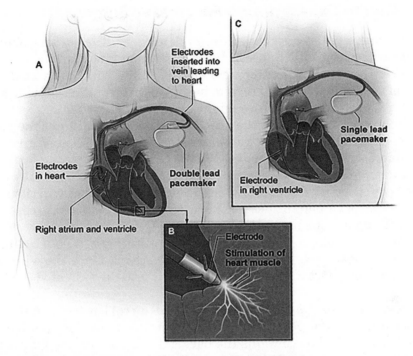

Figure 50.1. *Cross-Section of a Chest with a Pacemaker*

The image shows a cross-section of a chest with a pacemaker. Figure A shows the location and general size of a double-lead, or dual-chamber, pacemaker in the upper chest. The wires with electrodes are inserted into the heart's right atrium and ventricle through a vein in the upper chest. Figure B shows an electrode electrically stimulating the heart muscle. Figure C shows the location and general size of a single-lead, or single-chamber, pacemaker in the upper chest.

Types of Pacemaker Programming

The two main types of programming for pacemakers are demand pacing and rate-responsive pacing.

A demand pacemaker monitors your heart rhythm. It only sends electrical pulses to your heart if your heart is beating too slow or if it misses a beat.

A rate-responsive pacemaker will speed up or slow down your heart rate, depending on how active you are. To do this, the device monitors your sinus node rate, breathing, blood temperature, and other factors to determine your activity level.

Your doctor will work with you to decide which type of pacemaker is best for you.

What to Expect during Pacemaker Surgery

Placing a pacemaker requires minor surgery. The surgery usually is done in a hospital or special heart treatment laboratory.

Before the surgery, an intravenous (IV) line will be inserted into one of your veins. You will receive medicine through the IV line to help you relax. The medicine also might make you sleepy.

Your doctor will numb the area where she or he will put the pacemaker so you do not feel any pain. Your doctor also may give you antibiotics to prevent infection.

First, your doctor will insert a needle into a large vein, usually near the shoulder opposite your dominant hand. Your doctor will then use the needle to thread the pacemaker wires into the vein and to correctly place them in your heart.

An X-ray "movie" of the wires as they pass through your vein and into your heart will help your doctor place them. Once the wires are in place, your doctor will make a small cut into the skin of your chest or abdomen.

She or he will slip the pacemaker's small metal box through the cut, place it just under your skin, and connect it to the wires that lead to your heart. The box contains the pacemaker's battery and generator.

Once the pacemaker is in place, your doctor will test it to make sure it works properly. She or he will then sew up the cut. The entire surgery takes a few hours.

What to Expect after Pacemaker Surgery

Expect to stay in the hospital overnight so your healthcare team can check your heartbeat and make sure your pacemaker is working well. You will likely have to arrange for a ride to and from the hospital because your doctor may not want you to drive yourself.

For a few days to weeks after surgery, you may have pain, swelling, or tenderness in the area where your pacemaker was placed. The pain usually is mild; over-the-counter (OTC) medicines often can relieve it. Talk to your doctor before taking any pain medicines.

Your doctor may ask you to avoid vigorous activities and heavy lifting for about a month after pacemaker surgery. Most people return to their normal activities within a few days of having the surgery.

What Are the Risks of Pacemaker Surgery?

Pacemaker surgery generally is safe. If problems do occur, they may include:

- Swelling, bleeding, bruising, or infection in the area where the pacemaker was placed

- Blood vessel or nerve damage

- A collapsed lung

- A bad reaction to the medicine used during the procedure

Talk with your doctor about the benefits and risks of pacemaker surgery.

How Will a Pacemaker Affect Your Lifestyle?

Once you have a pacemaker, you have to avoid close or prolonged contact with electrical devices or devices that have strong magnetic fields. Devices that can interfere with a pacemaker include:

- Cell phones and MP3 players (for example, iPods)

- Household appliances, such as microwave ovens

- High-tension wires

- Metal detectors

- Industrial welders

- Electrical generators

These devices can disrupt the electrical signaling of your pacemaker and stop it from working properly. You may not be able to tell whether your pacemaker has been affected.

How likely a device is to disrupt your pacemaker depends on how long you are exposed to it and how close it is to your pacemaker.

To be safe, some experts recommend not putting your cell phone or MP3 player in a shirt pocket over your pacemaker (if the devices are turned on).

You may want to hold your cell phone up to the ear that is opposite the site where your pacemaker is implanted. If you strap your MP3 player to your arm while listening to it, put it on the arm that is farther from your pacemaker.

You can still use household appliances, but avoid close and prolonged exposure, as it may interfere with your pacemaker.

You can walk through security system metal detectors at your normal pace. Security staff can check you with a metal detector wand as long as it is not held for too long over your pacemaker site. You should avoid sitting or standing close to a security system metal detector. Notify security staff if you have a pacemaker.

Also, stay at least two feet away from industrial welders and electrical generators.

Some medical procedures can disrupt your pacemaker. These procedures include:

- Magnetic resonance imaging, or MRI

- Shock-wave lithotripsy to get rid of kidney stones

- Electrocauterization to stop bleeding during surgery

Let all of your doctors, dentists, and medical technicians know that you have a pacemaker. Your doctor can give you a card that states what kind of pacemaker you have. Carry this card in your wallet. You may want to wear a medical ID bracelet or necklace that states that you have a pacemaker.

Physical Activity

In most cases, having a pacemaker will not limit you from doing sports and exercise, including strenuous activities.

You may need to avoid full-contact sports, such as football. Such contact could damage your pacemaker or shake loose the wires in your heart. Ask your doctor how much and what kinds of physical activity are safe for you.

Ongoing Care

Your doctor will want to check your pacemaker regularly (about every three months). Over time, a pacemaker can stop working properly because:

- Its wires get dislodged or broken

- Its battery gets weak or fails

- Your heart disease progresses

- Other devices have disrupted its electrical signaling

To check your pacemaker, your doctor may ask you to come in for an office visit several times a year. Some pacemaker functions can be checked remotely by using a phone or the Internet.

Your doctor also may ask you to have an EKG to check for changes in your heart's electrical activity.

Battery Replacement

Pacemaker batteries last between 5 and 15 years (with an average around 6 to 7 years), depending on how active the pacemaker is. Your doctor will replace the generator along with the battery before the battery starts to run down.

Replacing the generator and battery is less-involved surgery than the original surgery to implant the pacemaker. Your pacemaker wires also may need to be replaced eventually.

Your doctor can tell you whether your pacemaker or its wires need to be replaced when you see her or him for follow-up visits.

Chapter 51

Procedures to Treat Heart Valve Problems

No medicines can cure heart valve disease. However, lifestyle changes and medicines often can treat symptoms successfully and delay problems for many years. Eventually, though, you may need surgery to repair or replace a faulty heart valve.

Heart-Healthy Lifestyle Changes to Treat Other Related Heart Conditions

To help treat heart conditions related to heart valve disease, your doctor may advise you to make heart-healthy lifestyle changes, such as:

- Heart-healthy eating
- Aiming for a healthy weight
- Managing stress
- Physical activity
- Quitting smoking

This chapter includes text excerpted from "Heart Valve Disease," National Heart, Lung, and Blood Institute (NHLBI), November 18, 2013. Reviewed May 2019.

Medicines for Treating Heart Valve Disease

In addition to heart-healthy lifestyle changes, your doctor may prescribe medicines to:

- Lower high blood pressure or high blood cholesterol

- Prevent arrhythmias (irregular heartbeats)

- Thin the blood and prevent clots (if you have a human-made replacement valve). Doctors also prescribe these medicines for mitral stenosis (MS) or other valve defects that raise the risk of blood clots.

- Treat coronary heart disease (CHD). Medicines for coronary heart disease can reduce your heart's workload and relieve symptoms.

- Treat heart failure. Heart failure medicines widen blood vessels and rid the body of excess fluid.

Repairing or Replacing Heart Valves

Your doctor may recommend repairing or replacing your heart valve(s), even if your heart valve disease is not causing symptoms. Repairing or replacing a valve can prevent lasting damage to your heart and sudden death.

The decision to repair or replace heart valves depends on many factors, including:

- The severity of your valve disease

- Whether you need heart surgery for other conditions, such as bypass surgery to treat coronary heart disease. Bypass surgery and valve surgery can be performed at the same time.

- Your age and general health

When possible, heart valve repair is preferred over heart valve replacement. Valve repair preserves the strength and function of the heart muscle. People who have valve repair also have a lower risk of infective endocarditis after the surgery, and they do not need to take blood-thinning medicines for the rest of their lives.

However, heart valve repair surgery is harder to do than valve replacement. Also, not all valves can be repaired. Mitral valves often can be repaired. Aortic and pulmonary valves often have to be replaced.

Repairing Heart Valves

Heart surgeons can repair heart valves by:

- Adding tissue to patch holes or tears or to increase the support at the base of the valve

- Removing or reshaping tissue so the valve can close tighter

- Separating fused valve flaps

Sometimes, cardiologists repair heart valves using cardiac catheterization. Although catheter procedures are less invasive than surgery, they may not work as well for some patients. Work with your doctor to decide whether repair is appropriate. If so, your doctor can advise you on the best procedure.

Heart valves that cannot open fully (stenosis) can be repaired with surgery or with a less invasive catheter procedure called "balloon valvuloplasty." This procedure also is called "balloon valvotomy."

During the procedure, a catheter (thin tube) with a balloon at its tip is threaded through a blood vessel to the faulty valve in your heart. The balloon is inflated to help widen the opening of the valve. Your doctor then deflates the balloon and removes both it and the tube. You are awake during the procedure, which usually requires an overnight stay in a hospital.

Balloon valvuloplasty relieves many symptoms of heart valve disease, but it may not cure it. The condition can worsen over time. You still may need medicines to treat symptoms or surgery to repair or replace the faulty valve. Balloon valvuloplasty has a shorter recovery time than surgery. The procedure may work as well as surgery for some patients who have mitral valve stenosis (MVS). For these people, balloon valvuloplasty often is preferred over surgical repair or replacement.

Balloon valvuloplasty does not work as well as surgery for adults who have aortic valve stenosis (AVS). Doctors often use balloon valvuloplasty to repair valve stenosis in infants and children.

Replacing Heart Valves

Sometimes, heart valves cannot be repaired and must be replaced. This surgery involves removing the faulty valve and replacing it with a human-made or biological valve.

Biological valves are made from pig, cow, or human heart tissue and may have human-made parts as well. These valves are specially treated, so you will not need medicines to stop your body from rejecting the valve.

Human-made valves last longer than biological valves and usually do not have to be replaced. Biological valves usually have to be replaced after about 10 years, although newer ones may last 15 years or longer. Unlike biological valves, however, human-made valves require you to take blood-thinning medicines for the rest of your life. These medicines prevent blood clots from forming on the valve. Blood clots can cause a heart attack or stroke. Human-made valves also raise your risk of infective endocarditis.

You and your doctor will decide together whether you should have a human-made or biological replacement valve.

If you are a woman of childbearing age or if you are athletic, you may prefer a biological valve so you do not have to take blood-thinning medicines. If you are elderly, you also may prefer a biological valve, as it will likely last for the rest of your life.

Ross Procedure

Doctors also can treat faulty aortic valves with the Ross procedure. During this surgery, your doctor removes your faulty aortic valve and replaces it with your pulmonary valve. Your pulmonary valve is then replaced with a pulmonary valve from a deceased human donor.

This is a more involved surgery than a typical valve replacement, and it has a greater risk of complications. The Ross procedure may be especially useful for children because the surgically replaced valves continue to grow with the child. Also, lifelong treatment with blood-thinning medicines is not required. But in some patients, one or both valves fail to work well within a few years of the surgery.

Other Approaches for Repairing and Replacing Heart Valves

Some forms of heart valve repair and replacement surgery are less invasive than traditional surgery. These procedures use smaller incisions (cuts) to reach the heart valves. Hospital stays for these newer types of surgery usually are three to five days, compared to a five-day stay for traditional heart valve surgery.

New surgeries tend to cause less pain and have a lower risk of infection. Recovery time also tends to be shorter—two to four weeks versus six to eight weeks for traditional surgery.

Transcatheter Valve Therapy

Interventional cardiologists perform procedures that involve threading clips or other devices to repair faulty heart valves by using a catheter inserted through a large blood vessel. The clips or devices are used to reshape the valves and stop the backflow of blood. People who receive these clips recover more easily than people who have surgery. However, the clips may not treat backflow as well as surgery.

Doctors also may use a catheter to replace faulty aortic valves. This procedure is called "transcatheter aortic valve replacement" (TAVR). For this procedure, the catheter usually is inserted into an artery in the groin (upper thigh) and threaded to the heart. A deflated balloon with a folded replacement valve around it is at the end of the catheter.

Once the replacement valve is placed properly, the balloon is used to expand the new valve so it fits securely within the old valve. The balloon is then deflated, and the balloon and catheter are removed.

A replacement valve also can be inserted in an existing replacement valve that is failing. This is called a "valve-in-valve (VIV) procedure."

Chapter 52

Aneurysm Repair

An aneurysm is a balloon-like bulge in an artery. Arteries are blood vessels that carry blood from your heart to your organs. Aortic aneurysms are aneurysms that occur in the aorta, the main artery carrying oxygen-rich blood to your body. This chapter focuses on two types of aneurysms that affect the aorta: abdominal and thoracic aortic aneurysms.

The aorta has thick walls that withstand normal blood pressure. However, certain medical problems, genetic conditions, and trauma can damage or weaken these walls. The force of blood pushing against the weakened or injured walls can cause an aneurysm.

Surgical Repair

Depending on the cause or size of an aneurysm or how quickly it is growing, your doctor may recommend surgery to repair it. A rupture or dissection of an aneurysm may require immediate surgical repair.

Open surgical repair is the most common type of surgery. You will be asleep during the procedure. Your surgical team first makes a large incision, or cut, in your abdomen or chest, depending on the location of the aneurysm, then removes the aneurysm and sews a graft in its place. This graft is typically a tube made of leak-proof polyester. Recovery time for open surgical repair is about a month.

This chapter includes text excerpted from "Aortic Aneurysm," National Institute of Neurological Disorders and Stroke (NINDS), March 29, 2012. Reviewed May 2019.

Endovascular aneurysm repair (EVAR) is less invasive than open surgical repair. This is because the surgical cut is smaller, and you usually need less recovery time. EVAR is used to repair abdominal aortic aneurysms more often than to repair thoracic aortic aneurysms. During the procedure, your surgical team makes a small cut, usually in the groin, then guides a stent graft—a tube covered with fabric— through your blood vessels and up to the aorta. The stent graft then expands and attaches to the aortic walls. A seal forms between the stent graft and the vessel wall to prevent blood from entering the aortic aneurysm.

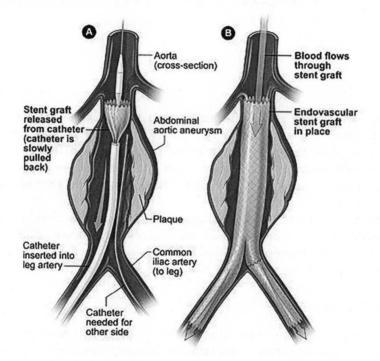

Figure 52.1. *Endovascular Repair*

The illustration shows the placement of a stent graft in an abdominal aortic aneurysm. In figure A, a catheter is inserted into an artery in the groin. The catheter is threaded to the abdominal aorta, and the stent graft is released from the catheter. In figure B, the stent graft is expanded and allows blood to flow through the aorta.

Possible Surgery-Related Complications

Complications of both types of aortic aneurysm repair can occur, and they may be life-threatening. These include:

- Bleeding and blood loss

- Blood clots in blood vessels, leading to the bowel, kidneys, legs, or in the graft

- Damage to blood vessels or walls of the aorta when placing the stent graft. The stent graft may also move after it is placed.

- Endoleak, which is a blood leak around the stent graft into the aneurysm. Endoleak may cause rupture of the aneurysm if not treated.

- Gastrointestinal bleeding, which rarely occurs if an abnormal connection forms between the aorta and your intestines after the repair. Blood may show up in your stool, or your stool may be black.

- Heart complications, such as heart attack or arrhythmia

- Decreased blood flow to the bowels, legs, kidneys or other organs during surgery. This may lead to injury to these organs.

- Infection of the incision or the graft

- Kidney damage

- Spinal cord injury, which may cause paralysis

- Stroke

Chapter 53

Total Artificial Heart

A total artificial heart (TAH) is a pump that is surgically installed to provide circulation and to replace heart ventricles that are diseased or damaged. The ventricles pump blood out of the heart to the lungs and other parts of the body. Machines outside the body control the implanted pumps, helping blood flow to and from the heart.

A doctor may recommend a TAH if you have heart failure caused by ventricles that no longer pump blood well enough, and you need long-term support. TAH surgery may be an alternative treatment in certain patients who are unable to receive a heart transplant.

As with any surgery, TAH surgery can lead to serious complications, such as blood clots or infection. You may have to stay in the hospital to prevent or manage these complications. In some cases, people with a TAH can leave the hospital to wait for a heart transplant.

How Does It Work?

The total artificial heart replaces the lower chambers of the heart, called "ventricles." Tubes connect the TAH to a power source that is outside the body. The TAH then pumps blood through the heart's major artery to the lungs and the rest of the body.

This chapter includes text excerpted from "Total Artificial Heart," National Heart, Lung, and Blood Institute (NHLBI), February 11, 2018.

The total artificial heart has 4 mechanical valves that work as the heart's own valves to control blood flow. These valves connect the TAH to your heart's upper chambers, called the "atrium," and to the major arteries, the pulmonary artery and the aorta. Once the TAH is connected, it duplicates the action of a normal heart, providing mechanical circulatory support and restoring normal blood flow through the body. The TAH is powered and controlled by a bedside console for patients in the hospital. After they leave the hospital, people with a TAH use a portable control device that fits in a shoulder bag or backpack and weighs about 14 pounds. It can be recharged at home or in a car.

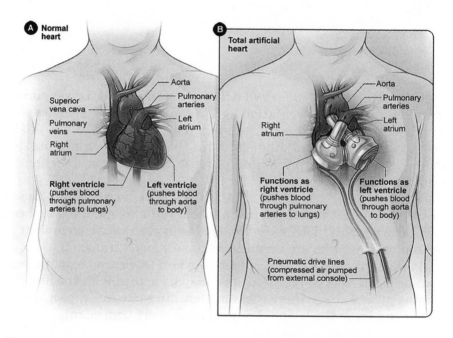

Figure 53.1. *Normal Heart and a Total Artificial Heart Device*

Figure A shows the normal structure and location of the heart. Figure B shows a total artificial heart, including the tubes that exit the body and connect to a machine that powers and controls the total artificial heart.

Who May Benefit from Total Artificial Heart Surgery?

You may benefit from a TAH if you have heart failure caused by ventricles that no longer pump blood well enough, and other treatments have not worked. If you are waiting for a heart transplant, a TAH can help prolong your life.

Talk to your doctor about whether you are eligible for a TAH and whether the benefits of the device outweigh the risks from surgery and possible complications from living with a TAH.

Who Is Eligible to Get a Total Artificial Heart?

You may be eligible for a TAH if you have heart failure and both of your ventricles are working poorly. The U.S. Food and Drug Administration (FDA) approved the TAH device as a bridge to a transplant; TAHs help keep people with heart failure alive while they wait for a heart transplant. In addition, artificial hearts have been given to a few patients as part of clinical research. Researchers are working on smaller TAHs that will fit infants, children, women, and smaller men who are waiting for a heart transplant, as well as devices that are alternative treatments for adults who are not eligible for a transplant.

Who Is Not Eligible to Get a Total Artificial Heart?

A total artificial heart should not be used if you have any of these characteristics or conditions:

- Are small. The device is too large to fit in the chests of children and some adults. Researchers are testing smaller TAHs in infants, children, women, and smaller men.

- Can benefit from other treatments, including medicines

- Have heart failure on only one side of your heart. In these cases, treatment with a ventricular assist device (VAD) may be more appropriate.

- Cannot take anticlotting medicines. These medicines are required as long as the TAH is in place.

Before Surgery

If you are not already in the hospital, you will likely spend at least a week in the hospital to prepare for the TAH surgery. You will continue to take any heart medicines your doctor gave you. During this time, you will learn about the TAH that you are getting and how to live with it.

You and your loved ones will meet with your surgeons, your cardiologist, and other doctors and nurses who specialize in the heart. The members of your healthcare team will provide you with the information that you need before surgery, including steps you need to take at home to prepare. You can ask to see what the device looks like and how it will be attached inside your body.

Your doctors will make sure that your body is strong enough for the surgery. You may need to get extra nutrition through a feeding tube.

You may have the following tests before your surgery:

- **Blood tests.** Doctors use these tests to determine your blood type for any blood you may need during surgery and to check how well your liver and kidneys are working. The tests will also show your blood cell levels, as well as important chemicals in your blood.

- **Chest computed tomography (CT) scan.** This test takes pictures of the inside of your chest. Doctors use these pictures to make sure that the TAH, which is large, will fit in your chest.

- **Chest magnetic resonance imaging (MRI).** This test creates detailed pictures of the organs in your chest, including your heart, lungs, and blood vessels.

- **Chest X-ray.** This test also takes pictures of the inside of your chest. Doctors use these pictures to check your lungs, your heart, and your major arteries.

- **Electrocardiogram (EKG).** Doctors use this test to monitor your heart's rhythm. It can show how well your ventricles are working before surgery.

- **Echocardiogram (Echo).** This test uses sound waves to create moving pictures of your heart. It shows the movement of the blood through your heart and major blood vessels to see, for example, whether there are any blockages.

- **Pulmonary function tests.** These tests measure how well your lungs work to help determine your risk for needing a ventilator for a long time after the surgery.

During Surgery

The surgery to connect the TAH is complex and can last from five to nine hours. Learn about the team that performs the surgery and the steps involved in connecting a TAH to your body.

Surgical Team

As many as 15 people might be in the operating room during the surgery, including:

- Surgeons, who do the operation

- Surgical nurses, who assist the surgeons

- Anesthesiologists, who give you medicine that makes you sleep during the surgery

- Perfusionists, who oversee the heart-lung bypass machine that keeps blood flowing through your body while the TAH is placed in your chest

- Engineers, who assemble the TAH and make sure that it is working well

Connecting the Total Artificial Heart Device

An anesthesiologist will give you medicine to make you sleep before the surgery. During the surgery, the anesthesiologist will check your heart rate, blood pressure, oxygen levels, and breathing.

A breathing tube is placed in your windpipe through your mouth. This tube is connected to a ventilator machine that will support your breathing during the surgery.

Medicines are used to stop your heart. This allows the surgeons to operate on your heart while it is not moving. A heart-lung bypass machine keeps oxygen-rich blood moving through your body during the surgery.

To perform the surgery, your surgeons will cut into your chest bone to get to your heart. Your surgeons will open your ribcage, remove your heart's ventricles, and attach the TAH to the upper chambers of your heart and to the aorta and the pulmonary artery. When everything is attached, the heart-lung bypass machine will be switched off and the surgical team will activate the TAH so it starts pumping. If the TAH is working properly and you are not bleeding abnormally, the surgeon will close your chest again. In some cases, it will remain partially closed for a few days. The medical team will fully close the chest once additional tests confirm that everything is working as it should.

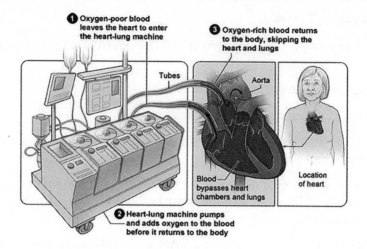

Figure 53.2. *Heart-Lung Bypass Machine*

The image shows how a heart-lung bypass machine works during surgery

After Surgery

After surgery you may have possible surgery-related complications, such as blood clots or infections.

Recovery from Surgery

Your hospital stay after surgery could last a month or more. Recovery time after TAH surgery will depend a lot on your health before the surgery.

Right after surgery, you will be moved to the hospital's intensive care unit (ICU). You may still need a ventilator to help you breathe. For a while, you may receive fluids and nutrition through a feeding tube or an intravenous (IV) line in your arm. Your healthcare team will monitor another IV line in your neck or your leg to evaluate how the TAH is working. You will also have a tube inserted into your urinary tract to drain urine and to evaluate how your kidneys are working.

After a few days or more, you will be moved to a regular hospital room. Nurses who have experience with TAHs and similar devices will take care of you. The nurses will help you sit, get out of bed, and walk around. Most patients are able to get up and move around after two weeks. Nurses and physical therapists will help you gain your strength through a slow increase in activity.

Medical staff will perform exams, such as blood tests, as well as chest imaging tests, including CT scans, X-rays, and echocardiograms. Since most of the heart has been removed, electrocardiograms; heart monitors; and procedures, such as cardiopulmonary resuscitation, (CPR) will no longer be useful.

Once you become stronger, your healthcare team will remove your feeding, IV, and urine tubes. You will be able to begin eating regular food, go to the bathroom on your own, and take a shower. You will also learn how to care for your TAH at home.

During your recovery time in the hospital, you may enjoy visits from family or friends. These visitors can help you with various activities. They can also learn how to care for the TAH so that they can help you when you go home.

Possible Surgery-Related Complications

As with any surgery, there are possible surgery-related complications after getting a TAH, such as blood clots, bleeding, or infection.

Blood Clots

Blood may clot more easily as a result of the contact with the manufactured parts of the TAH. Blood clots can block blood vessels that deliver oxygen to important organs in your body and can cause severe complications, such as stroke, a type of venous thromboembolism (VE) called "pulmonary embolism" (PE), or death. For this reason, you need to take anticlotting medicine as long as you have a TAH.

Bleeding

The surgery to connect a TAH to your heart is very complex. Bleeding can occur in your chest during and after the surgery. Anticlotting medicine also raises your risk of bleeding, because it thins your blood. Balancing the anticlotting medicine with the risk of bleeding can be hard. Be sure to take your medicine exactly as your doctor prescribes.

Infection

After surgery, you will be at risk for infection, so your doctor may prescribe medicine to reduce this risk. Your healthcare team will watch you closely for fever or other signs of infection.

Other Complications

The medical team will also watch you closely for the possibility of other complications including:

- High blood pressure

- Liver failure

- Kidney failure

- Anemia, which may require a blood transfusion

During the TAH surgery, there is a risk of dying. There is also a risk that your body may respond poorly to the medicine used to put you to sleep during the surgery.

Living with a Total Artificial Heart

Learn about going home after TAH surgery, ongoing medical care you need, and possible complications of living with a TAH. If you are on the waiting list for a heart transplant, you will stay in close contact with the transplant center.

Slowly Increase Your Activity Level

Your recovery will continue after you go home. Once you are at home, you will need to slowly increase your activity level, protect and care for your TAH, and get the right nutrition and exercise.

When you go home after TAH surgery, you will likely be able to do more activities than you could before the surgery. The machine with the power supply and device controls is portable, so you will probably be able to get out of bed, get dressed, and move around the house. You may even be able to drive. Your healthcare team will advise you on the level of activity that is safe for you.

Protect and Care for Your Total Artificial Heart

Your healthcare team will explain how to troubleshoot your TAH, change or charge the portable device's batteries, and respond to alarms.

A total artificial heart is attached to a power source outside your body through holes in your abdomen. These holes increase the risk of bacteria getting in and causing an infection. Your doctor may tell you how often to check your temperature as part of your routine care. You may also need to take special steps before you bathe, shower, or swim. Your healthcare team will explain how to make sure that the tubes going through your skin do not get wet. They also will recommend that you avoid steam baths and dry saunas, which can overheat the TAH driver.

Get the Right Nutrition and Physical Activity

While you recover from TAH surgery, it is important that you get good nutrition. Talk with your healthcare team about following a proper eating plan for recovery.

Your healthcare team may recommend a supervised physical activity program. Physical activity can give your body the strength that it needs to recover. During the months or years before surgery, when your heart was not working well, the muscles in your body may have weakened. Building up the muscles again will allow you to do more activities and feel less tired.

Ongoing Care

You will have regular checkups with your healthcare team to check your progress and make sure that your TAH is working well. There is a chance that you may have problems with your TAH. In some cases, you may need surgery again.

Medicines

You will need to take anticlotting medicine to prevent dangerous blood clots as long as you have a TAH. Regular blood tests will help determine the correct dose.

You also will need to take medicine to try to prevent infections. Your doctor may tell you how often to check your temperature to make sure you do not have a fever, which can be a warning sign of infection.

Make sure to take all your medicines as prescribed and report any side effects to your doctor.

Heart Transplant

If you are on the waiting list for a heart transplant, you will likely be in close contact with the transplant center. Most donor hearts must be transplanted within four hours after removal from the donor.

You need to be prepared to arrive at the hospital within two hours of being notified about a donor heart.

Emotional Health

Getting a total artificial heart may cause fear, anxiety, and stress. If you are waiting for a heart transplant, you may worry that the TAH will not keep you alive long enough to get a new heart. You may feel overwhelmed or depressed.

These feelings are common for someone going through major heart surgery. Talk with your healthcare team about how you feel. Talking to a professional counselor also can help. If you are very depressed, your doctor may recommend medicines or other treatments that can improve your quality of life (QOL).

Support from family and friends can help relieve stress and anxiety. Let your loved ones know how you feel and what they can do to help you.

Problems with Your Device

There is a risk that the TAH will have problems and not work properly. For example, the device may not have the correct pumping action, the power source may fail, or parts may stop working well. Talk with your healthcare team about how to spot potential problems and what to do if a problem occurs.

Chapter 54

Treating Congenital Heart Defect

Treatment will depend on which type of congenital heart defect (CHD) you have. Treatments for CHDs include medicines, surgery, and cardiac catheterization procedures. Many CHDs do not require treatment at all. However, children with critical CHDs will need surgery in their first year of life. Some people with CHDs may need treatment, including repeated surgery, throughout their lives. All people with CHDs should be followed by a cardiologist, a doctor who specializes in the heart, throughout their whole life.

Medicines

Your child's doctor may prescribe medicines to help close patent ductus arteriosus (PDA) in premature infants.

- **Indomethacin** or **ibuprofen** triggers the PDA to constrict or tighten, which closes the opening.

- **Acetaminophen** is sometimes used to close PDA.

This chapter includes text excerpted from "Congenital Heart Defects," National Heart, Lung, and Blood Institute (NHLBI), May 2, 2018.

Cardiac Catheterization

Cardiac catheterization is a common procedure that is sometimes used to repair simple heart defects, such as atrial septal defect (ASD) and PDA if they do not repair themselves. It may also be used to open up valves or blood vessels that are narrowed or have stenosis.

In this procedure, a thin, flexible tube called a "catheter" is put into a vein in the groin or neck. The tube is threaded to the heart. Possible complications include bleeding, infection, pain at the catheter insertion site, and damage to blood vessels.

Surgery

In heart surgery, a cardiac surgeon opens the chest to work directly on the heart.

Surgery may be done for these reasons:

- To repair a hole in the heart, such as a ventricular septal defect (VSD) or an atrial septal defect

- To repair a PDA

- To repair complex defects, such as problems with the location of blood vessels near the heart or how they are formed

- To repair or replace a valve

- To widen narrowed blood vessels

Surgeries that are sometimes needed to treat CHD include:

- **Heart transplant.** Children may receive a heart transplant if they have a complex CHD that cannot be repaired surgically or if the heart fails after surgery. Children may also receive a heart transplant if they are dependent on a ventilator or have severe symptoms of heart failure. Some adults with CHDs may eventually need a heart transplant.

- **Palliative surgery.** Some babies with only one ventricle are too weak or too small to have heart surgery. They must have palliative surgery, or temporary surgery, first to improve oxygen levels in the blood. In this surgery, the surgeon installs a shunt, a tube that creates an additional pathway for blood to travel to the lungs to get oxygen. The surgeon removes the shunt when the baby's heart defects are fixed during the full repair.

- **Ventricular assist device (VAD).** For people with heart failure from a CHD, this device supports the heart until a transplant occurs. These devices can be difficult to use in people who have CHDs because of the heart's abnormal structure.

- **Total artificial heart (TAH).** For some people with complex CHDs, a total artificial heart may be needed instead of a ventricular assist device.

Chapter 55

Heart Transplant

A heart transplant removes a damaged or diseased heart and replaces it with a healthy one. The healthy heart comes from a donor who has died. It is the last resort for people with heart failure when all other treatments have failed. The heart failure might have been caused by coronary heart disease (CHD), damaged heart valves or heart muscles, congenital heart defects, or viral infections of the heart.

Although heart transplant surgery is a life-saving measure, it has many risks. Careful monitoring, treatment, and regular medical care can prevent or help manage some of these risks.

After the surgery, most heart transplant patients can return to their normal levels of activity. However, fewer than 30 percent return to work for many different reasons.

Heart Transplant for Cardiovascular Disorder

Most heart transplants are done on patients who have end-stage heart failure, a condition in which your heart is severely damaged or weakened, and on people who have failed other treatment options. End-stage heart failure may be caused by conditions, such as CHD, viral infections, or hereditary conditions. In rare instances, a heart

This chapter contains text excerpted from the following sources: Text in this chapter begins with excerpts from "Heart Transplantation," MedlinePlus, National Institutes of Health (NIH), August 8, 2018; Text under the heading "Heart Transplant for Cardiovascular Disorder" is excerpted from "Heart Transplant," National Heart, Lung, and Blood Institute (NHLBI), July 25, 2011. Reviewed May 2019.

transplant may be performed at the same time as a lung transplant in patients who have severe heart and lung disease.

Who Can Undergo Heart Transplant Surgery?

You may be eligible for heart transplant surgery if you have severe heart disease that does not respond to other treatments. If you are otherwise healthy enough for surgery, you will be placed on the National Organ Procurement and Transplantation Network's (OPTN) waiting list. This national network handles the organ-sharing process for the United States. If a match is found, you will need to have your heart transplant surgery right away.

What Happens during a Heart Transplant Surgery

Heart transplant surgery will be done in a hospital. You will have general anesthesia and will not be awake during the surgery. You will receive medicine through an intravenous (IV) line in your arm. A breathing tube connected to a ventilator will help you breathe. A surgeon will open your chest, connect your heart's arteries and veins to a heart-lung bypass machine, and remove your diseased heart. The body's arteries and veins will be taken off the bypass machine and reconnected to the healthy donor heart. The heart transplant is complete after the surgeon closes your chest.

What Happens after a Heart Transplant Surgery

After the surgery, you will recover in the hospital's intensive care unit (ICU) and stay in the hospital for up to three weeks. During your recovery, you may start a cardiac rehabilitation program (CRP). Before leaving the hospital, you will learn how to keep track of your overall health; monitor your weight, blood pressure, pulse, and temperature; and learn the signs of heart transplant rejection and infection. For the first three months after leaving the hospital, you will return often for tests to check for infection or rejection of your new heart, to test your heart function, and to make sure that you are recovering well.

Living With

Practicing good hygiene, obtaining routine vaccines, and making healthy lifestyle choices are very important after a heart transplant to reduce your risk of infection. Regular dental care is also important. Your doctor or dentist may prescribe antibiotics before any dental work to prevent infection. Following your doctor's advice will help you recover and stay as healthy as possible.

Risks

A heart transplant has some serious risks. Primary graft dysfunction happens when the donor heart fails and cannot function. This is the most frequent cause of death for the first month after transplant. Your immune system also may reject your new heart. Rejection is most likely to occur within six months after the transplant. You will need to take medicines for the rest of your life to suppress your immune system and help prevent your body from rejecting your new heart. These medicines weaken your immune system and increase your chance for infection. Their long-term use also can increase your risk for cancer, cause diabetes and osteoporosis, and damage your kidneys. Cardiac allograft vasculopathy (CAV) is a common and serious complication of heart transplant. Cardiac allograft vasculopathy is an aggressive form of atherosclerosis that, over months or a few years, can quickly block the heart's arteries and cause the donor heart to fail. Over time, your new heart may fail due to the same reasons that caused your original heart to fail. Some patients who have a heart transplant that fails may be eligible for another transplant.

Despite these risks, heart transplant has a good success rate that has improved over many decades of research. Survival rates are about 85 percent at 1 year after surgery, with survival rates decreasing by about 3 to 4 percent each additional year after surgery because of serious complications. Mechanical circulatory support (MCS), possibly from left ventricular assist devices (VAD), may be an alternative to heart transplant. But, more research is needed to determine long-term survival rates for these new devices.

Chapter 56

Rehabilitation after Heart Attack or Stroke

Chapter Contents

Section 56.1

Cardiac Rehabilitation

This section includes text excerpted from "How Cardiac
Rehabilitation Can Help Heal Your Heart," Centers for Disease
Control and Prevention (CDC), July 10, 2017.

If you have a heart attack or other heart problem, cardiac rehabilitation (rehab) is an important part of your recovery. Cardiac rehab can help prevent another, perhaps more serious, heart attack and can help you build heart-healthy habits.

Nearly 800,000 people in the United States have a heart attack every year. About 1 in 4 of those people have already had a heart attack. Cardiac rehab not only can help a person recover from a heart problem, but it can also prevent another heart problem in the future.

What Is Cardiac Rehab?

Cardiac rehab is an important program for anyone recovering from a heart attack, heart failure, or other heart problem that required surgery or medical care.

Cardiac rehab is a supervised program that includes:

- Physical activity

- Education about healthy living, including healthy eating, taking medicine as prescribed, and ways to help you quit smoking

- Counseling to find ways to relieve stress and improve mental health

A team of people may help you through cardiac rehab, including your healthcare team, exercise and nutrition specialists, physical therapists, and counselors or mental-health professionals.

Who Needs Cardiac Rehab

Anyone who has had a heart problem, such as a heart attack, heart failure, or heart surgery, can benefit from cardiac rehab. Studies have found that cardiac rehab helps men and women; people of all ages; and people with mild, moderate, and severe heart problems. But, certain people are less likely to go to or finish a cardiac rehab program. These include:

- **Women.** Studies show that women, especially minority women, are less likely than men to go to or complete a cardiac rehab program. This may be because doctors may be less likely to suggest cardiac rehab to women.

- **Older adults.** Older adults are also less likely to join a cardiac rehab program following a heart problem. They may think they are unable to do the physical activity because of their age, or they may have other conditions that can make exercising harder, such as arthritis.

This makes cardiac rehabilitation especially useful for older adults since it can improve strength and mobility to help make daily tasks easier.

How Does Cardiac Rehab Help?

Cardiac rehab can have many benefits to your health in both the short and long-term, including:

- Strengthening your heart and body after a heart attack

- Relieving symptoms of heart problems, such as chest pain

- Building healthier habits, including getting more physical activity, quitting smoking, and eating a heart-healthy diet. A nutritionist or dietitian may work with you to help you limit foods with unhealthy fats and eat more fruits and vegetables that are high in vitamins, minerals, and fiber.

- Reducing stress

- Improving your mood. People are more likely to feel depressed after a heart attack. Cardiac rehab can help prevent and lessen depression.

- Increasing your energy and strength, making daily activities easier, such as carrying groceries and climbing stairs

- Making you more likely to take your prescribed medicines that help lower your risk for future heart problems

- Preventing future heart problems and death. Studies have found that cardiac rehab decreases the chances you will die in the 5 years following a heart attack or bypass surgery by around 20 to 30 percent.

Where Can You Get It?

Some programs are done in a hospital or rehabilitation center, while some programs can be done in the patient's home. Cardiac rehab may start while you are still in the hospital or right after you leave the hospital.

Cardiac rehab programs usually last about three months but can range anywhere from two to eight months.

Talk to your doctor about a cardiac rehab program. Many insurance plans, including Medicaid and Medicare, cover it but require your doctor to provide a referral for the program.

Section 56.2

Stroke Rehabilitation

This section includes text excerpted from "Recovering from Stroke," Centers for Disease Control and Prevention (CDC), March 27, 2018.

What to Expect after a Stroke

If you have had a stroke, you can make great progress in regaining your independence. However, some problems may continue:

- Paralysis (inability to move some parts of the body), weakness, or both on one side of the body

- Trouble with thinking, awareness, attention, learning, judgment, and memory

- Problems understanding or forming speech

- Trouble controlling or expressing emotions

- Numbness or strange sensations

- Pain in the hands and feet that worsens with movement and temperature changes

- Trouble with chewing and swallowing

- Problems with bladder and bowel control
- Depression

What Does Stroke Rehabilitation Include?

Rehab can include working with speech, physical, and occupational therapists.

- Speech therapy helps people who have problems producing or understanding speech.
- Physical therapy uses exercises to help you relearn movement and coordination skills you may have lost because of the stroke.
- Occupational therapy focuses on improving daily activities, such as eating, drinking, dressing, bathing, reading, and writing.
- Therapy and medicine may help with depression or other mental-health conditions following a stroke. Joining a patient support group may help you adjust to life after a stroke. Talk with your healthcare team about local support groups, or check with an area medical center.

Support from family and friends can also help relieve fear and anxiety following a stroke. Let your loved ones know how you feel and what they can do to help you.

Preventing Another Stroke

If you have had a stroke, you are at high risk for another stroke:

- 1 in 4 strokes each year are recurrent.
- The chance of stroke within 90 days of a transient ischemic attack (TIA) may be as high as 17 percent, with the greatest risk during the first week.

That is why it is important to treat the causes of stroke, including heart disease, high blood pressure, atrial fibrillation (AF) (fast, irregular heartbeat), high cholesterol, and diabetes. Your doctor may prescribe you medicine or tell you to change your diet, exercise, or adopt other healthy lifestyle habits. Surgery may also be helpful in some cases.

Part Seven

Preventing
Cardiovascular Disorders

Chapter 57

Preventing Heart Disease at Any Age

Chapter Contents

Section 57.1

Healthy Body, Happy Heart

This section includes text excerpted from "Healthy Body,
Happy Heart," *NIH News in Health*, National Institutes
of Health (NIH), November 2017.

Every moment of the day, your heart is pumping blood throughout your body. In silent moments, you can hear the thump-thump-thump of its demanding work. Do you take your heart for granted? Most of us will have heart trouble at some point in our lives. Heart disease is the number one killer of women and men in the United States. But, you can take steps now to lower your risk.

"About 1 out of 3 people in America will die of heart disease," says National Institutes of Health (NIH) heart disease expert Dr. David C. Goff, Jr. "And about 6 out of every 10 of us will have a major heart disease event before we die."

Heart disease develops when the blood vessels supplying the heart become clogged with fatty deposits or plaque. After the blood vessels narrow, blood flow to the heart is reduced. That means oxygen and nutrients cannot get to the heart as easily.

Eventually, an area of plaque can break open. This may cause a blood clot to form on the surface of the plaque. A blood clot can block blood flow to the heart. That can cause a heart attack.

A heart attack happens when a vessel supplying the heart is blocked and the heart cannot get enough oxygen, which leads to the death of heart muscle.

The three major risk factors for heart disease have been known since the 1960s: smoking, high blood pressure, and high cholesterol levels. These were identified in the NIH's Framingham Heart Study, a long-term study of people in Framingham, Massachusetts.

"If we could eliminate cigarette smoking, elevated blood pressure, and elevated cholesterol levels, we could eradicate about 9 out of 10 heart attacks in our country," says Dr. Daniel Levy, a heart specialist at the NIH who oversees the Framingham Heart Study currently.

The study has also uncovered other risk factors, including diabetes, obesity, and physical inactivity. Levy's research team is now hunting for genes that may be risk factors for heart disease. By understanding the factors that play a role in heart disease, scientists hope to find new ways to prevent and treat it.

Get Tested

Early heart disease may not cause any symptoms. That is why regular checkups with your doctor are so important. "The sad truth is that the vast majority of us have heart disease, and we do not know it," Goff says.

Blood pressure and cholesterol levels can provide early signs. "People should see their doctor, find out their cholesterol and blood pressure numbers, and if needed, take medication," advises Goff.

There are many other tests to detect heart disease. An electrocardiogram, also called an "EKG" or "ECG," measures electrical activity in your heart. It can show how well your heart is working and pick up signs of a previous heart attack.

Another test called an "echocardiogram" uses sound waves to detect problems. It shows the size, shape, and structures of your heart. It can also measure blood flow through your heart.

Although early heart disease might not cause symptoms, advanced heart disease may cause chest pressure, shortness of breath, or fatigue. Some people may feel light-headed, dizzy, or confused. Tell your doctor if you are experiencing any symptoms.

Make Healthy Choices

Talk with your doctor about your risk of heart disease and what you can do to keep your heart healthy. "The most important things for everyone to do to keep their heart healthy—to keep their entire body healthy—is to eat a healthy diet, get plenty of physical activity, maintain lean body weight, and avoid smoking and exposure to secondhand smoke," Goff says.

Following a heart-healthy eating plan is important for everyone. "When someone puts food on their plate, about half the plate should be fruits and vegetables. About a quarter of the plate should be whole grain. And about a quarter should be lean protein, like lean meat or seafood," says Goff.

If you have high blood pressure, you may want to follow the Dietary Approaches to Stop Hypertension (DASH) diet. This diet emphasizes fruits, vegetables, whole-grain foods, and low-fat dairy products.

Goff also advises, "Avoid foods that have a lot of salt in them. Salt is a major contributor to high blood pressure and risk of heart disease."

Ask Your Doctor

For some people, having a heart attack is the first sign of heart disease. Pain or discomfort in your chest or upper body, a cold sweat, or shortness of breath are all signs of a heart attack.

If you feel any of these signs, get medical help right away. Acting fast can save your life and prevent permanent damage.

Heart disease and heart attacks are major risk factors for cardiac arrest, which is when the heart suddenly stops beating. Blood stops flowing to the brain and other parts of the body. If not treated within minutes, cardiac arrest can lead to death.

Heart disease and heart attacks can also make it harder for your heart's electrical system to work. As a result, an irregular heartbeat, or arrhythmia, can occur. Your heart may beat too fast, too slow, or with an uneven rhythm. A dangerous arrhythmia can lead to cardiac arrest.

Regular checkups help ensure that a doctor will check your heart for problems. Heart disease and arrhythmias can be treated to lower the risk of cardiac arrest.

Be good to your heart. Do not take it for granted. Get tested for heart disease, and follow your doctor's suggestions.

Section 57.2

Preventing Heart Disease: Other Medical Conditions

This section includes text excerpted from "Preventing Heart Disease: Other Medical Conditions," Centers for Disease Control and Prevention (CDC), October 22, 2018.

Check Your Cholesterol

Your healthcare provider should test your blood levels of cholesterol at least once every five years. If you have already been diagnosed with high cholesterol or have a family history of the condition, you may have your cholesterol checked more frequently. Talk with your healthcare team about this simple blood test. If you have high cholesterol, medications and lifestyle changes can help reduce your risk for heart disease.

Control Your Blood Pressure

High blood pressure usually has no symptoms, so be sure to have it checked on a regular basis. Your healthcare team should measure your blood pressure at least once every two years if you have never had high blood pressure or other risk factors for heart disease. If you have been diagnosed with high blood pressure, also called "hypertension," your healthcare team will measure your blood pressure more frequently to ensure you have the condition under control. Talk to your healthcare team about how often you should check your blood pressure. You can check it at a doctors office, at a pharmacy, or at home.

If you have high blood pressure, your healthcare team might recommend some changes in your lifestyle or advise you to lower the sodium in your diet; your doctor may also prescribe medication when necessary to help lower your blood pressure.

Manage Diabetes

If your healthcare provider thinks you have symptoms of diabetes, she or he may recommend that you get tested. If you have diabetes, monitor your blood sugar levels carefully. Talk with your healthcare team about treatment options. Your doctor may recommend certain lifestyle changes to help keep your blood sugar under control—those actions will help reduce your risk for heart disease.

Take Your Medicine

If you take medication to treat high cholesterol, high blood pressure, or diabetes, follow your doctor's instructions carefully. Always ask questions if you do not understand something. Never stop taking your medication without talking to your doctor, nurse, or pharmacist.

Talk with Your Healthcare Team

You and your healthcare team can work together to prevent or treat the medical conditions that lead to heart disease. Discuss your treatment plan regularly, and bring a list of questions to your appointments.

If you have already had a heart attack, your healthcare team will work with you to prevent another heart attack. Your treatment plan may include medications or surgery and lifestyle changes to reduce your risk. Be sure to take your medications as directed and follow your doctor's instructions.

Chapter 58

How to Prevent High Blood Pressure

About one in three adults in the United States has high blood pressure or hypertension, but many do not realize it. High blood pressure usually has no warning signs, yet it can lead to life-threatening conditions, such as heart attack or stroke. The good news is that you can often prevent or treat high blood pressure. Early diagnosis and simple, healthy changes can keep high blood pressure from seriously damaging your health.

How Can I Prevent High Blood Pressure?

You can help prevent high blood pressure by having a healthy lifestyle. This includes:

- **Eating a healthy diet.** To help manage your blood pressure, you should limit the amount of sodium (salt) that you eat, and increase the amount of potassium in your diet. It is also important to eat foods that are lower in fat, as well as plenty of fruits, vegetables, and whole grains. The Dietary Approaches to Stop Hypertension (DASH) diet is an example of an eating plan that can help you to lower your blood pressure.

This chapter includes text excerpted from "How to Prevent High Blood Pressure," MedlinePlus, National Institutes of Health (NIH), February 13, 2019.

- **Getting regular exercise.** Exercise can help you maintain a healthy weight and lower your blood pressure. You should try to get moderate-intensity aerobic exercise at least 2 and a half hours per week, or vigorous-intensity aerobic exercise for 1 hour and 15 minutes per week. Aerobic exercise, such as brisk walking, is an exercise in which your heart beats harder and you use more oxygen than usual.

- **Being at a healthy weight.** Being overweight or obese increases your risk for high blood pressure. Maintaining a healthy weight can help you control high blood pressure and reduce your risk for other health problems.

- **Limiting alcohol.** Drinking too much alcohol can raise your blood pressure. It also adds extra calories, which may cause weight gain. Men should have no more than two drinks per day, and women only one.

- **Not smoking.** Cigarette smoking raises your blood pressure and puts you at higher risk for heart attack and stroke. If you do not smoke, do not start. If you do smoke, talk to your healthcare provider for help in finding the best way for you to quit.

- **Managing stress.** Learning how to relax and manage stress can improve your emotional and physical health and lower high blood pressure. Stress management techniques include exercising, listening to music, focusing on something calm or peaceful, and meditating.

If you already have high blood pressure, it is important to prevent it from getting worse or causing complications. You should get regular medical care and follow your prescribed treatment plan. Your plan will include healthy lifestyle habit recommendations and possibly medicines.

Chapter 59

Treating High Cholesterol

High blood cholesterol is treated with heart-healthy lifestyle changes and medicines to control or lower your high blood cholesterol. Lipoprotein apheresis (LA) is a procedure that can be used to treat familial hypercholesterolemia (FH).

Heart-Healthy Lifestyle Changes

To help you lower or control your high blood cholesterol, your doctor may recommend that you adopt the following lifelong heart-healthy lifestyle changes:

- **Heart-healthy eating.** As recommended in the 2015 to 2020 *Dietary Guidelines for Americans*, heart-healthy eating includes limiting the amount of saturated and trans fats that you eat. It also includes consuming fish high in omega-3 fatty acids and vegetable oils that can help lower blood cholesterol levels and the risk of cardiovascular disease (CVD). The Therapeutic Lifestyle Changes (TLC) diet and the Dietary Approaches to Stop Hypertension (DASH) eating plan can help you lower your "bad" low-density lipoprotein (LDL) cholesterol. These plans also encourage eating whole grains, fruits, and vegetables rather than refined carbohydrates, such as sugar. Talk to your doctor about other nutritional changes that you can make.

This chapter includes text excerpted from "High Blood Cholesterol," National Heart, Lung, and Blood Institute (NHLBI), January 30, 2019.

- **Being physically active.** There are many health benefits to being physically active and getting the recommended amount of physical activity each week. Studies have shown that physical activity can lower LDL cholesterol and triglycerides and increase "good" high-density lipoprotein (HDL) cholesterol. Before starting any exercise program, ask your doctor what level of physical activity is right for you.

- **Aiming for a healthy weight.** If you have high blood cholesterol and are overweight or obese, you can improve your health by aiming for a healthy weight. Research has shown that adults that are overweight or obese can reduce LDL cholesterol and increase HDL cholesterol by losing only 3 to 5 percent of their weight. Achieving 5 to 10 percent weight loss in 6 months is recommended.

- **Managing stress.** Research has shown that chronic stress can sometimes increase LDL cholesterol levels and decrease HDL cholesterol levels.

- **Quitting smoking.** For free help and support to quit smoking, you may call the National Cancer Institute's (NCI) Smoking Quitline at 877-448-7848.

Medicines

If you are unable to lower or control your high blood cholesterol levels with lifestyle changes alone, your doctor may prescribe medicine.

- **Statins** inhibit cholesterol synthesis in the liver by blocking the protein HMG-CoA reductase from making cholesterol. Liver cells try to compensate for the low cholesterol by synthesizing more LDL receptors on the cell surface to increase LDL uptake from the blood. Statins are the most common medicine used to treat high blood cholesterol in people who are 10 years of age or older. In certain cases, doctors may prescribe statins in people younger than 10 years of age.

- **PCSK9 inhibitors** lower LDL cholesterol by decreasing the destruction of LDL receptor in the liver, which helps remove and clear LDL cholesterol from the blood.

- **Bile acid sequestrants** block the reabsorption of bile acids and increase conversion of cholesterol to bile acids. This has the effect of lowering plasma cholesterol levels.

- **Ezetimibe** blocks dietary cholesterol from being absorbed in the intestine.

- **Fibrates** promote the removal of very low-density lipoprotein (VLDL) cholesterol, part of non-HDL.

- **Lomitapide** blocks the liver from releasing VLDL cholesterol into the blood. It is used only in patients who have familial hypercholesterolemia.

- **Mipomersen** decreases levels of non-HDL cholesterol in the blood. It is used only in patients who have familial hypercholesterolemia.

- **Niacin (nicotinic acid)** decreases LDL cholesterol and triglycerides and raises HDL cholesterol.

If your doctor prescribes medicines as part of your treatment plan, be sure to continue your healthy lifestyle changes. The combination of the medicines and the heart-healthy lifestyle changes helps to lower and control your high blood cholesterol. Talk to your doctor about possible side effects to help decide which medicine is best for you.

Lipoprotein Apheresis

Some patients with familial hypercholesterolemia may benefit from lipoprotein apheresis to lower their blood cholesterol levels. Lipoprotein apheresis is a dialysis-like process, in which LDL cholesterol is removed from the blood by a filtering machine, and the remainder of the blood is returned to the patient.

Chapter 60

Steps to Control Diabetes

Type 2 diabetes prevention is proven, possible, and powerful. Taking small steps, such as eating less and moving more to lose weight, can help you prevent or delay type 2 diabetes and related health problems. The information below is based on the National Institutes of Health (NIH)-sponsored Diabetes Prevention Program (DPP) research study, which showed that people could prevent or delay type 2 diabetes even if they were at high risk for the disease. Follow these steps to get started on your game plan.

Set a Weight Loss Goal

If you are overweight, the keys to preventing type 2 diabetes are to lose weight by choosing foods and drinks that are lower in calories, and to be more active. Set a weight-loss goal that you can reach. Try to lose at least 5 to 10 percent of your current weight within 6 months. For example, if you weigh 200 pounds, a 10 percent weight-loss goal means that you will try to lose 20 pounds. A good short-term goal is to lose 1 to 2 pounds per week.

Calculate your body mass index (BMI) by using the National Heart, Lung, and Blood Institute's (NHLBI) online BMI calculator to learn whether you are overweight.

This chapter includes text excerpted from "Your Game Plan to Prevent Type 2 Diabetes," National Institute of Diabetes and Digestive and Kidney Diseases (NIDDK), February 2017.

Use table 60.1 to find your current weight in the first column to see how much weight you would need to lose for a 5-, 7-, or 10-percent weight loss. For example, if you weigh 200 pounds and want to lose 5 percent of your current weight, then you would need to lose 10 pounds.

Table 60.1. Finding Your Weight-Loss Goal

Your Current Weight in Pounds	Pounds to Lose 5 Percent of Your Weight	Pounds to Lose 7 Percent of Your Weight	Pounds to Lose 10 Percent of Your Weight
150	8	11	15
175	9	12	18
200	10	14	20
225	11	16	23
250	13	18	25
275	14	19	28
300	15	21	30
325	16	23	33
350	18	25	35

Use the table below to learn how to calculate your exact weight-loss goal. In this example, the goal is for a 240-pound person to lose 5 percent of her or his weight.

Table 60.2. Calculating Your Weight-Loss Goal

Step Number	Action	Result
Step 1	Weigh yourself to get your current weight.	"My weight is 240 pounds."
Step 2	Multiply your weight by the percent you want to lose.	"I want to lose 5 percent of my weight." 240 pounds (current weight) x .05 (5 percent weight loss) 12 pounds to lose
Step 3	Subtract the answer in Step 2 from your current weight.	240 pounds (current weight) - 12 pounds (amount to lose) 228 pounds (weight-loss goal)

As shown in the table above, a 240-pound person who wants to lose 5 percent of her or his weight would lose 12 pounds and weigh 228 pounds.

Follow a Healthy Eating Plan for Weight Loss

Research shows that you can prevent or delay type 2 diabetes by losing weight by following a low-fat, reduced-calorie eating plan and by being more active. Following an eating plan can help you reach your weight-loss goal. There are many ways to do this. Remember that the key to losing weight and preventing type 2 diabetes is to make lifelong changes that work for you. Many popular weight-loss plans promise "quick fixes" and have not been proven to work long-term or to prevent type 2 diabetes.

The four most important steps to eating healthy for weight loss are:

- Eat smaller portions than you currently eat of foods that are high in calories, fat, and sugar.

- Eat healthier foods in place of less-healthy choices.

- Choose foods with less *trans*-fat, saturated fat, and added sugars.

- Drink water instead of drinks with sugar, such as soda, sports drinks, and fruit juice.

Pay Attention to Portion Sizes

Using the plate method can help you manage your portion sizes. Fill half of your plate with fruits and vegetables. Fill one quarter with a lean protein, such as chicken or turkey without the skin, or beans. Fill one quarter with a whole grain, such as brown rice or whole-wheat pasta.

You can use everyday objects or your hand to judge the size of a portion. For example:

- One serving of meat or poultry is about the size of the palm of your hand or a deck of cards.

- One three-ounce serving of fish is the size of a checkbook.

- One serving of cheese is equivalent to six die.

- Half of a cup of cooked rice or pasta is equivalent to a rounded handful or a tennis ball.

- Two tablespoons of peanut butter is equivalent to a ping-pong ball.

Recommended Daily Calories and Fat Grams

Table 60.3 below shows how many calories and fat grams you should eat each day in order to lose weight. Your needs may be different, but these are good starting points. The amounts are based on the eating patterns used in the Diabetes Prevention Program (DPP) research study.

You can also use the body weight planner from the National Institute of Diabetes and Digestive and Kidney Diseases (NIDDK) to make a calorie and activity plan that can help you reach your weight-loss goals within a set time frame.

Table 60.3. Intake of Calories and Fat Grams per Day

Current Weight	Calories Per Day*	Fat Grams Per Day
120 to 170 pounds	1,200	33
175 to 215 pounds	1,500	42
220 to 245 pounds	1,800	50
250 to 300 pounds	2,000	55

* Eating less than 1,200 calories a day is not advised.
(Source: Diabetes Prevention Program (DPP) Lifestyle Manual of Operations.)

How to Read the Food Label

When making food choices, use the nutrition facts label on food packages to see how many calories and fat grams are in the foods you choose.

Eat Foods from Each Food Group

Your eating plan should include a variety of foods from each food group. Use the below eating plan chart from the U.S. Department of Agriculture (USDA) to learn more about which foods to eat.

Eating tips for weight loss:

- Try to get as close as possible to your daily calorie and fat gram goals.

- Eat meals and snacks at about the same time each day to keep from getting too hungry.

- Eat your meals on smaller plates, and put your drinks in smaller glasses to make portions look bigger. Do not worry about cleaning your plate.

- Eat slowly. It takes 20 minutes for your stomach to send a signal to your brain that you are full.

- Limit alcoholic beverages. If you drink alcohol, choose a light beer or wine instead of mixed drinks.

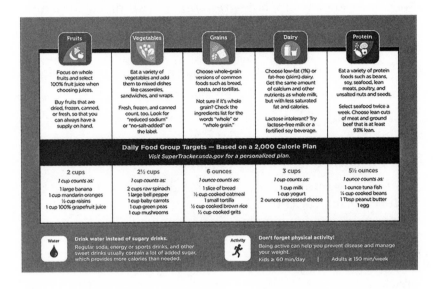

Figure 60.1. *Eating Plan Chart* (Source: U.S. Department of Agriculture (USDA).)

Tips for eating at home:

- Use low-fat, light, or fat-free sour cream, cream cheese, mayonnaise, cheese, and salad dressing.

- Cook with a mix of spices instead of salt.

- Refrigerate extra portions of food right after cooking so that you are less tempted to go back for seconds.

- Freeze extra portions of food to have meals ready on days when you are too busy or too tired to cook.

- Share a bowl of fruit with family and friends instead of cookies or chips.

- Eat fat-free or low-fat frozen yogurt or sherbet instead of ice cream.

Tips for eating at work or on the run:

- Take your lunch to work or meetings to stay in charge of what you eat.

- Pack your lunch the night before so it is ready to go when you are.

- Make a sandwich on whole-grain bread with turkey or lean beef.

- Use mustard or hummus instead of mayonnaise as a sandwich spread.

- Add carrots and celery sticks to your lunch instead of chips.

- Drink water instead of juice or regular soda.

- Pack a snack, such as an apple or fat-free yogurt, to eat if you get hungry.

Tips for eating in-between meals:

- Eat fruits, vegetables, or a small handful of unsalted nuts instead of chips or candy.

- To reduce calories, drink water instead of regular soda, sports drinks, or juice.

- Chew sugar-free gum between meals to help reduce your urge to snack.

Tips for food shopping:

- Make a list of what you need before going to the store, and stick to your list.

- Eat a healthy snack or meal before shopping for food. Do not shop on an empty stomach.

- Compare nutrition facts on food labels, and choose foods that are lower in calories, saturated fat, *trans* fats, and sodium.

- Buy a new fruit or vegetable to try each time you go to the store. Use it to add flavor and color to soups, stews, or salads.

- Buy reduced-fat or light versions of mayonnaise, cheese, and salad dressing.

- Buy fat-free, low-fat, or soy milk instead of whole milk.

Tips for eating when dining out:

- When possible, plan ahead by looking at the menu and nutrition information online.

- Take time when reading the menu to choose healthier meal options.

- Order from a menu instead of a buffet, where it is harder to control how much you eat.

- Ask about the portion size, amount of fat, and the number of calories in menu items when deciding what to order.

- Ask to have your meal prepared with less fat, salt, or added sugars.

- Choose foods that are baked, steamed, grilled, or broiled instead of fried.

- Choose healthier foods at fast food restaurants. Eat grilled chicken (without the skin) instead of a cheeseburger.

- Order a salad for starters, and share your main dish with a friend or have the other half wrapped to go.

- Order sauces, salad dressing, or spreads on the side to reduce the amount used on your meal.

- Ask to have the amount you do not want to eat put in a take-home container.

- It is okay to have a small portion of high-calorie foods once in a while. Just keep your weight-loss goal in mind.

Move More

When you move more every day, you will burn more calories. This can help you reach your weight-loss goal and keep the weight off. Even if you do not lose weight, being more active may help you prevent or delay type 2 diabetes.

Find ways to be active for at least 30 minutes, 5 days a week. Walking is recommended for most people. Check with your healthcare team about other exercise programs.

Use these tips to get started, and keep moving:

- **Dress to move.** Wear walking shoes that fit your feet and provide comfort and support. Your clothes should allow you to move and should keep you dry and comfortable. Look for fabrics that take sweat away from your skin to keep you cool.

- **Start slowly.** Start by taking a 5 to 10-minute walk (or doing another activity that you like) on most days of the week. Slowly, add more time until you reach at least 30 minutes of moderate-intensity activity 5 days a week. Moderate-intensity activity will increase your heart rate and breathing. To check your intensity, use the talk test: a person doing moderate-intensity activity is able to talk but not sing.

- **Add more movement to your day.** There are many ways you can add more movement to your day. If you have a dog, take your dog for a brisk walk in the morning or evening. When going shopping, park further away from the store's entrance to increase your walk time. If you ride the bus, get off one stop early and walk the rest of the way if it is safe.

- **Try to sit less in your day.** Get up every hour and move. When you watch TV, walk or dance around the room, march in place, or stretch.

- **Move more at work.** Take a "movement break" during the day. Go for a walk during lunchtime. Deliver a message in person to a coworker instead of sending an e-mail. Walk around your workplace while talking on the telephone. Take the stairs instead of the elevator to your workplace. Use the alarm on your phone, watch, or other devices to remind you to take "movement breaks."

- **Count your steps.** You may be surprised to learn how much walking you already do every day. Use a pedometer or other wearable device to keep track of your steps. A pedometer is a gadget that counts the number of steps you take. Work up to 7,000 to 10,000 steps per day.

- **Keep your muscles strong.** Do activities to strengthen your muscles, such as lifting weights or using resistance bands, two or more days a week.

- **Stretch it out.** If your body aches or is sore, you are less likely to move more. To reduce stiff or sore muscles or joints, consider stretching after being active. Do not bounce when you stretch. Perform slow movements and stretch only as far as you feel comfortable.

- **Make it social.** When you bring other people into your activities, you are more likely to stick to your plan. Make walking "dates" with friends or family members throughout the week. For family fun, play soccer, basketball, or tag with your children. Take a class at a local gym or recreation center to be active with other people. Start a walking group with your neighbors, at work, or where you worship.

- **Have fun.** Being active does not have to be boring or painful. Turn up the music and dance while cleaning the house. Go dancing with friends and family members. Play sports with your kids or grandkids. Try swimming, biking, walking, jogging, or any activity that you enjoy that gets you moving. Find different ways to be active so you would not get bored.

- **Keep at it.** Reward yourself with nonfood treats, such as watching a movie, to celebrate your small successes. The longer you keep at it, the better you will feel. Making changes is never easy, but being more active is one small step toward a big reward: a healthier life.

Track Your Progress

Research shows that people who keep track of their weight and activity reach their goals more often than those who do not. Weigh yourself at least once a week. Keep track of what you eat and drink, how many minutes of activity you get each day, and your weight.

The examples below show how to record your daily activity and food intake.

Table 60.4. Recording Your Daily Activity

Daily Activity	
Type of Activity	**Minutes**
Walking	10
Stationary bike	20
Daily Total	30
Daily Steps	
Number of Steps Taken	7,450

Table 60.5. Daily Food and Drink Intake

Time	Amount	Food Item	Calories	Fat Grams
8:00 a.m.	1 cup	Oatmeal	160	3.5
	½ cup	Strawberries	25	0
	6 oz.	Light yogurt	90	0
	1 cup	Tea with sugar-free sweetener	0	0
11:00 a.m.	10	Almonds	70	6

Table 60.5. Continued

Time	Amount	Food Item	Calories	Fat Grams
12:30 p.m.	2 slices	Wheat bread	160	2
	4 oz.	Ham	125	3
	2 tsp.	Mustard	5	0
	1 oz. slice	Cheese	110	9
	1 oz.	Potato chips	160	10
	10	Cherry tomatoes	30	0
4:00 p.m.	4 squares	Graham crackers	120	3
	1 tbsp.	Peanut butter	95	8
6:30 p.m.	3 oz. skinless	Chicken breast	140	3
	1 cup	Cooked broccoli	55	0
	½ cup	Brown rice	110	1
	1 cup	Pineapple chunks	80	0
	1 cup	Nonfat milk	90	0.5
Daily Total			1,625 calories	49.0 grams

You can also download an app to your smartphone or tablet that helps you track what you eat, your activity, and your weight.

Talk with Your Healthcare Team

People are usually more successful at weight loss and being more active if they have regular contact and support from health professionals. Talk with your healthcare team about the changes you want to make to prevent type 2 diabetes.

- Tell your healthcare team about your progress with weight loss and activity, and if you are having trouble sticking with your plan.

- Ask your healthcare team if you should take a medicine called "metformin." Research shows that taking metformin can help prevent or delay type 2 diabetes. It is most helpful in younger people who are overweight and have prediabetes, and for women that have had gestational diabetes, a type of diabetes that develops during pregnancy.

- Contact your health insurance provider to learn what benefits are offered for weight-loss programs, diabetes-prevention programs, nutrition counseling, or fitness programs.

  - Some people with Medicare may be eligible for intensive behavioral therapy for obesity. This service includes up to one year of in-person weight-loss counseling visits with a healthcare professional.

If you smoke or use other tobacco products, you should stop. Even though quitting smoking can make it hard to manage your weight, it is a very important step to improve your health. Ask your healthcare team to help you create a plan for quitting. You can start by calling the National Quitline at 800-784-8669.

Get Support for Changing Your Lifestyle

Making big changes in your life is hard. You do not have to change everything at once. You can make it easier by taking these steps:

- Think about what is important to your health. What are you willing and able to do? Example: I know that being more active can help me lose some weight.

- Decide what your goals are. Choose one goal to work on first. Example: I want to see if I can work up to getting 30 minutes of walking in a day on at least 5 days of the week.

- Decide what steps will help you reach your goal.

- Pick one step to try this week.

Table 60.6. Steps to Reach Your Goal with Examples

Steps to Reach Your Goal	Example
Set a time frame and deadline for making lifestyle changes.	I will start this week by walking for 10 minutes at lunchtime.
Plan what you need to get ready.	I need to take walking shoes to work.
Think about what might prevent you from reaching your goals.	In bad weather, I would not want to walk outside. I can walk inside instead.
Decide how you will reward yourself when you do what you have planned.	If I stick with my plans this week, I will watch a movie.

Add one or two healthy changes every week. Do not get upset with yourself if you have a setback or lose control of your plan. Everyone has slips. Injury, illness, or being too busy can make it hard to stick to your plan. It is not easy to make lifelong changes in what you eat and drink and in how often you are active. The important thing is to review your game plan and get back on track as soon as possible.

You Do Not Have to Do It Alone

Find family and friends who will support and encourage you in preventing type 2 diabetes. Join with a neighbor or coworker in changing your lifestyle. Talk with your healthcare team to learn about programs that may help, such as the National Diabetes Prevention Program (DPP).

The National Diabetes Prevention Program, led by the Centers for Disease Control and Prevention (CDC), the National DPP offers lifestyle change programs based on the DPP research study. Participants work with a lifestyle coach in a live group or online setting to receive a 1-year lifestyle change program that includes 16 core sessions (usually 1 per week) and 6 postcore sessions (1 per month). Find a program near you by visiting the CDC's website.

- Find a registered dietitian nutritionist (RDN) near you with the Academy of Nutrition and Dietetics' national referral service online.

- Find a diabetes educator near you with the online search tool offered by the American Association of Diabetes Educators (AADE).

- Local hospitals, health departments, libraries, senior centers, or faith-based organizations may offer additional programs or seminars about type 2 diabetes prevention.

Chapter 61

Heart-Healthy Lifestyle Changes

Heart-Healthy Eating

Heart-healthy eating involves consuming vegetables, fruits, whole grains, fat-free or low-fat dairy products, fish, lean meats, poultry, eggs, nuts, seeds, soy products, legumes, and vegetable oils (except coconut and palm oils). Also, it limits sodium, saturated and *trans* fats, added sugars, and alcohol.

Your doctor may recommend the heart-healthy Dietary Approaches to Stop Hypertension (DASH) eating plan because it has been proven to lower blood pressure and "bad" low-density lipoprotein (LDL) cholesterol in the blood.

Foods to Eat

The following foods are the foundation of a heart-healthy diet:

- **Vegetables,** such as greens (spinach, collard greens, kale), broccoli, cabbage, and carrots

This chapter contains text excerpted from the following sources: Text beginning with the heading "Heart-Healthy Eating" is excerpted from "Heart-Healthy Lifestyle Changes," National Heart, Lung, and Blood Institute (NHLBI), March 15, 2019. Text under the heading "Quitting Smoking" is excerpted from "Smoking and Your Heart," National Heart, Lung, and Blood Institute (NHLBI), March 12, 2013. Reviewed May 2019.

- **Fruits,** such as apples, bananas, oranges, pears, grapes, and prunes

- Whole **grains,** such as plain oatmeal, brown rice, and whole-grain bread or tortillas

- Fat-free or low-fat **dairy** foods, such as milk, cheese, or yogurt

- **Protein**-rich foods:

  - Fish high in omega-3 fatty acids, such as salmon, tuna, and trout, about 8 ounces a week

  - Lean meats, such as 95 percent lean ground beef or pork tenderloin

  - Poultry, such as skinless chicken or turkey

  - Eggs

  - Nuts, seeds, and soy products

  - Legumes, such as kidney beans, lentils, chickpeas, black-eyed peas, and lima beans

- Oils and foods containing high levels of monounsaturated and polyunsaturated fats can help lower blood cholesterol levels and the risk of cardiovascular disease (CVD). Some sources of these oils are:

  - Canola, corn, olive, safflower, sesame, sunflower, and soybean oils

  - Nuts, such as walnuts, almonds, and pine nuts

  - Nut and seed butter

  - Salmon and trout

  - Seeds, such as sesame, sunflower, pumpkin, or flax

  - Avocados

  - Tofu

How Much Should You Eat?

You should eat the right amount of calories for your body, which will vary based on your sex, age, and physical activity level. You can visit the U.S. Department of Health and Human Services (HHS) and U.S. Department of Agriculture (USDA) 2015–2020 *Dietary Guidelines for Americans* online for more information about healthy eating and to read about their recommendations for the following healthy eating patterns.

Nutrients to Limit

A heart-healthy diet limits sodium, saturated, and *trans* fats, added sugars, and alcohol.

Sodium

Adults and children over the age of 14 should eat less than 2,300 mg of sodium a day. Children younger than 14 years of age may need to eat even less sodium each day based on their sex and age. If you have high blood pressure, you may need to restrict your sodium intake even more. Talk to your doctor or healthcare provider about what amount of sodium is right for you or your child.

Try these shopping and cooking tips to help you choose and prepare foods that are lower in sodium.

- Read food labels, and choose products that have less sodium for the same serving size.

- Choose low-sodium, reduced sodium, or no-salt-added products.

- Choose fresh, frozen, or no-salt-added foods instead of preseasoned, sauce-marinated, brined, or processed meats, poultry, and vegetables.

- Eat at home more often, so you can cook food from scratch, which will allow you to control the amount of sodium in your meals.

- When cooking, limit your use of premade sauces, mixes, and "instant" products, such as rice, noodles, and ready-made pasta.

- Flavor foods with herbs and spices instead of salt.

Saturated and Trans Fats

When you follow a heart-healthy eating plan, you should:

- Eat less than ten percent of your daily calories from saturated fats found naturally in foods that come from animals and some plants.

- Limit intake of *trans* fats to as low as possible by limiting foods that contain high amounts of *trans* fats.

The following are examples of foods that are high in saturated or *trans* fats:

Saturated fats are found in high amounts in fatty cuts of meat, poultry with skin, whole-milk dairy foods, butter, lard, and coconut and palm oils.

Trans fats are found in high amounts in foods made with partially hydrogenated oils, such as some desserts, microwave popcorn, frozen pizza, stick margarine, and coffee creamers.

To help you limit your intake of saturated fats and *trans* fats:

- Read the nutrition labels, and replace foods high in saturated fats with leaner, lower-fat animal products or vegetable oils, such as olive or canola oil instead of butter. Foods that are higher in saturated fats, such as fatty meats and high-fat dairy products, tend to be higher in dietary cholesterol that should also be limited.

- Read the nutrition labels, and choose foods that do not contain *trans* fats. Some *trans* fats naturally occur in very small amounts in dairy products and meats. Foods containing these very low levels of natural *trans* fats do not need to be eliminated from your diet because they have other important nutrients.

Added Sugars

When you follow a heart-healthy eating plan, you should limit the number of calories you consume each day from added sugars. Because added sugars do not provide essential nutrients and are extra calories, limiting them can help you choose nutrient-rich foods and stay within your daily calorie limit.

Some foods, such as fruit, contain natural sugars. Added sugars do not occur naturally in foods but instead, are used to sweeten foods and drinks. Some examples of added sugars include brown sugar, corn syrup, dextrose, fructose, glucose, high-fructose corn syrup (HFCS), raw sugar, and sucrose.

In the United States, sweetened drinks, snacks, and sweets are the major sources of added sugars. Sweetened drinks account for about half of all added sugars consumed. The following are examples of foods and drinks with added sugars.

- **Sweetened drinks** include soft drinks or sodas, fruit drinks, sweetened coffee and tea, energy drinks, alcoholic drinks, and flavored waters.

- **Snacks** and sweets include grain-based desserts, such as cakes, pies, cookies, brownies, doughnuts; dairy desserts, such as ice cream, frozen desserts, and pudding; candies; sugars; jams; syrups; and sweet toppings.

To help you reduce the amount of added sugars in your diet:

- Choose unsweetened or whole fruits for snacks or dessert.

- Choose drinks without added sugar, such as water, low-fat or fat-free milk, or 100 percent fruit or vegetable juice.

- Limit intake of sweetened drinks, snacks, and desserts by eating them less often and in smaller amounts.

Alcohol

If you drink alcohol, you should limit your intake. Men should have no more than two alcoholic drinks per day. Women should have no more than one alcoholic drink per day. One drink is:

- 12 ounces of regular beer (5 percent alcohol)

- 5 ounces of wine (12 percent alcohol)

- 1½ ounces of 80-proof liquor (40 percent alcohol)

Talk to your doctor about how much alcohol you drink. Your doctor may recommend that you reduce the amount of alcohol you drink or that you stop drinking alcohol. Too much alcohol can:

- Raise your blood pressure and levels of triglyceride fats in your blood

- Add calories to your daily diet and possibly cause you to gain weight

- Worsen heart failure in some patients

- Contribute to heart failure in some people with cardiomyopathy

If you do not drink, you should not start drinking. You should not drink if you are pregnant; under the age of 21; taking certain medicines; or have certain medical conditions, including heart failure. It is important for people with heart failure to take in the correct amounts and types of liquids because too much liquid can worsen heart failure.

Remember that alcoholic drinks do contain calories and contribute to your daily calorie limits. The number of calories will vary by the type of alcoholic drink.

Aiming for a Healthy Weight

A healthy weight for adults is usually when your body mass index (BMI) is between 18.5 and 24.9. To figure out your BMI, use the National Heart, Lung, and Blood Institute's (NHLBI) online BMI calculator.

Always talk to your doctor or healthcare provider about what BMI is right for you. Talk to your child's doctor to determine if your growing child is a healthy weight because her or his BMI should be compared to growth charts specific for their age and sex. Following a heart-healthy eating plan and being physically active are some ways to help you achieve and maintain a healthy weight.

Health Risks of Being Overweight or Obese

The more body fat that you have and the more you weigh, the more likely you are to develop ischemic heart disease, high blood pressure, type 2 diabetes, breathing problems, and certain cancers.

Measuring Waist Circumference

If you are overweight or obese, your doctor may measure your waist circumference to help determine your risk of developing other health conditions. To correctly measure your waist circumference, stand and place a tape measure around your middle, above your hip bones. Measure your waist just after you breathe out.

If most of your fat is around your waist rather than at your hips, you are at a higher risk for heart disease and type 2 diabetes. This risk may be high with a waist circumference that is more than 35 inches for women or more than 40 inches for men.

Benefits of Maintaining a Healthy Weight

If you are overweight or obese, try to lose weight. Health professionals recommend losing 5 to 10 percent of your initial weight over the course of about 6 months. Even before you reach this goal, a loss of just 3 to 5 percent of your current weight can lower triglycerides and glucose levels in your blood, as well as your risk of developing type 2 diabetes. Losing more than 3 to 5 percent of your weight can improve blood pressure readings, lower "bad" LDL cholesterol, and increase "good" HDL cholesterol.

Managing Stress

Research suggests that an emotionally upsetting event—particularly one involving anger—can serve as a trigger for a heart attack or angina in some people. Stress can contribute to high blood pressure and other cardiovascular risks. Some of the ways people cope with stress—drinking alcohol, abusing other substances, smoking, or overeating—are not healthy ways to manage stress.

Learning how to manage stress and cope with problems can improve your emotional and physical health. Consider healthy stress-reducing activities such as:

- Visiting a qualified mental-healthcare provider
- Participating in a stress management program
- Practicing meditation
- Being physically active
- Trying relaxation therapy
- Talking with friends, family, and community or religious support systems

Physical Activity

Routine physical activity and reduction in sedentary lifestyle can improve physical fitness; lower many heart disease risk factors, such as LDL cholesterol levels, increase HDL cholesterol levels; control high blood pressure; and help you lose excess weight. Physical activity also can lower your risk for type 2 diabetes.

Everyone should try to participate in moderate-intensity aerobic exercise at least 2 hours and 30 minutes per week, or vigorous aerobic exercise for 1 hour and 15 minutes per week. Aerobic exercise, such as brisk walking, is an exercise in which your heart beats faster and you use more oxygen than usual. The more active you are, the more you will benefit. Participate in aerobic exercise for at least 10 minutes at a time spread throughout the week.

Talk to your doctor before you start a exercise plan. Ask your doctor how much and what kinds of physical activity are safe for you.

Another way you can begin to increase your activity level is by reducing how long you sit at a given time. People who sit for long periods of time have been found to have higher rates of heart disease, diabetes, and death. Reducing sedentary behavior by breaking up how long you sit will benefit your overall health.

Quitting Smoking

One of the best ways to reduce your risk of coronary heart disease is to avoid tobacco smoke. Do not ever start smoking. If you already smoke, quit. No matter how much or how long you have smoked, quitting will benefit you.

Also, try to avoid secondhand smoke. Do not go to places where smoking is allowed. Ask friends and family members to not smoke in the house and car.

Quitting smoking will benefit your heart and blood vessels. For example:

- Among persons diagnosed with coronary heart disease, quitting smoking greatly reduces the risk of recurrent heart attack and cardiovascular death. In many studies, this reduction in risk has been 50 percent or more.

- Heart disease risk associated with smoking begins to decrease soon after you quit, and for many people, it continues to decrease over time.

- Your risk of atherosclerosis and blood clots related to smoking declines over time after you quit smoking.

Quitting smoking can lower your risk of heart disease as much as, or more than, common medicines used to lower heart disease risk, including aspirin, statins, beta-blockers, and ACE inhibitors.

Strategies to Quit Smoking

Quitting smoking is possible, but it can be hard. Millions of people have successfully quit smoking and remain nonsmokers. Surveys of current adult smokers find that 70 percent say they want to quit.

There are a few ways to quit smoking, including quitting all at once (going "cold turkey") or slowly cutting back your number of cigarettes before quitting completely. Use the method that works best for you. Below are some strategies to help you quit.

Get Ready to Quit

If you want to quit smoking, try to get motivated. Make a list of your reasons for wanting to quit. Write a contract to yourself that outlines your plan for quitting.

If you have tried to quit smoking in the past, think about those attempts. What helped you during that time, and what made it harder?

Know what triggers you to smoke. For example, do you smoke after a meal, while driving, or when you have stressed? Develop a plan to handle each trigger.

Get Support

Set a quit date and let those close to you know about it. Ask your family and friends for support in your effort to quit smoking.

You also can get support from hotlines and websites. Examples include 800-QUIT-NOW (800-784-8669) and www.smokefree.gov. These resources can help you set up a plan for quitting smoking.

Get Medicine and Use It Correctly

Talk with your doctor and pharmacist about medicines and over-the-counter products that can help you quit smoking. These medicines and products are helpful for many people.

You can buy nicotine gum, patches, and lozenges from a drug store. Other medicines that can help you quit smoking are available by prescription.

Learn New Skills and Behaviors

Try new activities to replace smoking. For example, instead of smoking after a meal, take a brisk walk in your neighborhood or around your office building. Try to be physically active regularly.

Take up knitting, carpentry, or other hobbies and activities that keep your hands busy. Try to avoid other people who smoke. Ask those you cannot avoid to respect your efforts to stop smoking and not smoke around you.

Remove cigarettes, ashtrays, and lighters from your home, office, and car. Do not smoke at all—not even one puff. Also, try to avoid alcohol and caffeine. (People who drink alcohol are more likely to start smoking again after quitting.)

Be Prepared for Withdrawal and Relapse

Be prepared for the challenge of withdrawal. Withdrawal symptoms often lessen after only one or two weeks of not smoking, and each urge to smoke lasts only a few minutes.

You can take steps to cope with withdrawal symptoms. If you feel like smoking, wait a few minutes for the urge to pass. Remind yourself of the benefits of quitting. Do not get overwhelmed—take tasks one step at a time.

If you relapse (slip and smoke after you have quit), consider what caused the slip. Were you stressed out or unprepared for a situation that you associate with smoking? Make a plan to avoid or handle this situation in the future.

Getting frustrated with your slip will only make it harder to quit in the future. Accept that you slipped, learn from the slip, and recommit to quit smoking.

If you start smoking regularly again, do not get discouraged. Instead, find out what you need to do to get back on track so you can meet your goals. Set a new quit date, and ask your family and friends to help you. Most people who smoke make repeated attempts to quit before doing so successfully.

Many smokers gain weight after they quit, but the average weight gain is 10 pounds or less. You can control weight gain by following a heart-healthy eating plan and being physically active. Remember the bright side—food smells and tastes better if you are not smoking.

Chapter 62

Dietary Supplements and Heart Health

Chapter Contents

Section 62.1

Dietary Supplements: What You Need to Know

This section includes text excerpted from "Dietary
Supplements: What You Need to Know," U.S. Food and
Drug Administration (FDA), November 29, 2017.

What Are Dietary Supplements?

Dietary supplements include such ingredients as vitamins, minerals, herbs, amino acids, and enzymes. Dietary supplements are marketed in forms such as tablets, capsules, soft gels, gel caps, powders, and liquids.

What Are the Benefits of Dietary Supplements?

Some supplements can help assure that you get enough of the vital substances the body needs to function; others may help reduce the risk of disease. However supplements should not replace complete meals which are necessary for a healthful diet. Therefore, be sure you eat a variety of foods as well.

Unlike drugs, supplements are not permitted to be marketed for the purpose of treating, diagnosing, preventing, or curing diseases. That means supplements should not make disease claims, such as "lowers high cholesterol" or "treats heart disease." Claims similar to these cannot be legitimately made for dietary supplements.

Are There Any Risks in Taking Supplements?

Yes. Many supplements contain active ingredients that have strong biological effects in the body. This could make them unsafe in some situations and hurt or complicate your health. For example, the following actions could lead to harmful—even life-threatening—consequences.

- Combining supplements

- Using supplements with medicines (whether prescription or over-the-counter)

- Substituting supplements for prescription medicines

- Taking too much of some supplements, such as vitamin A, vitamin D, or iron. Some supplements can also have unwanted effects before, during, and after surgery. So, be sure to inform your healthcare provider, including your pharmacist about any supplements you are taking.

Some Common Dietary Supplements

- Calcium

- Echinacea

- Fish oil

- Ginseng

- Glucosamine and/or

- Chondroitin sulfate

- Garlic

- Vitamin D

- St. John's wort

- Saw palmetto

- Ginkgo

- Green tea

Who Is Responsible for the Safety of Dietary Supplements?

The U.S. Food and Drug Administration (FDA) is not authorized to review dietary supplement products for safety and effectiveness before they are marketed.

The manufacturers and distributors of dietary supplements are responsible for making sure their products are safe before they go to market.

If the dietary supplement contains a new ingredient, manufacturers must notify the FDA about that ingredient prior to marketing. However, the notification will only be reviewed by the FDA, not approved, and only for safety, not effectiveness.

Manufacturers are required to produce dietary supplements in a quality manner and ensure that they do not contain contaminants or impurities, and are accurately labeled according to current good manufacturing practice (cGMP) and labeling regulations.

If a serious problem associated with a dietary supplement occurs, manufacturers must report it to the FDA as an adverse event. The FDA can take dietary supplements off the market if they are found to be unsafe or if the claims on the products are false and misleading.

How Can I Find out More about the Dietary Supplement I Am Taking?

Dietary supplement labels must include name and location information for the manufacturer or distributor.

If you want to know more about the product that you are taking, check with the manufacturer or distributor about:

- Information to support the claims of the product

- Information on the safety and effectiveness of the ingredients in the product.

How Can I Be a Smart Supplement Shopper?

Be a savvy supplement user, and follow the tips listed below.

- When searching for supplements on the internet, use noncommercial sites (e.g., the National Institutes of Health (NIH), U.S. Food and Drug Administration (FDA), and the U.S. Department of Agriculture (USDA)) rather than depending on information from sellers.

- If claims sound too good to be true, they probably are. Be mindful of product claims such as "works better than [a prescription drug]," "totally safe," or has "no side effects."

- Be aware that the term natural does not always mean safe.

- Ask your healthcare provider if the supplement you are considering taking would be safe and beneficial for you.

- Always remember—safety first.

Report Problems to The U.S. Food and Drug Administration

Notify the FDA if the use of a dietary supplement caused you or a family member to have a serious reaction or illness (even if you are not certain that the product was the cause or you did not visit a doctor or clinic).

Follow these steps:

1. Stop using the product.

2. Contact your healthcare provider to find out how to take care of the problem

3. Report problems to the FDA in either of these ways:

   • Contact the Consumer Complaint Coordinator in your area.

   • File a safety report online through the Safety Reporting Portal.

Section 62.2

Omega-3 Fatty Acids for Prevention of Heart Disease

This section includes text excerpted from "5 Things to Know about Omega-3s for Heart Disease," National Center for Complementary and Integrative Health (NCCIH), September 24, 2015. Reviewed May 2019.

Omega-3 fatty acids are a group of polyunsaturated fatty acids that are important for a number of functions in the body. They are found in foods such as fatty fish and certain vegetable oils, and they are also available as dietary supplements. While experts agree that fish rich in omega-3 fatty acids should be included in a heart-healthy diet, there is no conclusive evidence that shows omega-3s have a protective effect against heart disease.

Experts agree that fish rich in omega-3 fatty acids should be included in a heart-healthy diet. Much research has been done on fish and heart disease, and the results provide strong, though not conclusive evidence that people who eat fish at least once a week are less likely to die of heart disease than those who rarely or never eat fish.

Omega-3s in supplement form has not been shown to protect against heart disease. While there has been a substantial amount of research on omega-3 supplements and heart disease, the findings of individual studies have been inconsistent. In 2012, two combined analyses of the results of these studies did not find convincing evidence that omega-3s protect against heart disease.

Omega-3 supplements may interact with drugs that affect blood clotting. Omega-3 supplements may extend the time it takes for a cut to stop bleeding. People who take drugs such as anticoagulants ("blood thinners") or nonsteroidal anti-inflammatory drugs should discuss the use of omega-3 fatty acid supplements with a healthcare provider.

Fish liver oils (which are not the same as fish oils) contain vitamins A and D, as well as omega-3 fatty acids; these vitamins can be toxic in high doses. Both of the vitamins A and D can be toxic in large doses. The amounts of vitamins in fish liver oil supplements vary from one product to another.

Talk to your healthcare provider before using omega-3 supplements. If you are pregnant or nursing a child, if you take medicine that affects blood clotting, if you are allergic to fish or shellfish, or if you are considering giving a child an omega-3 supplement, it is especially important to consult your (or your child's) healthcare provider.

Chapter 63

Other Interventions to Help Reduce Risk of Cardiovascular Disease

Chapter Contents

Section 63.1

Aspirin for Reducing Your Risk of Heart Attack and Stroke

This section includes text excerpted from "Aspirin for Reducing Your Risk of Heart Attack and Stroke: Know the Facts," U.S. Food and Drug Administration (FDA), November 16, 2017.

You can walk into any pharmacy, grocery store, or convenience store and buy aspirin without a prescription. The Drug Facts label on medication products will help you choose aspirin for relieving headache, pain, swelling, or fever. The Drug Facts label also gives directions that will help you use the aspirin so that it is safe and effective.

But what about using aspirin for a different use, time period, or in a manner that is not listed on the label? For example, using aspirin to lower the risk of heart attack and clot-related strokes. In these cases, the labeling information is not there to help you with how to choose and how to use the medicine safely. Since you do not have the labeling directions to help you, you need the medical knowledge of your doctor, nurse practitioner, or other healthcare professional.

You can increase the chance of having good effects and decrease the chance of having the bad effects of any medicine by choosing and using it wisely. When it comes to using aspirin to lower the risk of heart attack and stroke, choosing and using wisely means:

Know the Facts and Work with Your Health Professional

FACT: Daily use of aspirin is not right for everyone.

Aspirin has been shown to be helpful when used daily to lower the risk of heart attack, clot-related strokes and other blood flow problems in patients who have cardiovascular disease (CVD) or who have already had a heart attack or stroke. Many medical professionals prescribe aspirin for these uses. There may be a benefit to daily aspirin use for you if you have some kind of heart or blood vessel disease, or if you have evidence of poor blood flow to the brain. However, the risks of long-term aspirin use may be greater than the benefits if there are no signs of or risk factors for heart or blood vessel disease.

Every prescription and over-the-counter (OTC) medicine has benefits and risks—even such a common and familiar medicine as aspirin. Aspirin use can result in serious side effects, such as stomach bleeding,

bleeding in the brain, kidney failure, and some kinds of strokes. No medicine is completely safe. By carefully reviewing many different factors, your healthcare professional can help you make the best choice for you.

When you do not have the labeling directions to guide you, you need the medical knowledge of your doctor, nurse practitioner, or other healthcare professional.

FACT: Daily aspirin can be safest when prescribed by a medical healthcare professional

Before deciding if daily aspirin use is right for you, your healthcare professional will need to consider:

- Your medical history and the history of your family members

- Your use of other medicines, including prescription and over-the-counter

- Your use of other products, such as dietary supplements, including vitamins and herbals

- Your allergies or sensitivities, and anything that affects your ability to use the medicine

- What you have to gain, or the benefits, from the use of the medicine

- Other options and their risks and benefits

- What side effects you may experience

- What dosage, and what directions for use are best for you

- How to know when the medicine is working or not working for this use

Make sure to tell your healthcare professional all the medicines (prescription and over-the-counter) and dietary supplements, including vitamins and herbals, that you use—even if only occasionally.

FACT: Aspirin is a drug

If you are at risk for heart attack or stroke your doctor may prescribe aspirin to increase blood flow to the heart and brain. But any drug—including aspirin—can have harmful side effects, especially when mixed with other products. In fact, the chance of side effects increases with each new product you use.

611

New products include prescription and other over-the-counter medicines, dietary supplements (including vitamins and herbals), and sometimes foods and beverages. For instance, people who already use a prescribed medication to thin the blood should not use aspirin unless recommended by a healthcare professional. There are also dietary supplements known to thin the blood. Using aspirin with alcohol or with another product that also contains aspirin, such as a cough-sinus drug, can increase the chance of side effects.

Your healthcare professional will consider your current state of health. Some medical conditions, such as pregnancy, uncontrolled high blood pressure, bleeding disorders, asthma, peptic (stomach) ulcers, and liver and kidney disease, could make aspirin a bad choice for you.

Make sure that all your healthcare professionals are aware that you are using aspirin to reduce your risk of heart attack and clot-related strokes.

FACT: Once your doctor decides that daily use of aspirin is for you, safe use depends on following your doctor's directions.

There are no directions on the label for using aspirin to reduce the risk of heart attack or clot-related stroke. You may rely on your healthcare professional to provide the correct information on dose and directions for use. Using aspirin correctly gives you the best chance of getting the greatest benefits with the fewest unwanted side effects. Discuss with your healthcare professional the different forms of aspirin products that might be best suited for you.

Aspirin has been shown to lower the risk of heart attack and stroke in patients who have cardiovascular disease or who have already had a heart attack or stroke, but not all over-the-counter pain and fever reducers do that. Even though the directions on the aspirin label do not apply to this use of aspirin, you still need to read the label to confirm that the product you buy and use contains aspirin at the correct dose. Check the Drug Facts label for "active ingredients: aspirin" or "acetylsalicylic acid" at the dose that your healthcare professional has prescribed.

Remember, if you are using aspirin every day for weeks, months or years to prevent a heart attack, stroke, or for any use not listed on the label—without the guidance from your healthcare professional—you could be doing your body more harm than good.

Section 63.2

Heart Disease and Adult Vaccines

This section includes text excerpted from "What You Need to Know about Heart Disease and Adult Vaccines," Centers for Disease Control and Prevention (CDC), August 2018.

Each year thousands of adults in the United States get sick from diseases that could be prevented by vaccines—some people are hospitalized, and some even die. People with heart disease and those who have suffered a stroke are at higher risk for serious problems from certain diseases. Getting vaccinated is an important step in staying healthy.

Why Vaccines Are Important for You

Heart disease can make it harder for you to fight off certain diseases or make it more likely that you will have serious complications from certain diseases.

Some vaccine-preventable diseases, such as the flu, can increase the risk of another heart attack or stroke.

Immunization provides the best protection against vaccine-preventable diseases.

Vaccines are one of the safest ways to protect your health, even if you are taking prescription medications.

Vaccine side effects are usually mild and go away on their own. Severe side effects are very rare.

Getting Vaccinated

You may regularly see a cardiologist or your primary care provider. Either is a great place to start! If your healthcare professional does not offer the vaccines you need, ask for a referral so you can get the vaccines elsewhere.

Adults can get vaccines at doctors' offices, pharmacies, workplaces, community health clinics, health departments, and other locations.

To find a place near you to get a vaccine, go to vaccine.healthmap.org.

Most health insurance plans cover recommended vaccines. Check with your insurance provider for details and for a list of vaccine providers covered by your plan. If you do not have health insurance, visit www.healthcare.gov to learn more about health insurance options.

What Vaccines Do You Need?

Flu vaccine to protect against seasonal flu

Tdap vaccine to protect against tetanus, diphtheria, and pertussis (whooping cough) Pneumococcal vaccines to protect against serious pneumococcal diseases

Zoster vaccine to protect against shingles if you are 50 years or older

Section 63.3

Influenza Vaccine May Reduce Cardiovascular Disease Risk

This section includes text excerpted from "Flu and Heart Disease and Stroke," Centers for Disease Control and Prevention (CDC), February 5, 2019.

People with heart disease and those who have had a stroke are at high risk for developing serious complications from flu. Among adults hospitalized with flu during the 2017 to 2018 influenza season, heart disease was among the most commonly-occurring chronic conditions; about half of adults hospitalized with flu during the 2017 to 2018 flu season had heart disease. Studies have shown that influenza is associated with an increase of heart attacks and stroke.

Vaccination Is the Best Protection against Flu

Flu vaccination is especially important for people with heart disease or who have had a stroke because they are at high risk for complications from flu. Vaccination has been associated with lower rates of some cardiac events among people with heart disease, especially among those who had had a cardiac event in the past year. Flu vaccines are often updated each season to keep up with changing viruses, and immunity wanes over a year so annual vaccination is needed to ensure the best possible protection against influenza. A flu vaccine protects against the flu viruses that research indicates will be most common during the upcoming season.

Other Preventive Actions for People with Heart Disease or Who Have Had a Stroke

In addition to getting the flu shot, people with heart disease or who have had a stroke should take additional everyday preventive actions, including covering their coughs, washing their hands often, and avoiding people who are sick.

Specific health actions for people with heart disease or who have had a stroke:

- Maintain a two week supply of your regular medications during flu season.

- Do not stop taking your regular medications without first consulting your doctor, especially in the event that you get the flu or another respiratory infection.

- People with heart failure should be alert to changes in their breathing and should promptly report changes to their doctor.

When to Seek Emergency Medical Care

If you or your child have heart disease or have had a stroke and experience any of the following emergency warning signs of flu sickness, seek medical attention right away.

Emergency Warning Signs of Flu

People experiencing these warning signs should obtain medical care right away.

In Children

- Fast breathing or trouble breathing
- Bluish lips or face
- Ribs pulling in with each breath
- Chest pain
- Severe muscle pain (child refuses to walk)

615

- Dehydration (no urine for eight hours, dry mouth, and no tears when crying)
- Not alert or interacting when awake
- Seizures
- Fever above 104°F
- In children less than 12 weeks of age, any fever
- Fever or cough that improves but then returns or worsens
- Worsening of chronic medical conditions

In Adults

- Difficulty breathing or shortness of breath
- Persistent pain or pressure in the chest or abdomen
- Persistent dizziness, confusion, inability to arouse
- Seizures
- Not urinating
- Severe muscle pain
- Severe weakness or unsteadiness
- Fever or cough that improves but then returns or worsens
- Worsening of chronic medical conditions

These lists are not all inclusive. Please consult your medical provider for any other symptom that is severe or concerning.

Part Eight

Additional Help and Information

Chapter 64

Glossary of Terms Related to Cardiovascular Disease

abdomen: The part of the body between the ribs and pelvis that holds the stomach intestines liver and other organs.

aerobic exercise: A type of physical activity that burns fat, gets your heart rate going (you will be able to feel it beating faster), and makes your heart muscle stronger.

anemia: When the total amount of red blood cells or hemoglobin is below normal. Anemia can cause severe fatigue and other health problems.

anesthesia: A drug that makes you sleepy or can numb a part of your body before surgery so that you do not feel pain.

aneurysm: A thin or weak spot in an artery that balloons out and can burst.

angina: A recurring pain or discomfort in the chest that happens when some part of the heart does not receive enough blood.

angioplasty: A medical procedure used to open a blocked artery.

anorexia nervosa: An illness in which people do not eat enough, and therefore, cannot stay at a healthy body weight. Anorexia nervosa can result in life-threatening weight loss and amenorrhea.

This glossary contains terms excerpted from documents produced by several sources deemed reliable.

antibiotic: Medicine used to fight bacterial infections by killing bacteria or stopping it from growing. Antibiotics can help your body's immune system fight off infections.

antidepressant: Drugs given by your doctor to treat depression.

arrhythmia: A problem with the rate or rhythm of the heartbeat. During an arrhythmia, the heart can beat too fast, too slow, or with an irregular rhythm.

artery: Any of the thick-walled blood vessels that carry blood away from the heart to other parts of the body.

atherosclerosis: It occurs when plaque builds up in the arteries that supply blood to the heart (called "coronary arteries").

atrial fibrillation (AF): A type of arrhythmia that can cause rapid, irregular beating of the heart's upper chambers.

biopsy: When a doctor takes a very small piece of your body, such as some skin, to look at under a microscope.

birth defect: A problem that happens while a baby is forming in the mother's body. Most birth defects happen during the first three months of pregnancy and may affect how the baby's body looks, works, or both.

blood glucose level: The amount of glucose in the blood.

blood pressure: The force of blood against the walls of arteries.

blood test: This is either done by using a finger prick to get a few drops or by inserting a needle into a vein to get a larger amount of blood. Blood tests are used to check for many different diseases and viruses.

blood vessel: A tube-shaped part of the circulatory system which helps blood move through the body.

broken heart syndrome: A condition in which extreme stress can lead to heart muscle failure.

calorie: When talking about food, a calorie is a measure of the amount of energy you get from eating a certain amount of food. When talking about physical activity, a calorie is a measure of the energy that your body uses in performing the activity.

capillary: Any of the tiny blood vessels that branch through body tissues to deliver oxygen and nutrients and carry away waste products.

cardiac rehabilitation: A medically supervised program that helps improve the health and well-being of people who have heart problems.

cardiogenic shock: A condition in which a suddenly weakened heart is not able to pump enough blood to meet the body's needs.

cardiomyopathy: It occurs when the heart muscle becomes enlarged or stiff. This can lead to inadequate heart pumping (or weak heart pump) or other problems.

cardiovascular disease (CVD): Disease of the heart and blood vessels.

carotid artery disease: A disease in which a waxy substance called plaque builds up inside the carotid arteries.

cholesterol: A soft, waxy substance that is present in all parts of the body.

congenital heart defects: Problems with the heart that are present at birth. They are the most common type of major birth defect.

coronary heart disease (CHD): A disease in which a waxy substance called "plaque" builds up inside the coronary arteries.

coronary microvascular disease: A heart disease that affects the tiny coronary (heart) arteries. In coronary MVD, the walls of the heart's tiny arteries are damaged or diseased.

DASH (Dietary Approaches to Stop Hypertension) eating plan: A flexible and balanced eating plan that helps creates a heart-healthy eating style for life.

deep vein thrombosis (DVT): A blood clot that forms in a vein deep in the body. Blood clots occur when blood thickens and clumps together.

depression: An illness that involves the body, mood, and thoughts. It affects the way a person functions, eats and sleeps, feels about herself, and thinks about things.

electrocardiogram (ECG or EKG): An external, noninvasive test that records the electrical activity of the heart.

electrolyte imbalance: When the amounts of sodium and potassium in the body become too much or too little.

endocarditis: An infection of the inner lining of the heart chambers and valves.

endurance: The measure of your body's ability to keep up an activity without getting tired. The more endurance you have, the longer you can swim, bike, run, or play a sport before tiring out.

fat: A source of energy used by the body to make substances it needs.

fatigue: A feeling of lack of energy, weariness or tiredness.

heart: A muscular organ that pumps blood to your body.

heart attack: Happens when the flow of oxygen-rich blood to a section of heart muscle suddenly becomes blocked and the heart cannot get oxygen.

heart block: A problem that occurs with the heart's electrical system.

heart failure: A serious condition that occurs when the heart cannot pump enough blood to meet the body's needs. It does not mean that the heart has stopped but that muscle is too weak to pump enough blood.

heart murmur: An extra or unusual sound heard during a heartbeat. Murmurs range from very faint to very loud.

heart valve disease: It occurs if one or more of your heart valves do not work well.

hemochromatosis: A disease in which too much iron builds up in your body (iron overload). Iron is a mineral found in many foods.

high blood pressure: A common disease in which blood flows through blood vessels (arteries) at higher than normal pressures.

hypotension: Abnormally low blood pressure.

ischemia: A decrease in the blood supply to an organ, tissue, or other part caused by the narrowing or blockage of the blood vessels.

ischemic stroke: A blockage of blood vessels supplying blood to the brain, causing a decrease in blood supply.

Kawasaki disease: A rare childhood disease. This condition involves inflammation of the blood vessels.

long QT syndrome (LQTS): A disorder of the heart's electrical activity. It can cause sudden, uncontrollable, dangerous arrhythmias in response to exercise or stress.

lupus: One of a type of chronic diseases that causes the immune system to attack healthy tissues in the body. Lupus can affect many body parts including joints, skin, the heart, lungs, kidneys, and the nervous system.

Marfan syndrome: A condition in which your body's connective tissue is abnormal.

metabolic syndrome: A group of risk factors that raises your risk for heart disease and other health problems, such as diabetes and stroke.

obesity: Having too much body fat. Obesity is more extreme than being overweight, which means weighing too much.

palpitations: Feelings that your heart is skipping a beat, fluttering, or beating too hard or too fast.

patent ductus arteriosus (PDA): A heart problem that occurs soon after birth in some babies. In PDA, abnormal blood flow occurs between two of the major arteries connected to the heart.

pericarditis: A condition in which the membrane, or sac, around your heart is inflamed.

peripheral artery disease (PAD): It occurs when the arteries that supply blood to the arms and legs (the periphery) become narrow or stiff.

plaque: A buildup of fat, cholesterol and other substances that accumulate in the walls of the arteries.

platelet: Any of the small cells in the blood that play a key role in blood clotting.

pulmonary embolism (PE): A sudden blockage in a lung artery. The blockage usually is caused by a blood clot that travels to the lung from a vein in the leg.

Raynaud phenomenon: A rare disorder that affects the arteries.

rheumatic heart disease (RHD): A damage to the heart valves caused by a bacterial (streptococcal) infection called rheumatic fever.

stroke: It occurs if the flow of oxygen-rich blood to a portion of the brain is blocked.

sudden cardiac arrest (SCA): A condition in which the heart suddenly and unexpectedly stops beating. If this happens, blood stops flowing to the brain and other vital organs.

***trans* fat:** A type of fat, usually made by food manufacturers so that foods last longer on shelves or in cans. Eating *trans* fats increases the risk of some illnesses, like heart disease.

varicose veins: Swollen, twisted veins that you can see just under the surface of the skin.

vasculitis: A condition that involves inflammation in the blood vessels.

vein: Any of the thin-walled blood vessels that receive blood from capillaries and return it to the heart.

X-ray: A type of high-energy radiation. In low doses, X-rays are used to diagnose diseases by making pictures of the inside of the body.

Chapter 65

Directory of Resources Providing Information about Cardiovascular Disease

General

AboutKidsHealth
The Hospital for Sick Children
555 University Ave.
Toronto, ON M5G 1X8
Phone: 416-813-7474
Website: www.aboutkidshealth.ca
E-mail: privacy.office@sickkids.ca

American Academy of Family Physicians (AAFP)
11400 Tomahawk Creek Pkwy
Leawood, KS 66211-2680
Toll-Free: 800-274-2237
Phone: 913-906-6000
Fax: 913-906-6075
Website: www.aafp.org

American Academy of Pediatrics (AAP)
345 Park Blvd.
Itasca, IL 60143
Toll-Free: 800-433-9016
Fax: 847-434-8000
Website: www.aap.org
E-mail: csc@aap.org

American Association for Clinical Chemistry (AACC)
900 Seventh St. N.W.
Ste. 400
Washington, DC 20001
Toll-Free: 800-892-1400
Phone: 202-857-0717
Fax: 202-833-4576
Website: www.aacc.org

Resources in this chapter were compiled from several sources deemed reliable; all contact information was verified and updated in May 2019.

American Association of Cardiovascular and Pulmonary Rehabilitation (AACVPR)
330 N. Wabash Ave.
Ste. 2000
Chicago, IL 60611
Phone: 312-321-5146
Fax: 312-673-6924
Website: www.aacvpr.org
E-mail: aacvpr@aacvpr.org

American College of Cardiology (ACC)
2400 N. St. N.W.
Washington, DC 20037
Toll-Free: 800-253-4636
Phone: 202-375-6000
Fax: 202-375-7000
Website: www.acc.org
E-mail: resource@aac.org

American College of Chest Physicians (CHEST)
2595 Patriot Blvd.
Glenview, IL 60026
Toll-Free: 800-343-2227
Phone: 224-521-9800
Fax: 224-521-9801
Website: www.chestnet.org

American College of Rheumatology (ACR)
Association of Rheumatology Professionals Rheumatology Research Foundation
2200 Lake Blvd. N.E.
Atlanta, GA 30319
Phone: 404-633-3777
Fax: 404-633-1870
Website: www.rheumatology.org

American Heart Association (AHA)
7272 Greenville Ave.
Dallas, TX 75231
Toll-Free: 800-AHA-USA-1
(800-242-8721)
Phone: 214-570-5978
Website: www.heart.org

American Society of Echocardiography (ASE)
The Society for Cardiovascular Ultrasound Professionals
2530 Meridian Pkwy
Ste. 450
Durham, NC 27713
Phone: 919-861-5574
Fax: 919-882-9900
Website: www.asecho.org
E-mail: ASE@ASEcho.org

American Stroke Association (ASA)
American Heart Association (AHA)
7272 Greenville Ave.
Dallas, TX 75231
Toll-Free: 888-4-STROKE
(888-478-7653)
Website: www.strokeassociation.org

Brain Aneurysm Foundation (BAF)
269 Hanover St.
Bldg. 3
Hanover, MA 02339
Toll-Free: 888-272-4602
Phone: 781-826-5556
Fax: 781-826-5566
Website: bafound.org
E-mail: office@bafound.org

Cardiovascular Research Foundation (CRF)
1700 Bdwy.
Ninth Fl.
New York, NY 10019
Phone: 646-434-4500
Website: www.crf.org
E-mail: info@crf.org

Center for Prevention of Heart and Vascular Disease
535 Mission Bay Blvd. S.
San Francisco, CA 94158
Phone: 415-353-2873
Fax: 415-353-2528
Website: www.healthyheart.ucsf.edu
E-mail: Cardio-NewReferrals@ucsf.edu

Centers for Disease Control and Prevention (CDC)
1600 Clifton Rd.
Atlanta, GA 30329-4027
Toll-Free: 800-CDC-INFO
(800-232-4636)
Toll-Free TTY: 888-232-6348
Website: www.cdc.gov

Children's Cardiomyopathy Foundation (CCF)
P.O. Box 547
Tenafly, NJ 07670
Toll-Free: 866-808-CURE
(866-808-2873)
Fax: 201-227-7016
Website: dev.childrenscardiomyopathy.org
E-mail: info@childrenscardiomyopathy.org

Children's Hemiplegia and Stroke Association (CHASA)
4101 W. Green Oaks
Ste. 305-149
Arlington, TX 76016
Website: www.chasa.org

Cleveland Clinic
9500 Euclid Ave.
Cleveland, OH 44195
Toll-Free: 800-223-2273
Phone: 216-444-2200
Website: my.clevelandclinic.org

Heart and Stroke Foundation of Canada
110-1525 Carling Ave.
Ottawa, ON K1Z 8R9
Toll-Free: 888-473-4636
Fax: 613-727-1895
Website: www.heartandstroke.ca

Heart Failure Society of America (HFSA)
9211 Corporate Blvd., Ste. 270
Rockville, MD 20850
Phone: 301-312-8635
Toll-Free Fax: 888-213-4417
Website: www.hfsa.org
E-mail: info@hfsa.org

Hypertrophic Cardiomyopathy Association (HCMA)
18 E. Main St.
Ste. 202
Denville, NJ 07834
Phone: 973-983-7429
Fax: 973-983-7870
Website: www.4hcm.org
E-mail: support@4hcm.org

The Mended Hearts, Inc.
Resource Center
Merry Acres Executive Bldg.
1500 Dawson Rd.
Albany, GA 31707
Toll-Free: 888-HEART99
(888-432-7899)
Phone: 229-518-2680
Fax: 229-518-3879
Website: mendedhearts.org
E-mail: info@mendedhearts.org

Minneapolis Heart Institute Foundation (MHIF)
920 E. 28th St.
Ste. 100
Minneapolis, MN 55407
Toll-Free: 877-800-2729
Phone: 612-863-3833
Fax: 612-863-3801
Website: mplsheart.org
E-mail: info@mhif.org

National Center for Complementary and Integrative Health (NCCIH)
NCCIH Clearinghouse
9000 Rockville Pike
Bethesda, MD 20892
Toll-Free: 888-644-6226
Toll-Free TTY: 866-464-3615
Website: nccih.nih.gov

National Heart, Lung, and Blood Institute (NHLBI)
31 Center Dr.
Bldg. 31
Bethesda, MD 20892
Phone: 301-592-8573
Website: www.nhlbi.nih.gov
E-mail: nhlbiinfo@nhlbi.nih.gov

National Human Genome Research Institute (NHGRI)
Communications and Public
Liaison Branch (CPLB)
9000 Rockville Pike, 31 Center
Dr., MSC 2152
Bldg. 31, Rm. 4B09
Bethesda, MD 20892-2152
Phone: 301-402-0911
Fax: 301-402-2218
Website: www.genome.gov

National Institute of Arthritis and Musculoskeletal and Skin Diseases (NIAMS)
NIAMS Information
Clearinghouse
1 AMS Cir.
Bethesda, MD 20892-3675
Toll-Free: 877-22-NIAMS
(877-226-4267)
Phone: 301-495-4484
TTY: 301-565-2966
Fax: 301-718-6366
Website: www.niams.nih.gov
E-mail: NIAMSinfo@mail.nih.gov

National Institute of Diabetes, Digestive, and Kidney Diseases (NIDDK)
Health Information Center
Toll-Free: 800-860-8747
Phone: 301-496-3583
Toll-Free TTY: 866-569-1162
Website: www.niddk.nih.gov
E-mail: healthinfo@niddk.nih.gov

National Institute of Neurological Disorders and Stroke (NINDS)
NIH Neurological Institute
P.O. Box 5801
Bethesda, MD 20824
Toll-Free: 800-352-9424
Website: www.ninds.nih.gov

National Institute on Aging (NIA)
NIA Information Center
31 Center Dr., MSC 2292
Bldg. 31, Rm. 5C27
Bethesda, MD 20892
Toll-Free: 800-222-2225
Toll-Free TTY: 800-222-4225
Website: www.nia.nih.gov
E-mail: niaic@nia.nih.gov

National Institutes of Health (NIH)
9000 Rockville Pike
Bethesda, MD 20892
Phone: 301-496-4000
TTY: 301-402-9612
Website: www.nih.gov

The Nemours Foundation / KidsHealth®
Website: kidshealth.org

Office of Minority Health (OMH)
OMH Resource Center
Tower Oaks Bldg., 1101 Wootton Pkwy
Ste. 600
Rockville, MD 20852
Toll-Free: 800-444-6472
Phone: 240-453-2882
TDD: 301-251-1432
Fax: 301-251-2160
Website: minorityhealth.hhs.gov
E-mail: info@minorityhealth.hhs.gov

Office on Women's Health (OWH)
U.S. Department of Health and Human Services (HHS)
200 Independence Ave. S.W.
Rm. 712E
Washington, DC 20201
Toll-Free: 800-994-9662
Phone: 202-690-7650
Fax: 202-205-2631
Website: www.womenshealth.gov

Society for Vascular Surgery (SVS)
9400 W. Higgins Rd.
Ste. 315
Rosemont, IL 60018-4975
Toll-Free: 800-258-7188
Phone: 312-334-2300
Fax: 312-334-2320
Website: vascular.org
E-mail: vascular@vascularsociety.org

The Society of Thoracic Surgeons (STS)
633 N. Saint Clair St., Ste. 2100
Chicago, IL 60611
Phone: 312-202-5800
Fax: 312-202-5801
Website: www.sts.org

Texas Heart Institute (THI)
6770 Bertner Ave.
Houston, TX 77030
Phone: 832-355-4011
Website: www.texasheart.org

U.S. Food and Drug Administration (FDA)
10903 New Hampshire Ave.
Silver Spring, MD 20993-0002
Toll-Free: 888-INFO-FDA
(888-463-6332)
Phone: 301-796-8240
Toll-Free TTY: 866-300-4374
Website: www.fda.gov

Vascular Disease Foundation (VDF)
1075 S. Yukon, Ste. 320
Lakewood, CO 80226
Toll-Free: 866-PAD-INFO
(866-723-4636)
Phone: 303-989-0500
Fax: 303-989-0200
Website: www.vdf.org
E-mail: info@vdf.org

Women's Heart Foundation
P.O. Box 7827
West Trenton, NJ 08628
Phone: 609-771-9600
Website: www.womensheart.org
E-mail: bonnie@womensheart.org

World Heart Federation (WHF)
32, rue de Malatrex
1201 Geneva, Switzerland
Phone: 41-22-807-03-20
Fax: 41-22-807-03-39
Website: www.world-heart-federation.org
E-mail: info@worldheart.org

Arrhythmias

Heart Rhythm Society (HRS)
1325 G St. N.W.
Ste. 400
Washington, DC 20005
Phone: 202-464-3400
Fax: 202-464-3401
Website: www.hrsonline.org
E-mail: info@HRSonline.org

Washington Heart Rhythm Associates, LLC.
10230 New Hampshire Ave.
Ste. 204
Silver Spring, MD 20903
Phone: 301-408-7890
Fax: 301-408-7892
Website: www.washingtonhra.com

Congenital Disorders

March of Dimes
National Office
1550 Crystal Dr.
Ste. 1300
Arlington, VA 22202
Toll-Free: 888-MODIMES
(888-663-4637)
Website: www.marchofdimes.org

Myocarditis

Myocarditis Foundation
3518 Echo Mountain Dr.
Kingwood, TX 77345
Phone: 281-713-2962
Website: www.
myocarditisfoundation.org
E-mail: info@
myocarditisfoundation.org

Peripheral Arterial Disorders

The Erythromelalgia Association (TEA)
200 Old Castle Ln.
Wallingford, PA 19086
Phone: 610-566-0797
Website: erythromelalgia.org

Fibromuscular Dysplasia Society of America (FMDSA)
26777 Lorain Rd., Ste. 408
North Olmsted, OH 44070
Toll-Free: 888-709-7089
Phone: 216-834-2410
Website: www.fmdsa.org
E-mail: admin@fmdsa.org

Sudden Cardiac Arrest

Sudden Cardiac Arrest Association (SCAA)
910 17th St. N.W., Ste. 800
Washington, DC 20006
Toll-Free: 866-972-SCAA
(866-972-7222)
Website: www.
suddencardiacarrest.org
E-mail: info@
suddencardiacarrest.org

Sudden Cardiac Arrest (SCA) Foundation
7500 Brooktree Rd.
Wexford, PA 15090
Toll-Free: 877-722-8641
Website: www.sca-aware.org
E-mail: info@sca-aware.org

Valvular Disorders

The Howard Gilman Institute for Heart Valve Disease
635 Madison Ave.
Third Fl.
New York, NY 10022
Phone: 212-289-7777
Website: www.gilmanheartvalve.
org
E-mail: info@gilmanheartvalve.
us

Vasculitis

Vasculitis Foundation (VF)
P.O. Box 28660
Kansas City, MO 64188
Toll-Free: 800-277-9474
Phone: 816-436-8211
Fax: 816-656-3838
Website: www.
vasculitisfoundation.org

Index

Index

For Reference

Not to be taken from this room

LINDENHURST MEMORIAL LIBRARY
One Lee Avenue
Lindenhurst, New York 11757